SpringerWienNewYork

I. Mader, P. R. Fürst-Weger,
R. M. Mader, E. Nogler-Semenitz,
S. Wassertheurer

Extravasation of Cytotoxic Agents

Compendium for Prevention and Management

Second edition

SpringerWienNewYork

Ines Mader, MD
CRETA - Cancer Research & Trial Agency GmbH, Bad Sauerbrunn, Österreich

Mag. pharm. Patrizia Fürst-Weger
SMZ Floridsdorf, Krankenhaus und Geriatriezentrum, Wien, Österreich

Univ.-Prof. Dr. Robert Mader
Univ.-Klinik für Innere Medizin I, Klinische Abteilung für Onkologie, Wien, Österreich

Mag. pharm. Dr. Elisabeth Nogler-Semenitz
Anstaltsapotheke, Landeskrankenhaus - Universitätskliniken Innsbruck, Österreich

Mag. pharm. Sabine Wassertheurer
Apotheke LKH-Univ.-Klinikum Graz, Österreich

Translated from German by Birte Twisselmann

Softcover re-print of the Hardcover 2nd edition 2010

SpringerWienNewYork is a part of Springer Science + Business Media
springer.at

Typesetting: Integra Software Services Pvt. Limited, India

SPIN: 12325764

Cover photo: from Alfons Schilling „Ich/Auge/Welt - The Art of Vision" (Springer-Verlag Wien New York 1997, S. 156)

With 4 Figures and 5 Working sheets

Additional material to this book can be downloaded from http://extras.springer.com.

ISBN 978-3-7091-1667-8 SpringerWienNewYork
ISBN 3-211-83859-7 1st edn. SpringerWienNewYork
DOI 10.1007/978-3-211-88893-3 ISBN 978-3-211-88893-3 (eBook)

Preface for the 2nd edition

"Scientific work on the topic of extravasation of cytotoxic drugs is faced with many limitations." This sentence, the introduction to the preface of the 1st edition of this book, is still fully valid for the revised 2nd edition. The reasons are partly to do with the difficulty and complexity of the problem—but only partly.

The research question is a priori excluded from systematic work—prospective clinical studies, for example. Consequently, the knowledge gleaned is by necessity limited. Further difficulties include the lack of standardised processes in dealing with extravasation events, non-standardised documentation, case studies with imprecise data, and uncertainty in predicting the expected extent of the damage.

Knowing this state of affairs, the authors decided to update their original volume; the main emphasis of this revision was on original clinical articles. For the 51 most commonly used substances, an instruction manual was set out that can be translated into practice wherever, whenever, and as soon as the clinical emergency extravasation occurs. The substances bortezomib and permetrexed are new additions to the list of drugs. Some revisions include more recent insights into drugs such as docetaxel, paclitaxel, oxaliplatin, vinorelbine, and the anthracyclines. Moreover, the market authorization obtained for the first antidote, dexrazoxane, urged us to include an update on this newly introduced compound. For this antidote, only sporadic clinical data were available during the writing of the 2nd German edition. Adhering to the academic tradition, we have critically reviewed this data and implemented them in the text body. With the exception of this update, the rest of the text was left without change.

The two-part structure—a general part and a substance specific part—was retained as in the first edition. The structure of the general part was updated, as were the chapters "Type of damage", "Predisposition and prevention", Clinical practice" (including pathogenesis and differential diagnosis), and "Surgical intervention" (including "flushout technique" and liposuction). New chapters include "The formation of clinical working groups", "Quality assurance", "Unanswered questions", new antidotes such as dexrazoxane, and problems associated with central venous catheters.

As in the 1st edition, we laid emphasis on the chapter on "Prevention". We would therefore ask our readers to pay particular attention to this chapter.

Since it is important to the authors to spread quality standards, supporting materials may be found not only in the book itself but also on the internet (www.extravasation.at or www.paravasate.at). Further to forms and tables we also offer training materials, which provide an introduction to the topic.

The medical emergency that is extravasation continues to require an interdisciplinary approach in order to do justice to the multiple layers of the problem.

This volume was created with interdisciplinarity in mind. Without active cooperation from some colleagues we would not have succeeded in concluding this project, which took several years.

We thank in particular the following parties for their help in compiling this new edition:

Robert Terkola (DSc and Master's degree in pharmacy), from the pharmacy at the Social Medical Centre South in Vienna, Austria, whose detailed and committed revisions of the 1st chapter in the general part in the 1st edition formed the foundations for further revisions in the 2nd edition.

Professor Pietro Giovanoli MD and Matthias Rab MD, at the Department of Surgery, Clinical Department of Plastic and Reconstructive Surgery, at the Medical University of Vienna, who updated the surgical sections for the 2nd edition. They have succeeded in making a difficult chapter accessible for all conservative disciplines, and we can only express our deepest admiration for such an outstanding achievement.

Mrs Brigitte Spicker, EBEWE Pharma, Austria, whose organisational and logistical skills were supreme and without whom this project could not have succeeded.

This preface would not be complete without our mentioning EBEWE Pharma, Austria, whose generous support for many years has crucially contributed to the success of the project, in every way.

We conclude by expressing the same hope as for our 1st edition: We would like as many people as possible to read this book, but we hope that the occasions when its information may have to be used clinical practice may remain few and far between.

Vienna, August 2009

Ines Mader
Patrizia Fürst-Weger
Robert M. Mader
Elisabeth Nogler-Semenitz
Sabine Wassertheurer

Preface of the 1st Edition

Scientific work on the topic of extravasation of cytotoxic drugs is faced with many limitations.
The problem is excluded a priori from any form of systematic approach, such as prospective clinical trials. Poorly standardised methods of dealing with extravasation and its occasionally patchy documentation are a hinderance to comparing and assessing successful treatments. In the case of some substances, the number of documented cases is extremely small or no clinical data are available at all. In these cases, the interpretation of data from animal experiments was unavoidable, with all its limitations. In spite of all these hurdles the authors have attempted to set out an instruction manual for the 49 most widely used substances, based on a review of all available literature with an emphasis on original clinical studies, which in the clinical emergency "extravasation" can be put into practice without further ado.
In the general section, a comprehensive chapter deals with prevention. It includes a list of all factors that should be taken into consideration to avoid extravasations. This was of particular importance to the authors, as the current discussion still focuses mainly on interventions after extravasation. In view of the severe symptoms of extravasation and the impaired quality of life of patients with cancer, a new orientation towards prevention is a major goal.
In spite of all care, extravasations cannot be avoided entirely, and we have included documentation sheets with this book. The aim is to collect and evaluate information about the course and management of extravasations. Particularly with new cytotoxic agents, this will help to reduce the current uncertainties. To make these documentation sheets available for everyone, they can be accessed on the internet, together with the lists for the extravasation kit, and printed off (www.extravasation.net, www.extravasation.at, or www.springer.at).
Since the problem of extravasation necessitates an interdisciplinary approach, this book is the result of interdisciplinary thinking. Without the active collaboration of several colleagues, it would not have been possible to finish such a wide-ranging undertaking.

Our special thanks go to:
Beata Laszloffy MSc, pharmacy of the Kaiser-Franz-Josef-Hospital in Vienna, Austria, for her research into numerous substances that posed difficulties for us.

Catherina Pietrzak MD, Hospital Rudolfstiftung, III Medical Department, Vienna, Austria, for her clinical-oncological expertise, which she firmly committed to our project. Her medical contributions, her experience with clinical studies in oncology, and her bibliographical research have been extremely helpful.

Mrs. Maria Schmidmair, oncology nurse, Hospital Vöcklabruck, Department of Internal Medicine, Vöcklabruck, Austria, for accompanying and supporting this project with a wealth of experience from patient care in oncology wards and for her practical help in compiling this book.

Mrs Brigitte Spicker, EBEWE Pharma, Austria, for spending innumerable hours of putting our scribbles into a legible format and for her fabulous organisational skills.

Stefanie Chromy MD, Hospital Rudolfstiftung, II Surgical Department, Vienna, Austria, took care of the surgical section of this book. We thank her for making time for this important aspect in spite of her many responsibilities and obligations.

Birte Twisselmann PhD, London, UK, for the concise and accurate translation of the manuscript originally written in German. We are very obliged to her for numerous useful remarks and her prompt support.

Thanks also to the essential contribution of EBEWE Pharma (Austria), which has generously supported us in every way and thus helped the project to succeed.

This only leaves one wish open for the authors: We hope that our book will be read by many, but used in clinical practice only rarely!

Vienna, December 2002

Ines Mader
Patrizia Fürst-Weger
Robert Mader
Elisabeth Semenitz
Robert Terkola
Sabine Wassertheurer

Contents

Substance-specific part

We dedicate this book to
our Brigitte Spicker,
for 7 years full of big intentions,
plans,
ideas,
words,
laughter and
hard work
in order to achieve our final objective.

Problem outline

In everyday haemato-oncological practice, many cytostatic or cytotoxic drugs are being used, whose mechanisms of action are diverse. It is therefore essential to know some of the possible local complications associated with parenteral administration of these drugs, and familiarity with preventive and treatment measures is highly desirable.

Hyperosmolar solutions, vasopressors, and cytotoxic agents are the main causative agents of damage in cases of extravasation.

In the development of extravasations several factors such as tissue toxicity, osmolarity, vasospasticity, infusion pressure, tissue pressure, and regional anatomical conditions play a part.

Clinical evaluation is difficult because the involvement of the skin does not provide a reliable indication of the damage to the subcutaneous fatty and muscle tissues. Even when prevention guidelines are carefully adhered to and the venipuncture is placed correctly, extravasations will occasionally occur.

Standard treatment for such occasions is available for only a few cytotoxic agents.

As classic randomised studies for the treatment of extravasations are unthinkable because of ethical reasons, recommendations for prophylaxis and management of extravasations are mainly empirical, or based on clinical case reports, guidelines from the pharmaceutical manufacturers, and animal studies.

Additionally, theoretical considerations still have an important role in treating extravasations—another sure sign for the lack of clinical evidence.

The available data are often contradictory or cannot be reproduced. Many authors have, however, published guidelines for the prevention and treatment of extravasations.

This book aims to evaluate these data critically and separate confirmed facts from unprovable assumptions. The results of this analysis are supposed to serve as knowledge base to foster new investigations, which will be necessary in the future to answer open questions.

Literature search methods

Like the first edition, this second edition of the book contains a critical review of the literature about extravasations of cytotoxic agents and their treatment. Overviews with more or less representative articles are available in large numbers, and the authors have therefore attempted, as their foremost task, to compile a complete listing of original source materials and reviews of all investigations and documented case studies. Wherever that was possible, we used exclusively clinical studies to evaluate the potential dangers of different agents and the effectiveness of therapeutic interventions after extravasation. This literature is referred to as "original articles," since it shows the personal clinical experience of the author. "Secondary literature" comprises overviews and book articles. Data from animal studies were included as "original articles" for evaluation only in cases where the clinical literature was insufficient or not meaningful. References whose contents do not include anything notably new were included as "further reading," for completeness's sake. In all chapters, the following standard works were taken into consideration, which will not be always cited hereafter:

Barth J: Paravasate und deren Behandlung. In: Barth J (ed) Zytostatika-Herstellung in der Apotheke. Deutscher Apotheker Verlag, chapter VI-3: 1–9, 2000.

Bertelli G: Prevention and management of extravasation of cytotoxic drugs. Drug Safety 12: 245–255, 1995.

Dorr RT: Antidotes to vesicant chemotherapy extravasations. Blood Rev 4: 41–60, 1990.

Dorr RT: Pharmacologic management of vesicant chemotherapy extravasations. In: Dorr RT, Von Hoff DD (eds) Cancer Chemotherapy Handbook. Appleton & Lange, 2nd edition: 109–118, 1994.

Gain M, Melzer S, Meyer-Jürshof A, et al: Allgemeiner Teil: Behandlung von Paravasaten. In: Gain M, et al (eds) ADKA-Zytostatika-Handbuch, Pharmazeutisch-wissenschaftliche Monographien. Verlag Heiner Biller, vol 1, 2nd edition: A42–44, 1997.

Ignoffo RJ, Friedman MA: Therapy of local toxicities caused by extravasation of cancer chemotherapeutic drugs. Cancer Treat Rev 7: 17–27, 1980.

Krämer I, Stützle M: Zytostatika-Paravasation – Wie ist vorzugehen? Krankenhauspharmazie 23: 261–268, 2002.

Mullin S, Beckwith MC, Tyler LS: Prevention and management of antineoplastic extravasation injury. Hosp Pharm 35: 57–76, 2000.

Schneider G: Paravasate von Zytostatika. Diagnostik und Therapie. Aina S. Schneider Verlag, 6th edition: 1–17, 1999.

Stanley A: Managing complications of chemotherapy administration. In: Allwood M, Stanley A, Wright P (eds) The Cytotoxics Handbook. Radcliffe Medical Press, 4th edition: 119–193, 2002.

Jordan K, Grothe W, Schmoll HJ: Paravasation von Zytostatika: Prävention und Therapie. Dtsch Med Wochenschr 130: 33–37, 2005.

After discussing the many unanswered questions, we wrote up the information gained in the form of a consensus. Because of the incomplete information relating to some of the cytotoxic agents, a final evaluation remained impossible. In order to find a practical solution, however, we have attempted to provide clear and generally comprehensible recommendations for treating extravasations and thus create a volume that can be used easily and reliably in clinical emergencies.

General part

Introduction and definitions

Robert Mader

There is hardly an area in haemato-oncology in which as little progress has been achieved in recent years as the treatment of extravasation of cytotoxic drugs. Many medical doctors and pharmacists worldwide have focused intensely on this subject and have always reached the same conclusion: we have a certain amount of knowledge about risk factors, clinical course, and intervention strategies, but as far as the crucial questions are concerned, clinical certainty and clinical evidence are lacking. Despite all attempts to collect data systematically, instructions for action are usually based on a small number of case reports. A genuine systematic review of clinical cases has not gone any further than initial steps; important clinical information is often lacking.

Incidence of extravasations

In clinical practice, the emergency of an extravasated cytotoxic drug is more common than is often assumed. The percentage of patients affected by extravasations is estimated at 0.45–6.4% [1, 2]. In relation to the number of infusions this means a proportion of 0.01% [3] to a maximum of 0.9% [2] in adults. In children, the frequency and clinical severity of extravasations is clearly more pronounced: in 16,380 intravenous injections of different substances, no less than 1800 extravasations occurred over 6 months, corresponding to a proportion of 11%. Of these, 4 (0.24%) resulted in necroses [4].

These numbers do not include asymptomatic extravasations. These may occur often, for example, where, owing to (previous) damage to the endothelial tissue, an intravenously administered substance extravasates from the vessel in small quantities or where no serious consequences ensue owing to the lack of tissue toxicity [3]. The wide range of incidence data can undoubtedly be explained with the different patient populations, venipuncture techniques, different degrees of supervision during the infusion, and the subjective reports of extravasations [5]. Unfortunately, extravasations are not only relevant for peripheral venous infusions; they occur in central venous administration more often than might be assumed, where the consequences may be particularly serious. The reported incidence of these extravasations is 7.5% of all administrations [6].

Definition

Extravasation of cytotoxic agents is the unintentional instillation or leakage of these agents into the perivascular and subcutaneous spaces during their administration [3].

Type of damage

The type and extent of local damage depend primarily on the attributes of the cytotoxic agent and the absolute amount of extravasated substance [7-9]. This is defined by the concentration of the cytotoxic drug in the infusion solution and its extravasated volume. Secondary contributing factors that can increase local toxicity include carrier substances, unphysiological pH, and osmolarity. The extent of the damage also has a strong individual component. This is defined by pharmacokinetic variables such as velocity and extent of redistribution from the tissue into the systemic circulation and the ratio of the substance volume of interstitial to intercellular space. Individual pharmacodynamic variables include toxicity for the different cell types of the affected tissue and patient's varying individual sensitivities.

- **Non-vesicant**

This includes substances that do not cause a notable local reaction after extravasation.

- **Irritant**

A local irritant produces – with or without visible extravasation – swelling, local pain at the injection site, a burning sensation, and/or signs of local inflammation extending to phlebitis, reversible skin toxicity, blistering, but no necrosis.

- **Vesicant**

A vesicant agent may cause intravascular irritation, ulceration, and tissue necrosis during extravasation. The final result can be dystrophy or atrophy, scar formation, damage to nerves, muscles, ligaments, joints, and loss of limb function. Débridement, skin grafts, and amputation may be necessary [10].
Although this classification is broad, it relates closely to clinical practice, and we will therefore continue to use it. In the recent English language literature, it was suggested to refine the classification further, which is a justifiable idea [11]. The five suggested classes comprise the following categories, some of which are defined in very vague terms: "neutrals", "inflammatory agents", "irritants", "exfoliants", and "vesicants". Apart from the fact that these suggestions require more solid scientific

foundations, there are practical reasons to question such a classification. For some substances we do not have sufficient data to enable a final classification; and the focus of this compendium is on clinical measures in a scenario of extravasation, not on academic discussion. We will therefore continue to use the term "vesicant" as a clearly recognisable warning signal that requires immediate and undivided attention from doctors and nursing staff.

Potential damage mechanisms

The literature mentions five different mechanisms to describe the damage mechanism of medical drugs in the tissue at the cellular level [12]. Four have been discussed in connection with extravasation of cytotoxic drugs: direct cellular toxicity, hyperosmolarity, mechanical compression, and bacterial colonisation as a secondary effect. The fifth mechanism, ischaemic tissue necrosis, is observed more often in connection with vasopressor agents and electrolyte solutions.

Direct cellular toxicity

The damage mechanism that is most important for extravasation is undoubtedly the direct damage to the affected tissues. Cytotoxic agents have a multitude of mechanisms of action at the molecular or cellular level. Attempts to classify these mechanisms have not yielded a satisfactory result thus far. In the literature, the most important distinguishing feature in connection with extravasation is reported to be DNA binding, which does indeed constitute an important pharmacological aspect, but, although it is important, it is still only one of many. The effects on healthy tissue are defined by a multitude of variables, including the amount and concentration of the cytotoxic agent, cellular absorption, inactivation owing to metabolic reactions, tissue anatomy, and mean length of stay in the tissue/tissue clearance.
Many antimetabolites are administered in high dosages and incorporated into DNA, but they are subject to a high inactivation rate and tissue clearance. Doxorubicin, by contrast, is incorporated into the cell nucleus, where it intercalates the DNA and inhibits topoisomerase II as the parent drug. If the cell dies because of the inhibition of essential functions, the anthracycline is released, incorporated into adjacent cells, and in turn cause these to die [7, 9]. The result: the agent remains in the tissue for an extremely long time—several weeks—as has been documented after extravasation of anthracyclines [13, 14]. The concentrations observed in these studies of up to 8 μg doxorubicin/g tissue weeks after extravasation suggest that the time of residence in the tissue probably runs to months.

Pure topoisomerase inhibitors—such as irinotecan or topotecan—are not considered problematic with regard to extravasation. Their toxicity seems to increase exponentially, however, if, as is the case for the anthracyclines, several mechanisms of action accumulate: intercalation of DNA, toposiomerase inhibition, and formation of free radicals, paired with a high tissue affinity. Free radicals can cause devastating damage in certain settings and can thoroughly disrupt the balance of the entire cellular architecture owing to peroxidation of the cellular membrane. In addition to the anthracyclines, this mechanism has been described as characteristic for the podophyllotoxins etoposide and teniposide, as well as for bleomycin.

Other DNA binding agents are the alkylating cytotoxic drugs, which are consumed during this reaction and are therefore not able to damage further cells directly. The primary damage to the DNA can be repaired by repair enzymes, which contributes to tissue restoration. However, such a repair takes time, which, in some of the alkylating cytotoxic agents—such as bendamustine, busulfan, carmustine, dacarbazine, fotemustine, and melphalan—contributes to their irritant attributes.

This summary of possible mechanisms of action shows that there is no simple explanation for tissue toxicity. The coincidence of several unfavourable factors is responsible for the cases of massive damage that have been observed after extravasation. The pharmacological insights from experimental oncology cannot be extrapolated to extravasation because, owing to a totally different experimental design, the mechanisms of action are mostly studied in tumour cells and not healthy tissue.

Hyperosmolarity

If owing to instillation of hyperosmolaric fluids the equilibrium between intra- and extracellular fluids is disturbed, this in turn alters the cell tonus. To compensate for this, fluid will move from the intracellular space to the extracellular space; the tissue interstitial space. In turn, the resulting progressive formation of oedema may lead to ischaemia and tissue necrosis [15, 16]. A similar development may be expected for protein containing exudates as a tissue reaction to the extravasation, although the underlying mechanism is different. This damage mechanism is not of primary importance in clinical practice, because cytotoxic drugs are rarely given in undiluted form; without exception, today's infusion solutions are manufactured in isotonic carrier fluids.

Mechanical compression

Increased hydrostatic pressure is usually caused by a mechanical infusion pump. A vicious circle ensues whereby interstitial pressure is raised, venous compression develops, and arterial function is impaired as a result [12]. This type of damage can become important during permanent infusion of undiluted preparations, of the combination of mechanical compression and hyperosmolarity result in underperfusion of the tissue. If this process lasts for a longer time period, cell death and skin breakdown may be the result [17].

Bacterial colonisation

This is an additional risk factor that occurs only in case of tissue breakdown (ulceration, necrosis) as a secondary development or may occur in early invasive surgical interventions such as the "flush-out" technique and liposuction. Bacterial colonisation can increase the extent and depth of tissue loss. In extreme cases the result may be a 1000-fold increase in germs, which meets the criteria of wound sepsis [12].

The damage mechanisms mentioned here can be cumulative during the clinical course of an extravasation so that in the worst case scenario, several negative components intensify each other. In individual cases, the resultant tissue damage can therefore vastly exceed the expected extent, which has been observed sporadically after administrations of small amounts of doxorubicin.

Damage mechanisms of the anthracyclines

Extravasations of anthracyclines range among the most feared complications in the the context of cytotoxic therapy [18]. Because of different types of reactions to extravasations of anthracyclines [19-21], we want to discuss the pathogenesis in greater detail. Four different types of reactions have to be distinguished over time:

The most common form is the **paravenous reaction type.** The following sequence of symptoms has been described for this type:

- **Immediately:** Burning pains, swelling, erythema
- **After days and weeks:** Capillary thromboses, necrobiosis of collagen fibres, induration, ulceration, skin necroses leading to exposed tendons, ulcers heal only after more than 6 months
- **Permanent damage:** Persistent pain, contractures, impaired movement of the affected limb, immediate damage enables no predictions about long term damage

Thrombophlebitis type: This is a hypersensitivity reaction of the vessel chosen as the injection site for the cytotoxic medication. Hypersensitivity may occur even when only minute amounts of the anthracycline penetrate into the vascular wall during the injection process.

Clinical course:

- **Immediately:** Venospasm, pain on injection site
- **Hours later:** Painful swelling around the injection site, degenerative changes to the endothelial tissue
- **Days later:** Hardening and thrombosing of the vessel, discolouration of the skin, development of collateral circulation, no skin ulcers

Capillary type: Anthracyclines penetrate into the capillary bed as a result of stasis or reversal of the blood flow. Injection is possible only against resistance.

Clinical course:

- **Immediately:** Pain, discolouration along the affected vessel and the associated capillary region
- **Hours and days later:** Damages unfolds to its full extent after extravasation of anthracyclines, without any inflammatory reaction at the injection site

The **allergic type** is an extremely rare from of anthracycline damage, but it is accompanied by the most extensive necroses. The reaction is due to a hyperallergic reaction to the cytotoxic agent. A tiny amount of extravasated drug is sufficient for this reaction, which may have escaped the attention of patient and doctor.

Clinical course:

- **Immediately:** No symptoms!
- **Days later:** Increasing pain around the injection site and its environs
- **Weeks later:** Erythema, induration, and exulceration

Necrosis potential of individual cytotoxic agents

The following classification is an orientation aid and based on a consensus among the authors. In part, the allocation to the type of damage is being controversially discussed in the literature (see chapter "Type of damage").

Vesicant	
Amsacrine	Mitoxantrone
Cisplatin (≥0.4 mg/ml)	Oxaliplatin
Dactinomycin	Paclitaxel

Daunorubicin
Doxorubicin
Epirubicin
Idarubicin
Mitomycin C
Vinblastine
Vincristine
Vindesine
Vinorelbine

Irritant

Bendamustine[1]
Bortezomib[1]
Busulfan[1]
Carmustine
Cisplatin (<0.4 mg/ml)
Dacarbazine
Daunorubicin liposomal[1]
Docetaxel
Doxorubicin liposomal[1]
Etoposide
5-Fluorouracil (undiluted)
Fotemustine
Gemcitabine
Melphalan
Streptozocin[1]
Teniposide
Treosulfan[1]
Trimetrexate[1]

Non-vesicant

Asparaginase
Bleomycin
Carboplatin
Cladribine
Cyclophosphamide
Cytarabine
Estramustine[1]
Etoposide phosphate[1]
Fludarabine
5-Fluorouracil (diluted)
Ifosfamide
Irinotecan[1]
Methotrexate
Nimustine[1]
Pegaspargase
Pemetrexed[1]
Pentostatin
Raltitrexed
Thiotepa
Topotecan

[1] Owing to little experience with extravasations no final classification possible.

Predisposition and prevention

Ines Mader

Risk factors

An increased risk for damage caused by extravasation may be patient associated, caused by drugs, or iatrogenic. It also depends on the type of access that has been selected (peripheral venous or central venous). By strictly adhering to the measures described in the chapter "Prevention", this risk can be minimised.

Risk factors associated with patients

1. Anatomical factors:

- Fragile veins or veins with a small diameter, for example in older patients and children [22]
- Sclerosed veins [23]
- Narrow vascular lumen [23]
- Damaged veins owing to previous treatments
- Multiple venipunctures [24,25]

2. Pathophysiological factors:

- Venospasm at the puncture site [21,24]
- (Thrombo-) phlebitis [24,26]
- Reduced perfusion or stasis, or raised intravenous pressure, owing to cardiovascular disorders (for example, right heart failure, superior vena cava syndrome, [10,21,22,27], thromboembolic events [28], or mediastinal tumours [29].
- Vascular obstruction by locally infiltrating tumour [26]
- Lymphoedema, for example after dissection of the axillary lymph nodes in the ipsilateral arm [9, 10] or radiotherapy [23].
- Generalised vascular disorders (for example, Raynaud's syndrome) [22,30].

3. Patient characteristics:

- Polyneuropathy, for example due to diabetes mellitus or previous therapy with vinca alkaloids [23,31]
- Clotting disorders with delayed clotting around the puncture site [27]
- Prior radiotherapy [32]
- Motor unrest

- Impaired communication, for example in children [12], comatose patients or dementia patients, and in patients receiving antiemetic or antidepressant drugs [23]

Medication-related risk factors

- Vesicant potential of effective or carrier substance(s) [28]
- Concentration of effective or carrier substance(s) [28]
  In formulations that contain benzyl alcohol, extravasation may initially remain undetected and painless, owing to the local anaesthetic effect [33]
- Osmolarity [7,8,10,34]
- pH [7,8,10,34]
  Undiluted solutions of 5-fluorouracil have a pH of almost 9 and constitute an increased risk in permanent infusions administered through a central venous catheter
- Length of exposure [7,8,34]
- Hypersensitivity to the substance [10]
- Amount of substance that has been administered [10]

Iatrogenic risk factors

- Choice of unsuitable puncture site (for example, the dorsum of the hand) [10,16,21,24]
- Poor venipuncture technique [9,21,35]
- Multiple punctures [22,31,35]
- Inexperienced and insufficiently trained staff [23]
- Insufficient information given to patients [35]
- Not enough attention paid to complaints voiced by patients [10,35]
- Delayed diagnosis [36]
- Carelessness [10], for example by underestimating potential later harms [12], insufficient monitoring of infusions [4,35]
- Covering the puncture site with non-transparent material [23]
- Infusion characteristics, such as great speed of infusion, large volumes, and a long infusion period [23]
- Time pressure during administration [12,24]
- Overtired staff [37]

Risk factors associated with central venous catheter systems

The following aspects have been identified as problems in recent scientific discussion [38,39]:

- Formation of fibrin thrombi or deposits along the catheter or at the catheter tip, thereby occlusion or backflow in the catheter system
- Infections
- Spontaneous retraction of the catheter tip from the subclavian vein or another venous access
- Dislocation, migration of catheter tip or catheter
- Penetration of the catheter into adjacent organs or structures
- Mechanical compression of the catheter with intravascular catheter fracture or formation of fissures on the catheter caused by the costoclavicular ligament, which results in compression of the first rib and the clavicle ("pinch-off syndrome") [29,40–44].
- Faulty material
- Disconnection of catheter and chamber in port-systems
- Damage or rupture of port septum
- Incomplete penetration of the injection syringe through the port septum
- Inappropriate venipuncture and implantation technique [40]
- Inappropriate care for the system (for example, flushing under excessively high pressure) [40]
- Lack of experience in inserting central venous catheter systems
- Forced injection into a blocked catheter with resultant catheter fracture

CONSENSUS

Risk factors

Patient associated:

- Vascular condition/state
- Impaired lymphatic flow or venous circulation
- Polyneuropathy—for example, owing to diabetes mellitus or previous therapy using vinca alkaloids
- Impaired consciousness

Medication related:

- Vesicant potential of effective and/or carrier substance(s)
- Concentration of effective and/or carrier substance(s)
- Duration of exposure

Iatrogenic:

- Lacking training and experience
- Venipuncture and application technique
- Insufficient patient information given

Central venous catheters:

- Thromboses or fibrin deposits
- Infections
- Faulty material
- Dislocation and migration of the catheter tip, for example
- Penetration into neighbouring organs or structures
- "Pinch-off" syndrome
- Venipuncture and application technique

Prevention

Adherence to general guidelines for the administration of cytotoxic drugs can contribute to reducing the risk of extravasation. Before the application of these substances, it is important to familiarise oneself with their risk potential regarding extravasation (see chapter "Vesicant potential of individual cytotoxic agents").
The following preventive measures have been discussed in the literature:

1. **Application by well-trained personnel only** [12,21,24,35]
2. **Patients' medical histories** should include details on any of these factors:
   - Cardiovascular disorders with reduced venous backflow
   - Upper inflow stasis with increase in venous pressure (for example, owing to mediastinal tumours)
   - Polyneuropathy causing comorbidities, such as diabetes or previous therapy with vinca alkaloids (reduced sensation of pain and other symptoms)
   - Long term medication with antidepressive drugs, anxiolytics, sedatives, and antiemetics (impaired consciousness)
   - Previous radiotherapy
   - Previous extravasations
3. **Patient education and instruction:**
   - Use of patient information leaflets
   - Encourage immediate reporting of symptoms such as pain, burning, stinging, swelling, or erythema [45]
   - Immobilise limb during application [21]

Educating patients about possible extravasations, their risks and their symptoms, is extremely important (see chapter "Patient education") [21,28]

4. **i.v. Access:**
   - If using vesicant substances, establish new access site [25]
   - Choose adequate venous access (central? peripheral? which catheter or port system?) [10]
   - Preferred access site: large veins in middle of forearm (sufficient soft issue to protect nerves, vessels, and tendons) [9,12,34, 45,46]
   - Access sites to be avoided: dorsum of hand, wrist, elbow crease, owing to notably raised morbidity (closeness to joints and other structures) [25,26,34,46]
   - Multiple punctures should be avoided
   - Punctured vein should not be used for at least 24 hours after attempted venipuncture or end of application [23,47]
   - Use thin venflons if possible
   - Cave! no steel cannulas (for example, Butterfly® cannulas)
   - Immobilise limb

   Option: if vascular condition is poor, be generous at defining an indication for a central venous catheter [48]

WHERE?

Large veins in the middle of the forearm

WHERE NOT?

Dorsum of hand, wrist, antecubital fossa of arm
In patients with arteriovenous shunts, do not puncture the vein distal to the fistula but only the venous segment proximal to the fistula (otherwise risk of necrosis via rediffusion) [45,49]

HOW NOT?

Multiple punctures, in particular distal to an already punctured vessel [12,26]

USING WHAT?

- If possible use thin venflons; no steel cannulas (for example, Butterfly® cannulas)!
- Consider early on use of central venous catheter [24,50]
- Immobilise the limb, with the application site clearly visible [12]

Steel cannulas such as Butterfly® cannulas double the risk of extravasation [34,51]. Butterfly® cannulas often penetrate the back wall of the vessel with their sharp tip if the patient moves [24].

The strength of catheter is important. The Intravenous Nurses Society and the Oncology Nursing Society recommend thin catheters (20–23 Gauge) to guarantee sufficient blood flow around the catheter and thus adequate dilution of the substance [30,52,53].

5. **Position control:**
   - Aspiration of blood [27]
   - Flushing with agent-free carrier solution should be possible without resistance
   - In patients with central venous access, where there is doubt about positioning, this should be controlled radiologically [54], and a venogram should be ordered in suspected thrombus formation [53]
   - Visual control of venous access [48]

The correct aspiration of blood does not fully exclude the possibility of an extravasation as the vascular wall may have been damaged during venipuncture [26].

6. **Application:**
   - Avoid pressure on the injection site [12]
   - Do not use infusion pumps for peripheral venous application (of vesicant agents) - this would raise the pressure [48,53]
   - Minimum duration of application 3 minutes or a maximal infusion rate of 5 ml per minute [22]
   - Aspiration of blood after application of 1–2 ml of the cytotoxic agent; process to be repeated after a further 1–2 ml [22]
   - Do not inject against resistance [21]
   - Careful monitoring [4,15,21,35,46]
   - Cytotoxic agents should not be administered in a hurry [12]
   - Avoid direct i.v. application with cannula and syringe [16,21]

7. **Flushing:**

After applying a potentially vesicant substance the i.v. access should be flushed. This helps to avoid remaining cytotoxic agent reaching the surrounding tissues during removal of the catheter, and resulting in necrosis [27].
It is important to use a compatible injection solution (normally NaCl 0.9% or glucose 5%) [21,45].
Especially central venous access sites should be flushed using at least 10 ml syringes and with great care as syringes with a lower volume may produce higher pressure. This in turn increases the risk of a catheter rupture or disconnection [55].

8. **Vesicant substances:**
   - Avoid permanent infusion via peripheral venous access [23]
   - Do not use infusion pumps in peripheral venous application [23]
   - In peripheral venous application, use 2-syringe technique or "sidearm" technique [23,53]
   - In polychemotherapy, aim to administer the vesicant substance first [22]
   - If several vesicant agents are applied, administer sequentially, starting with the substance with the lowest application volume

A technique, which may be questioned for reasons of practicability is the 2 syringe technique: one syringe is used to administer the cytotoxic agent, whereas the second syringe is used for flushing the infusion line, aspirating blood after each 1–2 ml of cytotoxic agent administered, and to finally flush the peripheral access after the bolus injection of the drug is completed [23,53].
In the "sidearm" technique, a compatible infusion solution is applied through peripheral venous access, and an attempt is made to aspirate blood. If the short infusion of 50–100 ml is unproblematic and the aspiration attempt positive, then a Y piece is used to apply the vesicant substance slowly and simultaneously to the ongoing application of NaCl 0.9%, for example [23].

9. **Central venous access (port systems or central venous catheters):**
   - Take care to use the correct venipuncture technique [29]
   - Do not inject the cytotoxic drug against resistance [29]
   - Order a venogram if thrombosis is suspected [29]
   - Order contrast medium imaging of the catheter system in suspected "pinch-off" syndrome [29]
   - Control the position of the central venous access regularly [56]
   - Central venous catheters should not have a wider lumen than is strictly necessary [48]
   - Sports activities of the upper extremities are to be avoided, as is wearing a backpack in patients with implanted catheter systems [40,57]

CONSENSUS

Prevention of extravasations

1. **Application** by well-trained personnel only, haste is to be avoided
2. **Medical history** regarding:
   - Cardiovascular disorders
   - Upper blockage and backflow
   - Polyneuropathy causing comorbidities and previous therapy with vinca alkaloids
   - Permanent medication with antidepressive drugs, anxiolytic drugs, sedatives, and antiemetics
   - Prior radiotherapy
3. Patient **education** and instruction
   - Use of patient information leaflets
   - Immobilise limb during application
   - Encourage immediate reporting of symptoms such as pain, burning, stinging, swelling, or erythema
4. **i.v. Access:**
   - Choose adequate venous access
   - If possible establish new access site for each application
   - Preferred access site: large veins in middle of forearm
   - Access sites to be avoided: dorsum of hand, wrist, antecubital fossa
   - Multiple punctures, especially distal to an already punctured vein, should be avoided
   - Do not use punctured vein for at least 24 hours
   - Use thin venflons if possible
   - Cave! no steel cannulas (for example, Butterfly® cannulas)
   - Consider early on use of implantable Port-a-cath system
   - Immobilise limb, with application site clearly visible
5. **Positioning:**
   - Aspirate blood
   - Flushing has to be possible without resistance
   - Central venous access: if in doubt control positioning radiologically
   - Visual control of positioning
6. **Application:**
   - Do not use infusion pumps for peripheral venous application of vesicants
   - Minimum application time 3 minutes or maximal flow rate of 5 ml per minute
   - Do not inject against resistance
   - Careful monitoring

7. **Flushing** only with carrier solution of the cytotoxic agent injected last
8. **Vesicant substances:**
   - Avoid permanent infusion via peripheral venous access [23]
   - In peripheral venous application, use 2-syringe technique or "sidearm" technique
   - If several vesicants are applied, administer sequentially, starting with the substance with the lowest application volume and flush with carrier solution between the individual cytotoxic agents
9. **Central venous access:**
   - Take care to use the correct venipuncture technique
   - The position of the catheter should be controlled at regular intervals
   - Order contrast medium imaging of the catheter system in suspected "pinch-off" syndrome
   - Order a venogram if thrombosis is suspected [29]
   - Choose venipuncture site lateral to the medioclavicular line (to avoid "pinch-off" syndrome)
   - Wearing a backpack and fitness programmes for the upper extremities are to be avoided

Patient education/information

Dear patient,

The most efficient method of giving you the drug you require for your treatment is an intravenous injection. This means that the drug has to be administered via a vein to reach the blood circulation and finally the site of action.

What may happen during this injection is that the drug does not flow directly into the vein but into the tissue underneath the skin. Doctors call this phenomenon **"extravasation"**. On rare occasions this may result in damage to healthy tissue at the injection site.

Extravasations may be favoured by veins that are difficult to access or by a change on the positioning of the injection needle, caused, for example, by frequent arm movement during the infusion.

To avoid possible disadvantageous effects of an extravasation, please tell the nursing staff or doctor immediately if you notice

- **Pain** or a **burning** sensation at the injection site
- **Swelling** at the injection site
- **Reddening** skin at the injection site
- Or **pain** caused by the needle

If this is the case, the doctor will examine the injection site and, if required, position a new needle.

Please note that in some cases the preliminary signs such as pain, burning, reddening, swelling may be hardly noticeable during the infusion and increase only over time.

/__/__/./__/__/./__/__/ ____________________

Day Month Year Patient's signature

Clinical practice

Ines Mader

Peripheral venous extravasations

The clinical course of an extravasation depends mainly on the necrotic potential of the administered cytotoxic drug. Further, the extent of the damage is directly related to the administered volume of the drug; early detection and stopping the infusion immediately are therefore of utmost importance [25].

Langstein described a mean timespan from the onset of an extravasation to its detection of about 40 (!) days (1–45 days) [39]. The associated delay in therapeutic intervention makes for a poorer prognosis in the context of extravasation, especially for vesicant substances.

Initially, the following symptoms are usually described [11,32,38]:

- A burning and stabbing sensation at the venipuncture site
- Swelling
- Erythema (sometimes with delayed onset)
- Pain
- No aspiration of blood is possible
- Reduced infusion rate
- Increased resistance to the injection

After days, the pain may worsen, induration may develop, and blisters may be observed. In vesicant substances, ulcerations or necroses follow over the next 1–3 weeks; in individual cases these affect neighbouring structures such as tendons and muscles, as well as the periostium.

Sometimes, extravasations develop primarily asymptomatically, or the patients notice the symptoms only after a time delay.

Complications and permanent damage after extravasation:

- Paraesthesias/neuropathies after extravasation of vinca alkaloids [23, 32, 38]
- Super-infection with disruption to the wound healing process [23,58]
- Delayed occurrence of symptoms, sometimes only after weeks and months (for example, for mitomycin C or anthracyclines) [23,38]
- Squamous cell carcinoma of the skin after extravasation of doxorubicin [59]
- Fibroses, indurations [23]
- Skin discolourations [23]
- Functional impairment or loss of affected joints [23,32]

- Contractures [34]
- Scars [32]
- Amputation of the affected limb owing to progressive necrosis [32,38]
- Sudeck's disease [23]
- Recall reactions [23]

The authors differentiate between DNA binding cytotoxic agents (such as the anthracyclines) and non-DNA binding substances. Necroses that are induced by the latter take a similar course to "chemical burns" (for example, for the vinca alkaloids) [23].

The following **timeline** is typical for the **extravasation of anthracyclines** [21,29]:
It is postulated that extravasations of anthracyclines result in damage to normal tissues and disrupted wound healing mainly through DNA intercalation. According to this model, dead cells release new, reactive anthracycline molecules, which may then in turn damage adjacent cells [47]. This kind of local "anthracycline recycling" continues until the substance has been totally eliminated. The often observed, slowly progressing tissue damage/necrosis is supported by the fact that doxorubicin, for example, is detectable locally in the affected cells for weeks.
A second proposed mechanism is the formation of free oxygen radicals and associated tissue damage [58].
This is associated with slow wound healing and increase in ulcerations and necroses for weeks and months.
Anthracycline extravasation can be divided into the following phases:

- Immediately after extravasation
- Within days
- Within weeks
- Within weeks to months
- Persistent (permanent damage)

Immediately after extravasation:
- Burning or stabbing pain
- Local swelling
- Erythema
- Impaired movement has been observed
- An early, hard induration seems a reliable proof in predicting eventual ulceration [5]

Hours later (oedema phase):
- Vasodilatation
- Increasing pain
- Local erythema

- After days, transition from the oedema phase into a brown induration

Within days:
- Persistent pain
- Erythema
- Induration
- Capillary thromboses
- Necrobiosis of collagen (slow cell death in individual cells)

Within weeks:
- Varying extent of pain
- Sclerosing and skin atrophy in the wound region
- Stealthy development of ulcers or necrosis that includes all skin layers, with possible alteration of the underlying tendons and muscles and neurovascular structures—no spontaneous healing!
- Risk of super-infection of the ulcers or necroses

Within weeks to months:
- Ulcer formation stops after 3–5 months
- Slow healing of ulcers after about 6 months
- Pain and contractures often last for months [34]
- Skin transplants are rejected
- Super-infections with mostly gram positive bacteria [12]

Persistent (permanent damage):
- Permanent pain
- Contractures
- Impaired movement range or functional loss of affected extremity after extravasation near a joint [34]
- Joint stiffness
- Loss of extensor tendons after tissue necrosis
- Rarely amputation [12]

Systemic factors such as leucopenia, impaired immunological processes, and continued chemotherapy can delay the local healing process further [34].
Often, necrosis also affects the periostium, paratenon, and the fascias [8,9,16].
Without including the time it may take to perform necessary surgical reconstructions, the occurrence of an extravasation prolongs hospitalisation for an average 23 days [12].

Central venous extravasations

As a matter of principle, all patients with fragile veins who have had repeated chemotherapy should be provided with a safe venous access. Central venous catheter systems are increasingly used in the application of vesicant cytotoxic drugs [60].
Extravasations are rarer in central venous application than in peripheral venous application, but on the other hand they are associated with more severe complications [29]. The following chapter will focus on the advantages and disadvantages of central venous catheter systems. We have listed and described the possible complications in order to raise awareness of the problems associated with this application method.

The following types of central venous catheters need to be distinguished [60]:

- Peripherally or centrally applied **temporary** catheter
- **Permanent** central venous catheters
- Implantable port systems

Temporary central venous catheter systems:
Principally, because of a lower risk of infection, the recommendation is to puncture the jugular vein (ultrasound guided) or the subclavian vein.

Permanent central venous catheter systems:
The preferred access route is the subclavian vein. In case of unsuccessful venipuncture of the subclavian vein, the external jugular vein can also be used.
The tunnel originating from the trocar when implanting these catheter systems is sensitive with regard to the infection risk (tunnel infections) (see also: venous port systems).

Venous port systems:
These consist of a chamber and a catheter. The advantages lie in speedy access and a lower infection rate. Further, spontaneous opening of the catheter, as may occur in percutaneous catheter systems, can be ruled out. Because the port system is attached to the pectoral fascia below the clavicle, the subclavian vein is the preferred access route. The ipsilateral external jugular vein is an attractive alternative after unsuccessful venipuncture of the subclavian vein.
Care needs to be taken that only appropriate, non-coring cannulas are used since normal injection needles may cause micro-damage to the chamber membrane.
For intermittent cytotoxic therapy, the central venous port system is the preferred option [61].

The **advantages** of central venous catheter systems include [55, 60]:

- Uncomplicated implantation and removal
- Reduced risk of extravasations
- Possible outpatient care possible
- Long term use
- Avoidance of repeated, painful venipunctures
- No impairment of everyday activities

Complications for central venous catheters are observed more frequently since these systems are increasingly used for chemotherapy. The complications associated with central venous catheter systems fall into two categories—early and late complications. Their incidence is reported to be 1.8% and 14.4% [55, 61–69].

Early complications include:

- Arterial puncture
- Damage to neighbouring organs
- Pneumothorax
- Haemothorax (rarely)
- Disturbed cardiac rhythm
- Haemorrhages/haematomas
- Injury to the brachial plexus (rarely)
- Impaired aspiration of blood

Late complications are:

- Wound healing problems
- Infections (the most common port associated complication [55]; in neutropenic patients, the infection rate increases [68, 70])
- Catheter related sepsis
- Venous thrombosis
- Catheter related thrombosis
- Pulmonary embolism
- Catheter occlusion
- Catheter bend, fracture, tear, or rupture
- Malpositioning of the catheter
- Dislocation of the port needle or catheter
- Disconnection of catheter and chamber in port systems
- Penetration of port chamber
- Skin pressure necrosis in port systems
- **Extravasation**

In principle, central venous catheter systems reduce the risk of **extravasations**, but they cannot be regarded as offering 100% protection [10].

The incidence reported in the literature varies between 0.3%–7.5% [6,61,63,69,71–75].

In a retrospective study, Langstein and co-workers reported [39] that 27.3% of all observed extravasations occurred in the context of a central venous application of cytotoxic drugs. This observation thus confirms that central venous extravasations are a problem that requires to be taken seriously. Langstein and co-workers further assumed that some of these extravasation events go unnoticed. A possible cause is the confinement of the extravasated drug in the surrounding structures (muscles, soft tissues).

The infiltration of the vesicant substances into the thoracic wall or neck region is associated with higher morbidity.

The perceived **causes** of extravasations are:

- Poor positioning of the catheter syringe [62]
- Catheter separates from port body [55]
- Fracture of or fissures in the catheter [39,44,55,62]
- Backflow or reversed flow of the infusion subsequent to thromboses or fibrin deposits in the catheter or catheter tip [39,55,62]
- Dislocation, migration of the catheter tip or entire catheter [39,55,62]
- Mechanical compression of the catheter with subsequent catheter fracture and risk of embolisation of the central fragment ("pinch-off" syndrome (see also chapter "Predisposition and prevention") [29]
- Perforation of the vena cava superior or vena subclavia [39,62,76]
- Perforation of the membrane in implanted port systems [65]
- Escape of fluid from the port membrane or the joint between port and catheter

A particular problem in central venous extravasations is the fact that the diagnosis is delayed because of the uncommon complications in the context of central venous applications [36]. An aggravating factor is the fact that the symptoms usually manifest after a long delay (for example, in obese patients). Extravasations are therefore often noticed only when extensive tissue damage is present [62].

Initial clinical **symptoms**:

- (Thoracic) pain [36,44,53,76–80], headache [81]
- Burning, stabbing, itching, and/or prickling sensation [53, 55]
- Erythema [53,55,82,83]
- Haematoma [84]
- Palpable swelling, occasionally persistent [36,85,86]
- Facial oedema or oedema in the affected region [36, 82]
- Raised temperature/fever [36,53,77,81]

- Hyperthermia of the affected region [53,82,83]
- Coughing [44,87]
- Dyspnoea [81,87]
- Palpitations [44]
- Arrhythmias [77]

Symptoms/pathologies that occur with a time **delay:**

- Tissue damage, necrosis (for example, of the thoracic wall or fatty tissues) [62,67,83,84,88]
- Risk of abscess formation after extravasation into breast tissue [89]
- Thrombosis, for example, of the superior vena cava [36]
- Pleural effusion [76,79,80]
- Pericardial effusion [76,77,79]
- Mediastinitis [36]
- Pericarditis [77]
- Endocarditis [44]
- Pneumonitis [78]
- Pulmonary embolism [44]
- Cardiac perforation [44]
- Tracheal obstruction [90]
- Dysphagia [79]
- Hyperthyreosis [79]
- Collateral formation [78]
- Paraesthesias [48, 91]
- Paresis of the upper limb [91]
- Indurations [53]

The reason for all these potential complications is anatomical: there are no intrathoracal structures that form boundaries and could thus prevent the extravasated substances from spreading.

Possible **complications** and **long term damage:**

- Cardiac dysfunction
- Fibrosing of affected lung sections [78]
- Oesophageal dysfunction [76]
- Rejection reactions after skin transplants [62]
- Unilateral mastectomy after necrosis of the thoracic wall [62]
- Costophrenic adhesions [79]
- Migration of separated catheter fragments via the venous bloodstream into the right ventricle or lung, triggering sequelae [62, 92]
- Porto-bronchial fistula [87]
- Palpable swelling, induration, and fibrosing of affected area [85, 86]
- Skin discolourations [83, 86]

To date, **central venous extravasations** and other complications have been reported **in connection with the following cytotoxic agents:**

- Daunorubicin [79]
- Docetaxel [83]
- Doxorubicin [44,62,67,81,83]
- Epirubicin [65, 80]
- Epirubicin + 5-FU [76]
- Fluorouracil [44,75–78]
- Oxaliplatin [85,86]
- Paclitaxel [82]
- Vinblastine [36,62,93]
- Vincristine [62,81,84,88]

The application of vesicant substances through a central venous catheter can result in serious, occasionally even life threatening, complications if an extravasation occurs. Extreme care and experienced staff are therefore essential when central venous catheters are used.

Histopathological investigations

Are inflammatory alterations prominent events in extravasations?

The occurrence of inflammatory symptoms in the context of extravasations has resulted in widespread use of corticosteroids. In almost all review articles, the use of corticosteroids is listed as a possible intervention, in some even as an accompanying measure in any form of extravasation [11]. What is the evidence for their use?
The clinical symptoms after extravasation of cytotoxic drugs often match the criteria of an inflammatory process: erythema, local hyperthermia, swelling, and sometimes pain have been observed. Suppressing these clinical symptoms with corticosteroids—mostly hydrocortisone or dexamethasone—has often been described in the literature as an alleviating intervention for the benefit of the patient. However, the real question comes from a pathological perspective: what is really happening in the traumatised tissue after an extravasation? The sobering answer is: we have only a vague idea.
Histochemical **animal studies** have in the past described the infiltration of inflammatorty cells in the area of the extravasation and described a picture that rarely confirmed the immigration of immunocompetent cells. Even the first studies of doxorubicin in 1979, in rats and rabbits, described

inflammatory processes either as too low grade or entirely absent [94, 95]. Accordingly, the first studies of treating doxorubicin induced lesions in rabbits have not given proof of the efficacy of the intervention [96]. Studies in mice were ambiguous; low dose intradermal application showed a lowering of doxorubicin's necrotic effects, but systemic administration or high dosage intradermal hydrocortisone were not beneficial [97]. The use of hydrocortisone in rats was not found to be beneficial either, which prompted the authors to speak out very clearly against the use of corticosteroids after extravasation of doxorubicin [106].
Similar studies were subsequently conducted for several other substances (vincristine, actinomycin D, mitomycin C, and carmustine); administration of hydrocortisone in rats was not found to be beneficial here either [99].
However, the use of corticosteroids as an acute intervention has always had its place in clinical practice, even if the infiltration of inflammatory cells after extravasation of doxorubicin was observed in the animal model only after 7 days to a noticeable degree [100].
Similar observations have been made for individual pathological investigations in humans, in whom the inflammation was not the main issue either [12, 101, 102]. The conclusion: the occasional infiltration of inflammatory cells does not start immediately but—if at all—only days after the extravasation event.
Further to many reports of the low efficacy of corticosteroids, however, positive examples have been described—such as the application directly into the lesion of 70–80 mg triamcinolone acetonide after extravasation of vinorelbine, cisplatin, and doxorubicin in 10 cases [102].
The vinca alkaloids are a particular case in as far as the use of corticosteroids is strictly contraindicated. In the mouse model, a dramatic rise in tissue toxicity due to vinblastine, vincristine, and vindesine has been observed [103]. This precludes the use of corticosteroids for this indication, even though in the case of vinorelbine the inflammatory component is more pronounced than for the anthracyclines [104].

With all this in mind, several questions arise that bring us back to the original question asked in this chapter:

1. Is the acute reaction observed after extravasation an inflammatory reaction in the pathological sense?

2. Does this mechanism apply to all cytotoxic drugs or only some of them?

3. If the acute tissue reaction is not a genuine inflammatory response, does such a response occur later in the process? (For example, caused by the onset of tissue necrosis, which is always

followed by an inflammatory reaction with immunopathological involvement)

4. Does it make therapeutic sense to use corticosteroids to control symptoms, and if yes: what should the dosage be and what form should the administration take?
5. Does it make sense to suppress the local tissue reaction with corticosteroids, because the reaction may be a painful swelling, or could this be achieved by using a local anaesthetic?

Neither the literature nor clinical experience has thus far provided us with a satisfactory answer to these questions. However, it is important to stress that corticosteroids are exclusively a symptomatic treatment and their administration—if it is beneficial at all—is only one of many measures to be taken. In the absence of any real proof of their efficacy, it would be important to find answers for these questions so that a rationale for the treatment of extravasations could be laid out.

Conclusion:

Until further histopathological studies in humans have been published, a primary inflammatory reaction may not be assumed.

Differential diagnosis

Diagnostically, cytotoxic induced thrombophlebitides, local hypersensitivity reactions, allergic reactions, recall phenomena, and photosensitivity reactions need to be differentiated from extravasations of cytotoxic substances.

Thrombophlebitides

These are the most common complications associated with the application of cytotoxic drugs [23, 29].
They may be caused by local infections, if proceedings are not completely sterile, or by hypersensitivity to the carrier substances of cytotoxic drugs. The following symptoms are characteristic:

- Immediate pain on injection
- Swelling at injection site
- Venous thrombosis

Cutaneous hypersensitivity reactions

These are an immunologically mediated event and have to be differentiated from local toxicities. They are characterised by:

- Pain in the proximal course of the vein used for the injection
- Erythema
- Urticaria
- Pruritus

Local hypersensitivity symptoms usually cease spontaneously within the hour after stopping the infusion and flushing the vessel. They do not necessarily recur if the injection is repeated. Antihistamines are usually ineffective. The severity of symptoms can range from slight pruritus to severe erythema and anaphylaxis.
Immunologically, distinctions are made between 4 forms of hypersensitivity reactions; for the cutaneous manifestation, the so called type II has so far not been described for cytotoxic drugs (see also systemic hypersensitivity reactions).
Local hypersensitivity reactions occur mainly when the following drugs are used [105–109]:

- Asparaginase (type I, III)
- Bleomycin
- Busulfan (type III)
- Cyclophosphamide (type I, III)
- Cisplatin (type I)
- Daunorubicin (type I, IV after contamination of the skin surface)
- Docetaxel (type I)
- Doxorubicin (type I, IV after contamination of the skin surface)
- Etoposide (type I)
- 5-Fluorouracil (type IV in topical application)
- Gemcitabine (type I)
- Melphalan (type I)
- Methotrexate (type I)
- Mitomycin C (type IV)
- Mustargen (type III)
- Paclitaxel (type I)
- Teniposide (type I)
- Thiotepa (type I, III)
- Trimetrexate (type I)

A local allergic reaction is not a contraindication for continuing the chemotherapy [2].

Another local allergic reaction that has been described is the "**Adriamycin flare**," which occurs in 3% of all applications of doxorubicin. As per definition, the symptoms are erythema, indurations, and/or pruritus along the vein used for the infusion, necroses may develop [29]. The underlying pathomechanism under discussion is a hypoallergenic reaction to anthracyclines [21]. The symptoms remain even once the infusion has been stopped [110].

Systemic hypersensitivity reactions

Systemic hypersensitivity reactions are of great relevance for differential diagnosis in clinical practice [111, 112].
Principally, allergic reactions are categorised into 4 defined immunomechanisms (after Gell and Coombs). The type I reaction, with anaphylaxis, is the most important. However, the exact pathomechanisms and immunological processes underlying such reactions have been identified for very few cytotoxic drugs.

Type I (immediate type, anaphylactic type):

Mechanism:	Different mediators are released under mediating of cellular IgE antibodies (for example, histamine and vasoactive substances) from mast cells and basophils
Time to reaction:	Seconds to minutes; second reaction possible after 4–6 hours
Symptoms:	Urticaria, angio-oedema, exanthema, bronchospasm, hypotension, even allergic shock

Type II (cytotoxic type):

Mechanism:	Formation of immunocomplexes from cell wall antigens (such as cytotoxic agents) with circulating IgE, possible IgM, antibodies; cytolysis of the body's own cells through activation of complement or cytotoxic killer cells
Time to reaction:	6–12 hours
Symptoms:	Haemolytic anaemia, thrombopenia, agranulocytosis

Type III (immunocomplex type):

Mechanism:	Formation of tissue based or circulating immunocomplexes from IgG or IgM antibodies and antigens; phagocytosis or the immunocomplexes through granulocytes while releasing vesicant enzymes (for example, collagenase)
Time to reaction:	8–12 hours

Symptoms: Urticaria, erythema multiforme, vasculitis, angiooedema

Type IV (late type, cell mediated type):

Mechanism: Release of lymphokines from specifically sensitised T-lymphocytes on renewed antigen contact; promoting activation of macrophages and mononuclear cells

Time to reaction: 12–72 hours

Symptoms: Allergic contact dermatitis

The allergic reactions associated with asparaginase and taxane treatment have the greatest clinical relevance.
Since cytotoxic drugs are often combined with carrier substances to ensure better solubility and increase stability, hypersensitivity reactions may be due to those substances rather than the cytotoxic agent (examples include Cremophor® EL for paclitaxel, polysorbate 80 for etoposide and doxetaxel).

Substance	Reaction type	Frequency	Remarks
Asparaginase	Type I, III	10–35%	Up to 10% severe reactions
Paclitaxel	Type I	up to 40%	Rare for corticosteroids, severe in <2%
Teniposide	Type I	5–15%	Especially after rapid i.v. bolus administration
Docetaxel	Type I	5–10%	Rare for corticosteroids, mostly during 1st and 2nd applications
Cisplatin	Type I, II	5–10%	Intravascular =20%
Carboplatin	Type I, II	5–8%	
Melphalan	Type I	2–5%	
Daunorubicin	Type I	1–5%	
Doxorubicin	Type I	1–5%	
Etoposide	Type I	1–3%	Mostly after rapid i.v. administration
Bleomycin	Type I, IV	Rare	
Busulfan	Type III	Rare	
Cyclophosphamide	Type I	Rare	Even weeks or years after therapy
Cytarabine	Type I, cutaneous type III	Rare	
Dacarbazine	?	Rare	"Influenza-like" presentation with arthralgias and myalgias
Epirubicin	Type I	Rare	
5 FU	Type I	Rare	
Gemcitabine	Type I	Rare	
Methotrexate	Type I, III	Rare	Type I especially at high dosages, type III also at low dosages
Mitomycin C	Type IV	Rare	
Mitoxantrone	Type I	Rare	
Pentostatin	Type I	Rare	
Thiotepa	Type I, III	Rare	

[1] Substances listed by frequency of systemic hypersensitivity reactions.

Recall phenomena

In the context of cytotoxic agents, two recall reactions have to be differentiated:

- After previous chemotherapy
- After previous radiotherapy

A "recall", recurrence of skin toxicities **after preceding chemotherapy** with extravasation, has been described for:

- Docetaxel
- Doxorubicin [9,113]
- Epirubicin [114]
- 5-Fluorouracil
- Gemcitabine
- Idarubicin
- Mitomycin C
- Paclitaxel [115–117]

The symptoms worsen at the site of the original extravasation after repeated, correct application of the cytotoxic drug [118].

Radiation recall

D'Angio et al [119] first documented the "radiation recall phenomenon" in 1958 in connection with dactinomycin. It was described as a chemotherapy induced inflammatory reaction that developed at the site of the original radiotherapy 2 years after the radiotherapy had been completed. In the meantime, the "radiation recall phenomenon" has been described for several other cytotoxic agents, including:

- Bleomycin [109,120]
- Dactinomycin [109,111,119]
- Docetaxel [109,121–123]
- Doxorubicin [109,111,124,125]
- Etoposide [111,126]
- 5-Fluorouracil [109,111]
- Gemcitabine [109,128]
- Idarubicin [129]
- Methotrexate [109,111,130]
- Paclitaxel [109,111,131]
- Vinblastine [109,111,132]

The pathomechanism underlying this phenomenon is still not clear and is being discussed controversially [133, 134].

There are indications, however, that if these risk substances are applied within 10 days after radiotherapy the likelihood of a "radiation recall phenomenon" is reduced [109].
Characteristic for the radiation recall phenomenon is a pronounced skin reaction at the original radiation site. The clinical picture is one of severe sunburn.
The following symptoms have been described [109, 111]:

- Erythema
- Sensitivity to pressure and touch
- Swelling
- Inflammation
- Blistering
- Scaly skin
- Necrosis
- Skin discoloration

The "radiation recall phenomenon" can occur with a latency period of up to 15 years after completed radiotherapy [135].

Photosensitivity

Photosensitivity induced by cytotoxic drugs is an intensified skin reaction to sunlight. The clinical picture is characterised by erythema, oedema, and blister formation. Photosensitivity has been described after application of the following substances:

- Bleomycin
- Dactinomycin
- Dacarbazine
- 5-Fluorouracil
- Methotrexate
- Vinblastine

Severe toxic skin changes have been described especially for dacarbazine; avoiding sun exposure therefore constitutes causal prophylaxis [109].

Measures

Robert Mader

General unspecific measures in peripheral venous access

These general measures should be taken in cases of extravasation with **non-vesicant cytotoxic drugs:**

1. Stop injection/infusion immediately
2. Get extravasation kit
3. Put on (sterile) gloves
4. Replace infusion lead or syringe with 5 ml disposable syringe and aspirate slowly as much as possible of the extravasated drug; **Cave**! do not exert pressure on extravasation area
5. Remove i.v. access while aspirating
6. Elevate limb and immobilise
7. Complete extravasation documentation sheet (mention extent of extravasation)
8. Inform and instruct the patient and relatives
9. Regular control (aftercare)

The following general measures should be taken in cases of extravasation with **irritant cytotoxic drugs**:

1. Stop injection/infusion immediately
2. Get extravasation kit
3. Put on (sterile) gloves
4. Replace infusion lead or syringe with 5 ml disposable syringe and aspirate slowly as much as possible of the extravasated drug; **Cave**! do not exert pressure on extravasation area
5. Remove i.v. access while aspirating
6. If blisters occur: aspirate with 1 ml syringe and s.c. cannula, use new equipment for every new attempt at aspiration
7. Elevate limb and immobilise
8. Start **substance specific measures**
9. Complete extravasation documentation sheet (mention extent of extravasation)
10. Inform and instruct the patient and relatives
11. Regular control (aftercare)

The following general measures should be taken in cases of extravasation with **vesicant cytotoxic agents:**

1. Stop injection/infusion immediately
2. Get extravasation kit
3. Put on (sterile) gloves
4. Replace infusion lead or syringe with 5 ml disposable syringe and aspirate slowly as much as possible of the extravasated drug; **Cave!** do not exert pressure on extravasation area
5. Remove i.v. access while aspirating
6. If blisters occur: aspirate with 1 ml syringe and s.c. cannula, use new equipment for every new attempt at aspiration
7. Elevate limb and immobilise
8. Start **substance specific measures**
9. Ensure adequate analgesia
10. Complete extravasation documentation sheet (mention extent of extravasation)
11. Inform and instruct the patient and relatives
12. Regular control (aftercare)
13. Always consult a (plastic) surgeon within 24 hours

These measures are supported by a multitude of observations in the literature:

ad 1: Stop injection/infusion immediately:
The injection/infusion should be stopped immediately if the patient complains about a stinging or burning pain [15,21,28,45] or acute changes occur at the injection site [15, 139].
The responsible doctor should be informed immediately about an extravasation [139].
Possible other diagnoses should be excluded [45].
In case of an extravasation, disconnect the infusion lead or syringe from i.v. access [3].

ad 3: Put on (sterile) gloves [138]

ad 4: Replace infusion lead or syringe with 5 ml disposable syringe and aspirate slowly as much as possible of the extravasated drug [22, 139]:
The aspiration should be done with only slight suction as otherwise the opening of the catheter will adhere to the tissue. An attempt at aspiration is particularly promising if the catheter is positioned in the subfascia as the fluid is then collected in a defined space. In such cases the catheter should be left to facilitate the subsequent surgical exploration [37]. The syringe with content is disposed of as "hazardous waste" [138].

Do not exert pressure on extravasation area [37]:
Even minimal pressure in the area of the extravasation may distribute the vesicant agent widely [140].

ad 5: Remove i.v. access while aspirating:
Whether i.v. access should be maintained [22] or not [2, 28] is discussed controversially in the literature and depends on the kind of specific measures taken.
If access is maintained, then a stopper should be put on the catheter to keep the system sterile [138].

ad 6: If blisters occur: aspirate with 1 ml syringe and s.c. cannula, use new equipment for every new attempt at aspiration [22,27,141]:
This procedure is often described as painful and only rarely results in the removal of extravasated drug [3].

ad 7: Elevate limb and immobilise [15]:
In outpatients the arm may be put in a sling for two days [3].

ad 8: Start substance specific measures:
If i.v. access is maintained the literature offers the following measures: it has been attempted to dilute the drug with an infusion of 5–10 ml of NaCl 0.9% into the infiltrated area [139]. Alternatively, NaCl 0.9% may be mixed with hyaluronidase (150 IU in 1000 ml) [5].
If an antidote is known, it is infused through the existing i.v. access [25, 139]. This should guarantee for the antidote to reach the affected area. This technique is said to be much less traumatic for the patient than the multiple subcutaneous punctures. Immediate administration of the antidote is best [25].

It has been cited as a disadvantage that the original catheter through which the antidote is infused may still contain the cytotoxic agent [37].

After removing i.v. access the literature discusses s.c. injection of NaCl 0.9% at the extravasation site (for example, 20 ml into the wrist, 40 ml into the back of the hand, 60–90 ml into the lower arm and elbow crease). These injections were repeated three to a maximum of six times over the following days [142].
Other authors do not recommend the injection of NaCl 0.9% into the extravasation area as this might facilitate the diffusion of vesicant substance into the surrounding tissues [137].
Similar advantages [139] and disadvantages [28] have been described after administration of specific antidotes.
If no special measures are necessary, the affected region should merely be covered with sterile dressings [32].

ad 9: Ensure adequate analgesia:
This concerns not only any pain that is directly associated with the extravasation, but also comprehensive local analgesic medication during the s.c. application of the antidote hyaluronidase, which is perceived as painful [29].

ad 10: Complete extravasation documentation sheet (mention extent of extravasation!):
The extravasation and measures taken should be documented accordingly (documentation sheet, photo) [26, 28].
Areas underneath which an extravasation is suspected can be marked with a pen [28].

ad 13: After extravasation of a vesicant drug always consult a (plastic) surgeon within 24 hours:
Early consultation with a surgeon follows from the option of diluting the extravasated fluid in the tissue via flushout technique or liposuction [143-145]. The effectiveness of this invasive procedure is limited to 24 hours (see chapter "Surgical intervention).

General unspecific measures in central venous access

If an extravasation occurs at the site of the central venous access, the positioning of the catheter has to be examined radiographically or with a venogram. In addition to the general unspecific measures as in peripheral venous access [31], the following interventions have been described in the literature:

- Attempted aspiration [80]
- Dilution (described controversially)
- Use of antidotes (low evidence of efficacy in intrathoracal use)
- Drainage of pleural effusion [80]
- Surgical intervention [80]

Specific measures/antidotes

A number of substance specific measures to minimise the toxicity of extravasations is listed in the literature. The most important of these are:

- Application of topical cooling
- Application of dry heat
- Local application of dimethylsulfoxide (DMSO)
- Application of hyaluronidase

- Application of dexrazoxane
- Application of sodium bicarbonate (sodium hydrogen carbonate)
- Application of sodium thiosulfate ($Na_2S_2O_3 \times 5\ H_2O$)
- Application of dexamethasone or hydrocortisone cream

Although the measures mentioned are documented in many case reports and clinical studies, their number of observations and clinical relevance vary widely. The topical application of dimethylsulfoxide, for example, was tested in 144 patients with extravasations of cytotoxic agents. This means that the efficacy of DMSO is clearly better documented [146] than that of sodium thiosulfate, which has been described in a single case study as an antidote to inactivate mechlorethamine (mustargen) [147].
As the only approved antidote, dexrazoxane has recently been introduced. Similar to DMSO in combination with cooling, dexrazoxane is indicated after extravasation of anthracyclines if detected within six hours after the extravasation event [220].
Other antidotes mentioned in the literature are administered sporadically. Mostly they are mentioned in combination with antidotes that are known to be effective in isolation or tested in animal models exclusively so that their clinical efficacy as a single substance has not been proved. These antidotes include heparin [21,96,148], ascorbic acid (vitamin C) [149], N-acetylcysteine [150] and α-tocopherol (vitamin E) [151, 152].
The oxomorpholino derivative DHM3 has not been clinically tested in spite of promising animal experiments [153, 154].
The described efficacy of chondroitin sulfatase [155] may be explained with its functional similarity to hyaluronidase, which can be used to replace it in clinical practice. Interestingly, the use of hyaluronidase is a tried and tested measure in extravasations in dogs too [156]. The encapsulation of hyaluronidase in the sense of a liposomal depot has been described but not preclinically tested. There are therefore no data on the release and enzymatic activity of this formulation [157]. The use of Phlogenzym®, a mixture of the proteolytic enzymes trypsin, bromelain, and rutin, has been tested in 14 patients after extravasation of vinca alkaloids and/or anthracyclines. Although Phlogenzym® is well tolerated, its efficacy is not confirmed as two of the patients subsequently had to have surgery [158].
Other substances such as tetrachlordecaoxide were clinically tested after extravasation of doxorubicin and cisplatin but have not got any further than the trial stage despite positive initial reports [159].
Supportive measures such as the application of hyperbaric oxygene [160] or keratolytic cream with salicylic acid [161] remain anecdotal.
A possible new therapeutic concept is the discussion of growth factors such as basic fibroblast growth factor (bFGF) or keratinocyte growth

factor (KGF) [58]. It has to be borne in mind that extravasation is an acute event that requires swift action. Growth factors do, however, not become effective in minutes and hours and, even if further examination shows that they are sufficiently effective, would merely remain a supportive measure.

Intense studies of the mechanism of action of the anthracyclines have given prominence to the antidote dexrazoxane in the context of systematic studies. Because the anthracyclines suppress the activity of the target enzyme topoisomerase II in a sensitive phase, DNA strands break, which leads to cell death. This is due to formation of a complex of anthracycline enzyme DNA that poisons the enzyme ("cleavable complex"). As antagonists for this mechanism, the substance class of bisdioxopiperazines has been developed further for use after extravasations of anthracyclines. The antagonism is likely to consist of the competitive displacement of anthracyclines and the catalytic inhibition of topoisomerase II in a phase of the cycle where no DNA strand breakages occur [162].

In breast cancer therapy, dexrazoxane is licensed as a cardioprotective medication against doxorubicin associated cardiomyopathy. Studies have shown a protective effect after extravasation of anthracyclines in mice [163]. The efficacy as an antidote was observed for an application within three hours after the extravasation event. For daunorubicin, the effect was dose independent, but for doxorubicin this was not the case. Repeated application was superior to single application. The hypothesis that dexrazoxane protects against oxidative stress (subcutaneous administration of H_2O_2) has not been proved in vitro [164] nor in the mouse model [165].

Topical cooling

Discussed mechanism of action:

- Vasoconstriction
- Local demarcation of the extravasation area; simultaneously reduced transport from the affected region, which may be disadvantageous [140]
- Reduction of cellular absorption of doxorubicin in vitro [166]
- Reduction of cytotoxic effect of doxorubicin in mice [167], and of cisplatin, bleomycin, and carmustine in vitro [168]

Particular remarks:

- Limited effectiveness as single measure [28, 169]
- Synergistic effectiveness in combination with DMSO [146]

Examples of application:
Diverging information in the literature, hence no standardised procedure, for example:

- Ice packs 4 × daily for 15 minutes for a minimum of 3 days [28]
- Local cooling, to patient tolerance, for 24 hours [19]
- Application of a cold compress for 12 hours, to be interrupted every 3 hours for 20–30 minutes [139]

Advantages:
- Easy to use
- Non-invasive measure
- Hardly any side effects

Disadvantage:
- Enhanced toxicity of vinca alkaloids in mice! [103]

Cave!
- Moisture combined with cold can cause macerations (alcohol compresses should not be used)
- During treatment avoid pressure on the extravasation area

Administration:

Consensus:

1. Apply cold, dry pack immediately for at least 1 hour (for example, using a cold-hot pack)
2. Continue several times daily for 15 minutes each time

Application after extravasation of the following substances:

Topical cooling alone:	Daunorubicin liposomal Doxorubicin liposomal
Topical cooling in combination with DMSO:	Amsacrine Cisplatin Dactinomycin Daunorubicin Doxorubicin Epirubicin Idarubicin Mitomycin C Mitoxantrone

Dry heat

Discussed mechanism of action:
- Vasodilatation
- Increased local blood flow; this improves distribution and absorption from the affected tissue and simultaneously lowers the local concentration of cytotoxic drugs [140]

Particular remarks:
Although synergism with hyaluronidase has been discussed for vinca alkaloids [32], little evidence of this has been found in clinical or animal studies [103].

Examples of application:
- Warm compresses for 15 minutes every 6 hours for 48 hours [23]
- Dry heat for 1–2 hours [20]

Advantages:
- Ease of use
- Non-invasive measure
- No side effects

Disadvantage:
The remaining activity of some cytotoxic agents may be increased by heat. In vitro this has been shown for doxorubicin, cisplatin, bleomycin, and carmustine [168] and in mice for doxorubicin [167]; this means increased risk of severe tissue damage for some cytotoxic agents.

Cave!
- Moisture combined with heat can lead to macerations and favour the development of necroses [20, 170]
- During treatment avoid pressure on the extravasation area

Administration:

Consensus:

Application of dry heat in a subjectively agreeable manner (e.g., cold-hot pack, hot water bottle) 4 × daily over 20 minutes

Application after extravasation of the following substances:

Heat in combination with hyaluronidase:	Vinblastine Vincristine Vindesine Vinorelbine

Dimethylsulfoxide (DMSO)

Discussed mechanism of action:

- Vasodilatation [171]
- Fast penetration of tissue and high solubility for drugs [172]
- Increased permeability of skin caused by highly concentrated DMSO, which accelerates the systemic distribution of the extravasated drug [172]
- Anti-inflammatory effect [173]
- Radical scavenger (for example, for use in radical generating substances such as anthracyclines) [174]
- Reduced cytotoxicity of cisplatin in vitro [175] and nephrotoxicity in rats [176]

Particular remarks:

- In combination with intermittent topical cooling this is a very effective antidote to vesicant substances such as the anthracyclines [146]
- Concentrated DMSO (99%) seems to have superior efficacy to the diluted solution [177]
- DMSO additionally has a local anaesthetic effect [178]

Examples of application:

- Solution (99%) topical: start immediately, 4 drops per 10 cm^2 to be applied locally, every 8 hours for 1 week or until symptoms have subsided [146]
- Solution (99%) topical: to be applied locally every 6 hours over 14 days [179]

Advantages:

- Ease of use
- Non-invasive measure
- Effectiveness as antidote well documented
- Hardly any side effects [171]

Disadvantages:
- Characteristic garlic-like odour to the breath [146]
- Slight burning and erythema at treatment site [171], rarely urticaria [172], pain [180], or blistering [146,179]
- Drying out and scaling of skin [178]

Administration:

Consensus:

1. Apply DMSO (99%) every 8 hours (e.g. with a sterile gauze pad) without pressure
2. Allow to air-dry – **Cave!** do not cover
3. Continue for a minimum of 7 days

Application after extravasation of the following substances:

DMSO in combination with topical cooling:	Amsacrine Cisplatin Dactinomycin Daunorubicin Doxorubicin Epirubicin Idarubicin Mitomycin C Mitoxantrone

Hyaluronidase

Discussed mechanism of action:
- Enzymatic degradation of the connective tissue component hyaluronic acid, chondroitinic acid, and mucoitin sulfate results in a structural loosening of connective and supportive tissues and thus increased absorption of extravasated drug from the affected tissue [33, 181]
- Synergism with heat has been postulated [32] but proved neither clinically nor in animal studies [20,103]

Particular remarks:
- In animal experiments, contradictory findings were identified about the benefit of hyaluronidase in the extravasation of doxorubicin [182-184]

- After extravasation of vinorelbine, the combination of 1500 IU hyaluronidase with topical DMSO is recommended [178]
- As the s.c. application of hyaluronidase is usually associated with severe pain, local analgesia is recommended [29]

Examples of application:
- 300 IU (= 1 ml) s.c. to be injected in a star shape, from the periphery to the centre, around the affected area [33]
- 250 IU in 6 ml NaCl 0.9% to be infused through the indwelling intravenous access or 250 IU to be injected by six s.c. injections around the extravasation area [181]
- 1500 IU in 2 ml aqua ad inj. to be administered s.c. around the extravasation area [185]

Advantage:
- Hardly any side effects [186]

Disadvantage:
- Invasive measure

Administration:

> Consensus:
>
> Inject up to 1500 IU hyaluronidase s.c. around the affected area depending on size of extravasation. **Cave!** local analgesia is recommended

Application after extravasation of the following substances:

Hyaluronidase alone:	Paclitaxel
Hyaluronidase in combination with heat:	Vinblastine Vincristine Vindesine Vinorelbine

Dexrazoxane

Mechanism of action under discussion:

- Anthracycline antagonist as a catalytic inhibitor of topoisomerase II without causing DNA strand breaks [164, 187]
- Reduction of free radical formation from iron-anthracycline complexes as chelators of iron ions

Particular remarks:

- Based on the results of two relatively small randomized multicenter trials, dexrazoxane has been approved as antidote after extravasation of anthracyclines as proven by biopsy [221]. The application of dexrazoxane is supposed to start within 6 hours after the extravasation event. Data from animal studies suggest a better outcome when this interval is shorter (<3 hours) [165]. The mechanism of action has not been fully understood so far; especially the function as a radical scavenger needs to be proven *in vivo*
- As no comparison between the efficacy of dexrazoxane and that of DMSO/topical cooling has been performed so far, there is no clinical evidence proving the superiority of dexrazoxane over DMSO treatment (both randomized studies were done without the standard procedure DMSO/topical cooling as a control arm)
- In one case, a combination of DMSO/dexrazoxane was applied after extravasation of doxorubicin [188]
- In paediatric patients receiving chemotherapy for Hodgkin's disease, dexrazoxane was associated with an enhanced incidence to develop secondary malignancies; there was an increased relative risk >3 to develop a myelodysplastic syndrome or acute myeloic leukaemia after a cumulative dose of 3000 mg dexrazoxane/m^2 used as a cardiopulmonary protectant [222]

Application according to the marketing authorization:

- 1000 mg dexrazoxane /m^2 are administered i.v. within six hours after extravasation; the i.v. treatment is repeated on day 2 (1000 mg dexrazoxane /m^2) and on day 3 (500 mg dexrazoxane /m^2). For patients with a body surface area of more than 2 m^2 the single dose should not exceed 2000 mg [220]

Examples of application used in previous studies:

- I.v. infusion of 1000 mg dexrazoxane/m^2 within 48 hours after extravasation, followed by 500 mg dexrazoxane on day 3 [189, 190]
- I.v. infusion of 1500 mg dexrazoxane over 15 minutes withion 1 hour after extravasation. Repeat after 5 hours, followed by 750 mg dexrazoxane on the following day [191]

Advantage:
- Approved antidote after extravasation of anthracyclines

Disadvantages:
- Invasive measure
- Sometimes burning pain on injection site [220]
- Moderate nausea and vomiting [220]
- Increases chemotherapy induced leucopenia and thrombocytopenia [220]

Administration:

Consensus:

Dexrazoxane:
1. Administer 1000 mg dexrazoxane /m^2 i.v. within six hours after extravasation
2. Repeat the i.v. treatment on day 2 (1000 mg dexrazoxane /m^2) and on day 3 (500 mg dexrazoxane /m^2)

The substance may be considered after extravasation of the following substances:	Daunorubicin Doxorubicin Epirubicin Idarubicin

Sodium bicarbonate (sodium hydrogen carbonate)

Discussed mechanism of action:
- Increase of the local pH value reduces the binding of daunorubicin to DNA [192]
- In animal experiments, effective antidote to doxorubicin in rats [193], but not in swine [194]
- Chemical degradation of carmustine under alkaline conditions; observed *in vitro* [195, 196], but not proved *in vivo*

Examples of application:
- Sodium bicarbonate (8.4%) and NaCl 0.9% mixed 1:1, then 2–6 ml to be administered i.v. and s.c. perilesionally [197]
- 1–3 ml sodium bicarbonate (2.1%) to be infiltrated for 2 minutes and then aspirated [185]

Disadvantages:
- Invasive measure
- Sodium bicarbonate may cause tissue necrosis by itself and has to be dosed accurately [140]
- Severe tissue damage has been documented after s.c. administration of sodium bicarbonate (8.4%) [198, 199]
- By raising the pH value, the cellular absorption of anthracyclines [200] and their cytotoxicity were increased [201]

Cave!
In the literature the use of sodium bicarbonate is being discussed very controversially because of its potential to cause necrosis

Consensus:

Because of the danger of necrosis caused by sodium bicarbonate its use is not recommended!

Sodium thiosulfate ($Na_2S_2O_3 \times 5\ H_2O$)

Discussed mechanism of action:
- Chemical inactivation of cisplatin and chlormethin (mustargen) through nucleophilic reactions
- Radical scavenger: protection from oxygen radicals induced by cytotoxic drugs [202]
- Sodium thiosulfate inactivated cisplatin in animal experiments, but has never been clinically tested in extravasations of this substance [203]

Particular remarks:
- Preclinical studies in mice were unsuccessful in lesions with dactinomycin, vincristine, and cisplatin [204], but not with chlormethin [205]
- The use of sodium thiosulphate after extravasation of anthracyclines or vinca alkaloids was clinically successful [202]; case report describing a positive outcome in an incident with chlormethin (mustargen) [147]

Examples of application:
- Several ml of sodium thiosulfate (2%) s.c. combined with a gentle massage [202]
- 4 ml sodium thiosulfate (10%) via existing i.v. access [141]

Advantage:

- Hardly any side effects [206]

Disadvantage:

- Invasive measure

> Consensus:
>
> In the clinical setting the local effectiveness of sodium thiosulfate s.c. and i.v. is not sufficiently proved. At least the same result can be achieved with the application of DMSO, which is a non-invasive intervention. Hence, the application of sodium thiosulfate is not recommended.

Corticosteroids

Discussed mechanism of action:

- Anti-inflammatory effect

Examples of application:

- 100 mg hydrocortisone s.c. and i.v., hydrocortisone applied topically [185], 70–80 mg triamcinolone acetonide intralesionally, twice within one week [102]

Advantage:

- Topical application possible

Disadvantages:

- In animal models hydrocortisone increased the toxicity of vinca alkaloids [103]; corticosteroids influenced the effectiveness of doxorubicin only marginally [97, 98]
- The administration of corticosteroids is pharmacologically not indicated as extravasations are only rarely accompanied by inflammatory processes [20,47,95,146,207]
- Corticosteroids themselves are toxic for skin [58]

> Consensus:
>
> The use of corticosteroids is pharmacologically not indicated as extravasations are only rarely accompanied by inflammatory processes; usually, the immigration of inflammatory cells is a secondary event only.

Extravasation kit

To be able to react quickly if the clinical emergency of an extravasation occurs, an emergency kit should be to hand at an agreed location.
The kit contains, among others, the following 4 lists:

1. **List of substances:** the cytotoxic agents are listed alphabetically, by the name of their active substance; this offers an opportunity rapidly to obtain information about the possible dangers associated with an agent and about measures to be taken.

   It is recommended to set out a list specific to your hospital, in which the alphabetical listing is by trade name (example see appendix).
2. **List of general measures:** according to type of damage (non-vesicant/irritant/vesicant) 3 categories of general measures (I, II, III) are described.
3. **List of substance specific measures** with instructions on how to apply hyaluronidase, DMSO, dexrazoxane, topical cooling and heat, and measures to be avoided at all.
4. The individual components of the extravasation kit are listed under **"Contents of extravasation kit."**

The book's appendix contains A4 templates for photocopying of the following:

1. Information leaflet for outpatient/inpatient department
2. The preceding lists 1–4
3. An example of an internal list of substances
4. A suggestion for how to label the extravasation box

These documents can also be found on the accompanying CD-ROM or on the internet at <www.extravasation.at>, or <www.paravasate.at>.
The extravasation kit should be examined from time to time for completeness and up-to-date-ness, and after each use a new documentation sheet should be inserted. In clinical practice, a plastic box has proved useful (size approximately 20 cm × 15 cm) (Fig. 1).
Another option is a plastic emergency case from Rauscher (size about 30 cm × 20 cm). This option is slightly costlier but has the advantage of a wall mount, and both parts of the case can be used to store the extravasation kit in a safe and user friendly way (Fig. 2). This may sound trivial, but the literature has numerous examples of the effectiveness of organisational measures. The presence of an extravasation kit including a catalogue of measures on oncology wards has resulted in reduced morbidity and the frequency of cosmetic-plastic surgical procedures [136].

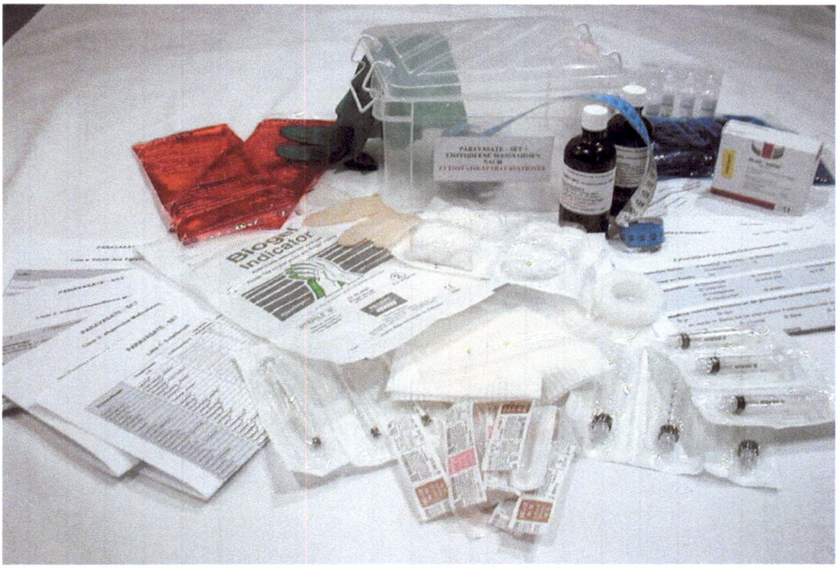

Fig. 1. Contents of extravasation kit

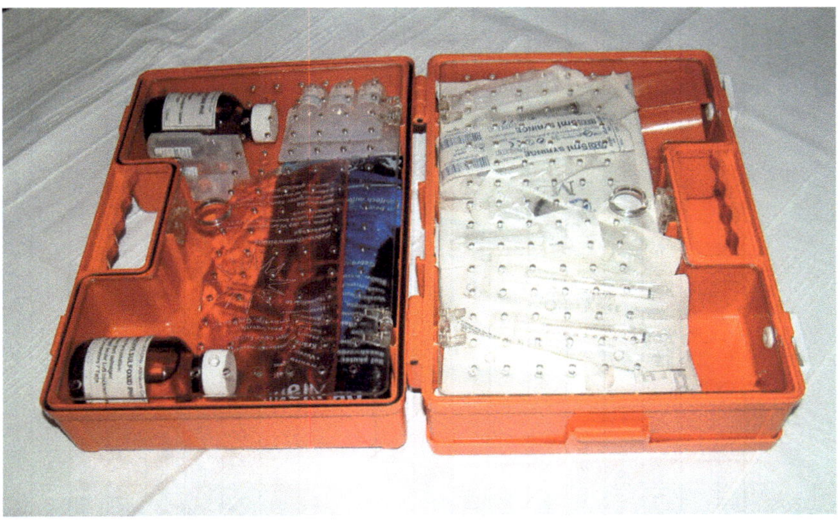

Fig. 2. Extravasation kit in emergency case

EXTRAVASATION KIT

List 1: Substances

Substance	Type of damage	General measures (see list 2)	Substance specific measures (see list 3)
Amsacrine	vesicant	III	+ topical DMSO/cooling
Asparaginase	non-vesicant	I	none
Bendamustine	irritant	II	none
Bleomycin	non-vesicant	I	none
Bortezomib	irritant	II	none
Busulfan	irritant	II	none
Carboplatin	non-vesicant	I	none
Carmustine	irritant	II	none
Cisplatin	vesicant ≥0.4 mg/ml	III	+ topical DMSO/cooling
	irritant		+ topical DMSO/cooling
Cladribine	non-vesicant	I	none
Cyclophosphamide	non-vesicant	I	none
Cytarabine	non-vesicant	I	none
Dacarbazine	irritant	II	**Cave!** no sunlight!
Dactinomycin	vesicant	III	+ topical DMSO/cooling
Daunorubicin	vesicant	III	+ topical DMSO/cooling *or* dexrazoxane i.v.
Daunorubicin liposomal	irritant	II	+ topical cooling

Substance	Type of damage	General measures (see list 2)	Substance specific measures (see list 3)
Docetaxel	irritant	II	none
Doxorubicin	vesicant	III	+ topical DMSO/cooling *or* dexrazoxane i.v.
Doxorubicin liposomal	irritant	II	+ topical cooling
Epirubicin	vesicant	III	+ topical DMSO/cooling *or* dexrazoxane i.v.
Estramustine	non-vesicant	I	none
Etoposide	irritant	II	none
Etoposide phosphate	non-vesicant	I	none
Fludarabine	non-vesicant	I	none
5-Fluorouracil	non-vesicant	I	none
	undiluted irritant	II	none
Fotemustine	irritant	II	none
Gemcitabine	irritant	II	none
Idarubicin	vesicant	III	+ topical DMSO/cooling *or* dexrazoxane i.v.
Ifosfamide	non-vesicant	I	none
Irinotecan	non-vesicant	I	none
Melphalan	irritant	II	none
Methotrexate	non-vesicant	I	none
Mitomycin C	vesicant	III	+ topical DMSO/cooling
Mitoxantrone	vesicant	III	+ topical DMSO/cooling

Substance	Type of damage	General measures (see list 2)	Substance specific measures (see list 3)
Nimustine	non-vesicant	I	none
Oxaliplatin	vesicant	III	**Cave!** no topical cooling
Paclitaxel	vesicant	III	+ hyaluronidase s.c.
Pegaspargase	non-vesicant	I	none
Pemetrexed	non-vesicant	I	none
Pentostatin	non-vesicant	I	none
Raltitrexed	non-vesicant	I	none
Streptozocin	irritant	II	none
Teniposide	irritant	II	none
Thiotepa	non-vesicant	I	none
Topotecan	non-vesicant	I	none
Treosulfan	irritant	II	none
Trimetrexate	irritant	II	none
Vinblastine	vesicant	III	+ hyaluronidase s.c./heat
Vincristine	vesicant	III	+ hyaluronidase s.c./heat
Vindesine	vesicant	III	+ hyaluronidase s.c./heat
Vinorelbine	vesicant	III	+ hyaluronidase s.c./heat

EXTRAVASATION KIT

List 2: General measures

In extravasations with non-vesicant cytotoxic agents (I):

1. Stop injection/infusion immediately
2. Get extravasation kit
3. Put on (sterile) gloves
4. Replace infusion lead or syringe with 5 ml disposable syringe and aspirate slowly as much as possible of the extravasated drug; **Cave!** do not exert pressure on extravasation area
5. Remove i.v. access while aspirating
6. Elevate limb and immobilise
7. Complete extravasation documentation sheet (mention extent of extravasation)
8. Inform and instruct the patient and relatives
9. Regular control (aftercare)

In extravasations with irritant cytotoxic agents (II):

1. Stop injection/infusion immediately
2. Get extravasation kit
3. Put on (sterile) gloves
4. Replace infusion lead or syringe with 5 ml disposable syringe and aspirate slowly as much as possible of the extravasated drug; **Cave!** do not exert pressure on extravasation area
5. Remove i.v. access while aspirating
6. If blisters occur: aspirate with 1 ml syringe and s.c. cannula, use new equipment for every new attempt at aspiration
7. Elevate limb and immobilise
8. Start **substance specific measures**
9. Complete extravasation documentation sheet (mention extent of extravasation)
10. Inform and instruct the patient and relatives
11. Regular control (aftercare)

In extravasations with vesicant cytotoxic agents (III):

1. Stop injection/infusion immediately
2. Get extravasation kit
3. Put on (sterile) gloves
4. Replace infusion lead or syringe with 5 ml disposable syringe and aspirate slowly as much as possible of the extravasated drug; **Cave!** do not exert pressure on extravasation area
5. Remove i.v. access while aspirating
6. If blisters occur: aspirate with 1 ml syringe and s.c. cannula, use new equipment for every new attempt at aspiration
7. Elevate limb and immobilise
8. Start **substance specific measures**
9. Ensure adequate analgesia
10. Complete extravasation documentation sheet (mention extent of extravasation)
11. Inform and instruct the patient and relatives
12. Regular control (aftercare)
13. Always consult a (plastic) surgeon within 24 hours

EXTRAVASATION KIT

List 3: Substance specific measures

+ Hyaluronidase s.c./dry heat
Hyaluronidase: Inject up to 1500 IU hyaluronidase s.c. around the affected area depending on size of extravasation; **Cave!** local analgesia is recommended **Immediately afterwards dry heat:** Application of dry heat in a subjectively agreeable manner (e.g., cold-hot pack, hot water bottle) 4 × daily over 20 minutes

+ Topical DMSO/topical cooling
DMSO: 1. Apply DMSO (99%) every 8 hours (e.g. with a sterile gauze pad) without pressure 2. Allow to air-dry – **Cave!** do not cover 3. Continue for a minimum of 7 days **Immediately afterwards topical cooling:** 1. Apply cold, dry pack immediately for at least 1 hour (for example, using a cold-hot pack) 2. Continue several times daily for 15 minutes each time

+ Dexrazoxane
Alternatively to DMSO and topical cooling **Dexrazoxane:** 1. Administer 1000 mg dexrazoxane /m² i.v. within six hours after extravasation 2. Repeat the i.v. treatment on day 2 (1000 mg dexrazoxane /m²) and on day 3 (500 mg dexrazoxane /m²)

In extravasations of all cytotoxic agents

Cave!	1. No flushing of i.v. access 2. No moist compresses 3. No alcohol compresses 4. No occlusive dressings

EXTRAVASATION KIT

List 4: Contents of extravasation kit

Product		Number	Conditions of storage
Disposable syringes	1 ml 2 ml 5 ml	3 3 3	Room temperature
Disposable cannulas	18 G (pink) 26 G (brown)	5 5	Room temperature
Cold-hot packs in-house product..		2 for warm compresses 2 for cold compresses	Room temperature Cold: 2–8°C
Gauze pads, sterile, plum size in-house product..		2 sets at 4 each	Room temperature
Gauze dressings, sterile, approx. 10×10 cm in-house product..		1 set at 5 pieces	Room temperature
Adhesive plaster in-house product..		1 roll	Room temperature
Gloves, sterile (medium and large) Protective gloves for handling cytotoxic agents, sterile (medium and large) in-house product..		1 pair each 1 pair each	Room temperature
Hyaluronidase in-house product..		1500 IU	Cold: 2–8°C
Dimethylsulfoxide (DMSO) 99% in-house product..		2 × 100 ml	Room temperature
List 1: Substances List 2: General measures List 3: Substance specific measures List 4: Contents of extravasation kit 1 Extravasation documentation form, 1 tape measure			

EXTRAVASATION KIT

Information leaflet for ward staff

Storage location and contents of extravasation kit

Storage location of extravasation kit (please define accordingly; for example: in-patient ward):		
1×10 ampoules hyaluronidase (in-house product) and 2 cold-hot packs in refrigerator:		
Product	**Number**	**Conditions of storage**
Disposable syringes 1 ml 2 ml 5 ml	3 3 3	Room temperature
Disposable cannulas 18 G 26 G	5 5	Room temperature
Cold-hot packs in-house product..	2 for warm compresses 2 for cold compresses	Room temperature Cold: 2–8°C
Gauze pads, sterile, plum size in-house product..	2 sets at 4 each	Room temperature
Gauze dressings, sterile, approx. 10 × 10 cm in-house product..	1 set at 5 pieces	Room temperature
Adhesive plaster in-house product..	1 roll	Room temperature
Gloves, sterile (medium and large) Protective gloves for handling cytotoxic agents, sterile (medium and large) in-house product..	1 pair each 1 pair each	Room temperature
Hyaluronidase in-house product..	1500 IU	Cold: 2–8°C
Dimethylsulfoxide (DMSO) 99% in-house product..	2 × 100 ml	Room temperature
List 1: Substances List 2: General measures List 3: Substance specific measures List 4: Contents of extravasation kit 1 Extravasation documentation form, 1 tape measure		

EXTRAVASATION KIT

Example of a list of in-house cytotoxic agents, in alphabetical order by trade name:

Cytotoxic agents in use	Name of substance	Type of damage	General measures	Substance specific measures

Label for extravasation emergency box:

EXTRAVASATION KIT +
RECOMMENDED MEASURES AFTER
EXTRAVASATION OF CYTOTOXIC AGENTS

Surgical intervention

In most patients conservative treatment is sufficient [142, 208]. In those patients, however, in whom conservative measures fail, surgical intervention is required. Langstein and colleagues reported 44 extravasations of vesicant substances in a six year observational study. 62% of the patients had to present to a plastic surgeon, and 24% had to undergo surgical treatment to achieve complete healing [39].

Consulting a plastic surgeon

The literature mentions consultations with plastic surgeons under the following circumstances:

- If extravasation of a cytotoxic agent is suspected [37]
- If conservative measures do not result in healing [25, 34, 209]

In addition to consulting a plastic surgeon, the literature recommends immediate surgical intervention in case of the following symptoms or indications:

- If a risk of compartment syndrome exists (caused by extravasation of infusion fluid or tissue oedema) [37]
- In persistent local pain [28,208,210]
- In case of extended or severe extravasations, if, for example, damage to neurovascular structures, tendons, etc. is to be expected [98, 209]
- If ulceration [210] or formation of eschar [211] occurs
- After extravasation of a vesicant, depending on the amount and localisation of the extravasated drug [37]

Although this is not yet commonly accepted in the literature, it seems reasonable to consult a plastic surgeon in those cases where permanent functional damage is suspected. In our experience, an absolute indication for immediate surgical intervention exists in all cases with symptoms of compartment syndrome on the extremities.

Opinions diverge about the moment when a plastic surgeon should be consulted:

- Within 4-24 hours [143, 145]

In severe extravasations as early as possible [209], in any case within 72 hours [28]

- 2–3 weeks after the initial damage [25]
- Between 1 day and 3 months after extravasation, on average within 2–3 weeks [5]

Timely consultation of a plastic surgeon after extravasation has the following advantages for the patient [28, 37]:

- A decision about acute intervention in the sense of the flushout technique or liposuction within 4 to 24 hours at the latest [143, 145]

Similar to the timing of the consultation with a plastic surgeon, the best time for a surgical intervention varies in the literature:

- 2 to 3 weeks after the initial damage [25]
- Several weeks after the extravasation [211]

We think that the ideal timing of the operation follows once the tissue necrosis is obviously demarcated against the surrounding tissues.
The literature does not make direct mention of this, but in the case of moist necroses, early débridement should be considered (danger of superinfections). In patients with dry necroses, a more conservative procedure may be considered—depending on the performance status and prognosis of the patient.
Because of the regularly observed recurrence of tissue damage in the area of the lesion after repeated administration of the cytotoxic agent, the literature recommends ceasing chemotherapy during wound healing [212]. After the wound has healed completely, the chemotherapy should be started immediately. On the basis of animal experiments (which have to be interpreted with caution) with doxorubicin [213–215], operations should be avoided within 7 days before the following course of chemotherapy or up to 5 days after an antineoplastic substance has been administered [28].

Surgical intervention methods

Flushout technique and liposuction

Whereas treatment of the lesion with plastic surgical techniques is usually done weeks after the extravasation event, the literature mentions two techniques that require rapid intervention. These are i) the flushout (also "washout") technique, also known as subcutaneous flushing, and ii) liposuction.
The **flushout technique** was first described in 1993 by Gault, on the basis of 96 patients with extravasations of different vesicant agents (cancer treatment and metabolic disorders), among them 39 receiving cytotoxic chemotherapy [143]. As a first step, 1500 IU hyaluronidase is applied to the affected area, and in a second step, the subcutaneous tissue is flushed with 500 ml of physiological saline. In a modified procedure, Khan et al applied a local anaesthetic with the hyaluronidase so the patients would suffer less [136]. The saline transports the cytotoxic drug to the outside through four incisions around the extravasation; the author refers to this as a "subcutaneous shower." To avoid injury to nerves and tendons, a blunt cannula with lateral infiltration holes (Verres needle) is used for the flushout procedure. Antibiotic protection and wound sterility are of particular importance in this invasive procedure. The author described the treatment as very successful; 39 of 44 patients did not suffer tissue damage. The procedure needs to be undertaken within 24 hours after the extravasation event are regarded.

In some of these patients, **liposuction** was performed under local or general anaesthesia. The rationale behind this procedure is to aspirate the extravasated drug with the subcutaneous fatty tissue because lipophilic cytotoxic agents spread rapidly in these. To help decision making about which technique to use, we refer to Gault's treatment algorithm of 1993. According to the algorithm, liposuction should always be the method of choice in extravasations that are surrounded by a thick layer of subcutaneous fat. If the subcutaneous fatty layer is thin (dorsum of hand, antecubital fossa), the washout technique should be used.

These recommendations have been adopted by plastic surgeons and tested after extravasation of contrast medium [216] and cytotoxic agents. The successful treatment of 3 patients by subcutaneous flushing in combination with hyaluronidase after extravasation of vinorelbine has been reported [144,145]. An animal study confirmed these findings partly for doxorubicin. Although the intervention was started within 2 hours of placing the intradermal doxorubicin lesion, necroses could not be avoided completely [217].

The evaluation of the reports cited earlier shows successful treatment after extravasation of vinorelbine when this invasive treatment was used. However, the successful treatment is being discussed controversially for liposuction because of further trauma to the tissues and the effects on the vessels [210]. The number of patients treated with subcutaneous flushing/liposuction within 24 hours who were receiving antineoplastic chemotherapy was not obvious from Gault's study. A final evaluation of this technique is therefore currently not possible. Because of the serious invasiveness of the treatment, this should be studied only for highly toxic substances such as the vinca alkaloids or the anthracyclines, but never for other vesicant substances such as paclitaxel or cisplatin.

The literature reflects a consensus on a two phase procedure, namely **débridement and later surgical covering** [5,15,25,34,37, 208]. According to more recent publications, however, wide excisional margins in the healthy tissue enable immediately surgical covering [212]. A direct grafting on to the ulcer has been described as not successful [34].

Débridement

The size of the lesion is often underestimated, which can necessitate repeated surgical revision [37]. Excision should be performed in healthy tissue [8,14,24,34,37,211,212]. It has to be borne in mind that after preceding conservative treatment the affected area may be smaller than originally assumed [208].

To locate anthracyclines in tissue their autofluorescence may be used. The intensity of this fluorescence is not high enough if the amount of extravasated drug is small [9, 218]. An additional injection of fluorescein to ascertain the extent of the extravasation may increase local toxicity through a potential synergistic effect with doxorubicin [208, 218].
Débridement is followed by either by immediate wound closure with split thickness skin grafting or, if necessary, pedicled or free flap, or by a period of conservative treatment, with temporary wound dressing. In our experience, sealing the wound with vacuum assisted closure (VAC) systems is the method of choice. Moist compresses have also been mentioned (for example, drenched in Ringer's solution) or paraffin gauze [37], as have newer local therapeutic measures to assist wound healing, such as the use of hydrocolloid or alginate dressings.
The literature also mentions the use of fibrin sealant in combination with α-aminocaproic acid (débridement, repeated application of fibrin sealant to the wound area and injection of it into the surrounding tissue). It remains to be seen whether the results can be improved by using a combination of débridement, skin grafting, and fibrin sealant [21].

Secondary skin grafting of the defect

The following interventions might be considered (ordered by increasing complexity):

- In smaller defects secondary covering may be omitted, for example, in granulation and healing after conservative treatment or delayed primary wound closure
- (Split thickness) skin graft [5,15,25], maybe in mesh graft technique [8,34,210]; if bones, tendons, larger nerves or blood vessels are exposed, skin grafts are not sufficient [8, 30, 112]

More complex techniques of covering should be assessed thoroughly in terms of their usefulness to the patient, bearing in mind the patient's underlying disease [5]. These include:

- Local pedicled flap graft (fasciocutaneous, myocutaneous, muscle flap with split thickness skin graft) [5,8,16,25,37,45]
- Distant pedicled flaps from other areas (loins, abdomen) [5]
- Free (microsurgical) flap reconstructions should be considered under the following conditions only:

  1. In defects that, because of their size and/or function, cannot be reconstructed by simpler methods
  2. If the underlying disease has a good prognosis
  3. In patients with curative chemotherapy

Case report of plastic surgical intervention

At her first presentation to the plastic surgery outpatient department, this 18 year old patient had extensive fatty tissue necrosis on the dorsum of her left hand, caused by anthracycline extravasation in the context of treatment for chronic myeloid leukaemia [219]. Initial débridement found extensive soft tissue damage (5 cm diameter) and exposed extensor tendons to the long fingers (Fig. 3A). Preoperative angiography was performed to determine the vascular architecture of arteria radialis and arteria ulnaris. Due to the lack of sufficient anastomosis between arteria radialis and arteria ulnaris at the level of the hand, a distally based radial forearm flap was not an option. Thus, the defect was repaired by a free musculus serratus anterior flap covered with a split-thickness skin graft from the thigh (Fig. 3B-D; Fig. 4A-D).

Possibly necessary tertiary or subsequent interventions

- If the skin graft does not heal (possibly also repeated débridement) [28]
- If contractures or other functional defects occur [16]

Before more extensive reconstructive surgery is undertaken, the patient's life expectancy should be taken into consideration [72]. In patients at progressive stages of disease early discharge from hospital with greater freedom in their everyday lives may balance out a less stable wound covering [16, 210].

Consensus:

- In every case of extravasation with vesicant cytotoxic agents, a plastic surgeon should be consulted within 24 hours
- Intervention with flushout technique or liposuction should be considered only for highly toxic substances such as the vinca alkaloids or the anthracyclines; further clinical evidence is needed
- If surgical intervention is necessary, a two phase approach should be considered (débridement and later wound covering)

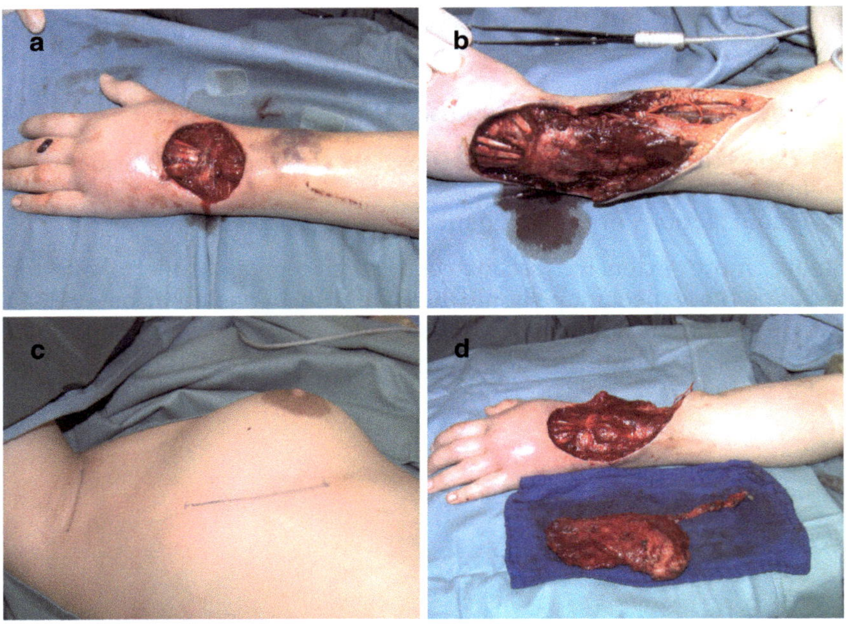

Fig. 3. Case report of a plastic surgical intervention **A** Soft tissue defect on the dorsum of the left hand after débridement of an extravasation necrosis with exposure of the extensor tendons of the 4th extensor tendon compartment. **B** After second débridement because of extensive damage to the soft tissues and preparation of the recipient vessels (radial artery and concomitant veins) for microsurgery. **C** Marked incision for harvesting of the serratus anterior muscle flap, paying particular attention to concealed scar in the axilla and inframammary fold in the 18 year old patient. **D** Muscle flap with long microvascular pedicle adjacent to the defect. The long vascular pedicle enables a reliable microanastomosis at a safe distance from the affected area

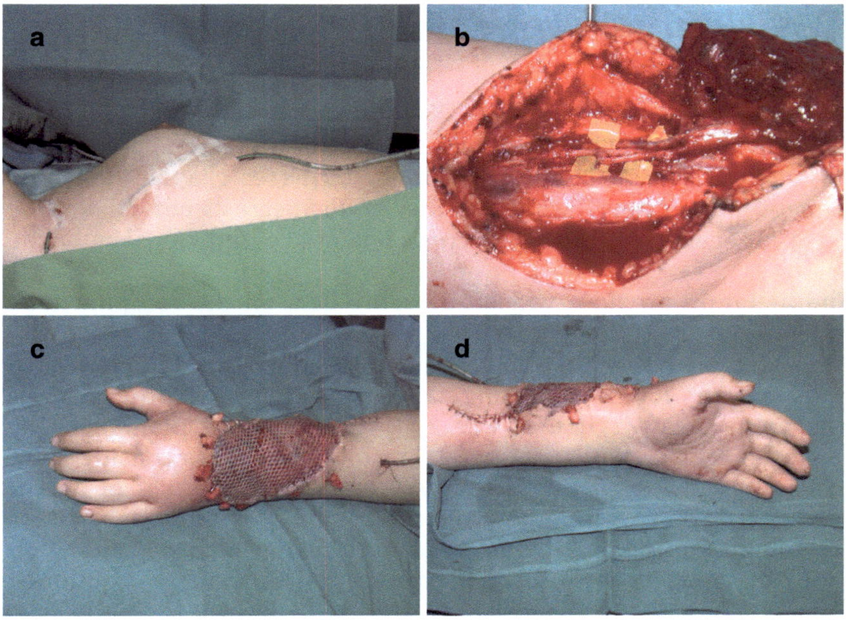

Fig. 4. Case report of a plastic surgical intervention (continued). **A** Donor region on the right submammary fold. **B** Microvascular anastomoses of the flap vessels end-to-side to the radial artery and end-to-end to a concomitant vein. **C** Defect covered with free serratus anterior muscle flap and meshed skin graft. **D** Closure of proximal incision proximal to the anastomosis of the flap vessels, at a safe distance from the affected area

Aftercare

Robert Mader

An individual adaptation of the intervals for aftercare appointments to the clinical presentation is recommended (see chapter "Potential damage mechanisms") while considering the necrosis potential of the cytotoxic agent (see chapter "Necrosis potential of individual cytotoxic agents").
The literature provides widely diverging data on the recommended timelines:
After acute treatment the site of the extravasation should be controlled every 4 hours for the following 24 hours [26]. The control intervals vary from a day [137] to a week [3]. In outpatients monitoring by request is seen as sufficient [137]. It has to be taken into consideration that extended subcutaneous necroses may occur in cases of absent erythema [21]. Therefore, after extravasation of vesicant substances, careful monitoring of patients is recommended, which, depending on the cytotoxic agent used and on the clinical course, should be continued for several months [3].
The patients should be instructed to contact the medical team without delay in case any unexpected problems occur [3].
If a patient is asymptomatic within 10 days after the extravasation event, further treatment is usually unnecessary. For patients who continue to have localised pain and do not respond to conservative treatment, surgical treatment should be considered.
The observation of the clinical course is done on the basis of the assessment of the following symptoms and necessary measures:

1. Progression of erythema
2. Intensity of pain and other complaints
3. Presence of ulcers or necroses
4. Necessity of surgical treatment
5. Functional loss

Aftercare is provided until complete cessation of the symptoms occurs [139].
To avoid contractures, support by physiotherapeutic treatments is recommended [28], especially if large areas are affected by the extravasation or if a risk of functional loss exists.

Documentation

Robert Mader

Extravasations that have occurred should be documented carefully, with all their developments and results of treatment and measures taken (taking photographs is recommended).
The literature mentions the following essential points for documentation:

- Date of administration [3]
- Time of administration [3]
- Site of administration [3,137]
- Administration technique [138]
- Size and type of cannula or catheter [138]
- Venipunctures in the past 24 hours [137]
- Drug administered [137]
- Concentration of drug in the injecting solution [3]
- Approximate dose administered [137]
- Sequence of drugs given [138]
- Volume of extravasated drug [3]
- Appearance of affected site after extravasation [3]
- Site of erythema or induration [139]
- Size (diameter) [139]
- Pain, discomfort, retrograde blood flow yes/no [139]
- Complaints and details reported by patient [138]
- Type of information and instructions given to patient [3]
- Treatment measures [139]
- Name of doctor who administered the drug [3]
- Names of people consulted after extravasation occurred [138]
- Signature of doctor [138]

To add to what is currently known about prevention and therapy of extravasations of cytotoxic agents, we are trying to set up a network in the German speaking areas. We would therefore ask you to complete the enclosed documentation sheets and return them for the purposes of anonymised data collection and evaluation to the following address:

Prof Dr. Robert Mader, Department of Medicine I, Division of Oncology, Währinger Gürtel 18–20, A-1090 Vienna, Austria,

Tel.: +43/1/40400-5466, Fax: +43/1/40400-6081
e-mail: robert.mader@meduniwien.ac.at

Patient's initials: |____|____|
First name Second name

Date of birth: |__:__|__:__|__:__|
Day Month Year

Extravasation of cytotoxic agents – Documentation (I)

Cannula used: ○ Butterfly® ○ Venflon® ○ Other. . . . .
Diameter . . . . G
Cannula fixated with: . . . .

Site of puncture: ○ Left arm ○ Right arm ○ Port-a-cath system
○ Forearm ○ Antecubital fossa ○ Central venous-catheter
○ Wrist ○ Dorsum of hand
○ Other: . . . .

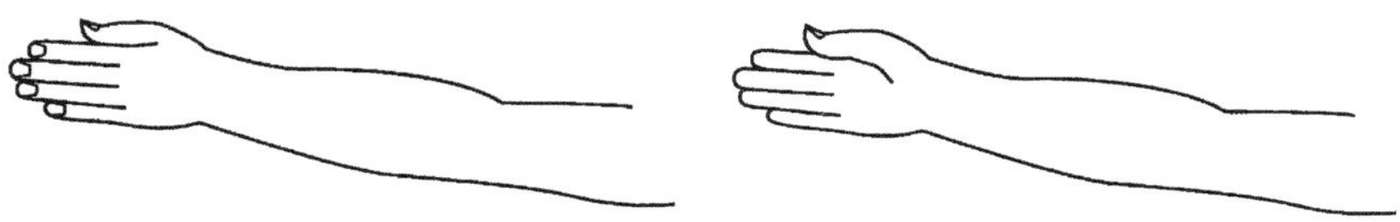

Was it necessary to puncture the same limb more than once?
○ Yes ○ No

Where – in relation to the original puncture site – was the vein punctured?
○ Proximal ○ Distal ○ Medial/lateral

Has the patient any of the following symptoms:
→ Upper blockage to inflow: ○ Yes ○ No
→ Lymphoedema (same arm): ○ Yes ○ No
→ Haematoma (same arm): ○ Yes ○ No

Sequence of application:

	Amount	Substance or trade name	Volume		
1.	mg		in	ml	○ extravascular
2.	mg		in	ml	○ extravascular
3.	mg		in	ml	○ extravascular
4.	mg		in	ml	○ extravascular
5.	mg		in	ml	○ extravascular

✎ **Estimated volume of extravasated drug:** . . . . ml
✎ **Type of administration:** ○ i.v. ○ i.a.
○ Bolus ○ Infusion ○ Infusion pump

Patient's initials: |_____|_____|
First name Second name

Date of birth: |__:__|__:__|__:__|
Day Month Year

Extravasation of cytotoxic agents – Documentation (II)

Extravasation recognised: Date |__:__|__:__|__:__| Time of day: . . . . . .
Day Month Year

- ○ During administration
- ○ Immediately after administration
- ○ . . . . . . hours after administration
- ○ . . . . . . days after administration

Measures:
- ✎ Aspiration of cytotoxic drug possible: ○ Yes ○ No
- ✎ Recommended general and substance specific measures taken: ○ Yes ○ No
- ✎ Additional measures taken: . . . .
. . . .
. . . .

Risk factors that may influence wound healing (for example, diabetes mellitus):
. . . .
. . . .

Information for/ instructions to patient: |__:__|__:__|__:__|
Day Month Year

(Plastic) surgeon consulted: ○ Yes |__:__|__:__|__:__| ○ No
Day Month Year

Next control appointment: |__:__|__:__|__:__| Time: . . . .
Day Month Year Ward: . . . .

Documented by: . . . .
Name in capital letters, please

E-mail: . . . .

Affiliation: . . . .

Patient's initials: |____|____|
First name Second name

Date of birth: |__:__|__:__|__:__|
Day Month Year

Extravasation of cytotoxic agents – Documentation (III)

	✓= Applies	↑ Deterioration		= No change		↓ Improvement	
	Status post paravasationem	1. Control	2. Control	3. Control	4. Control	5. Control	6. Control
Date							
Doctor's paragraph							
Symptoms after extravasation:							
Pain (burning, stinging)							
Oedema							
Erythema							
Blistering							
Discolouration							
Induration							
Functional impairment							
Ulceration							
Necrosis							
Demarcation							
Formation of eschar							
Infection							
Complete healing							

Extent of extravasation:

Two biggest diameters ↔ in cm							

Measures:

Conservative measures								
Surgical measures:	Excision							
	Transplantation							

Notes:

Forming clinical working groups

Robert Mader

Experience so far has clearly shown the limitations of conventional methods in dealing with extravasations. Especially splitting the intervention into disciplines that act independently from each other can result in contradictory therapeutic measures that will yield inconsistent documentation. The extent of knowledge also varies within the departments that administer chemotherapy. A possible solution to optimise knowledge and management in this difficult setting is the formation of interdisciplinary clinical working groups within the hospital. The working group would be tasked with the following:

1. The clinical colleagues in the working group are the first port of call within the hospital and help initiate immediate measures;
2. They coordinate the following treatment stages—especially with the plastic surgeons;
3. The working group members meet at regular intervals to discuss the cases of extravasation that have occurred and adapt the approaches with the aim to set out a standard operating procedure (SOP) that is adapted to each hospital; this includes defining what should be in the extravasation kit;
4. The working group members train all staff that will be involved in administering cytotoxic agents;
5. The working group evaluates the cases systematically, compares its own experiences with those described in the literature, and publishes its own data.

Such a working group has started at the university hospitals at Vienna General Hospital and has dedicated itself to the interdisciplinary management of extravasations. By systematically involving the working group in extravasation cases, it would be possible in a large hospital to gain expertise within very few years, which guarantees rapid and safe intervention in terms of quality assurance.

In the best-case scenario, the working group consists of oncologists, plastic surgeons, pharmacists (for example, colleagues responsible for the central preparation of cytotoxic agents), pathologists, nursing staff, and possibly colleagues from further disciplines, such as physiotherapists. In practice, a group of six has been found to be workable.

In the event of an extravasation, rapid assessment of the situation is crucial for the further clinical course (risk potential of the substance, volume and extent of the extravasation, symptoms). Once immediate measures have been initiated and a plastic surgeon has been consulted

if the extravasated drug is a vesicant substance, there is usually sufficient time to discuss further proceedings together. In this situation, seeking the opinions of colleagues from all disciplines are invaluable in helping to improve the patient's situation.
To clarify scientific questions in connection with extravasation, pathological analysis of skin samples has proved invaluable (infiltration of inflammatory cells, damage to the tissues adjacent to the necrosis, etc). For extravasations that require surgical intervention, this can be done from the tissue sample taken during the operation, without imposing further strain on the patient.
One of the objectives of the working group as the first port of call is to ensure immediate initiation of the correct measures as an essential step in patients' primary treatment. In addition to the already mentioned factors—such as the volume and extent of the extravasated substance—the time to intervention is the most relevant factor. In extravasations that have not been noticed or not treated for days, the effectiveness of antidotes is, in all experience, extremely limited. If even in optimal intervention—especially in large extravasations of substances such as the anthracyclines—serious damage cannot be excluded, all possible measures should be undertaken. In addition to the defects that the patient will have to tolerate in addition to his or her illness, there is also a risk of endangering the patient's prognosis by ceasing chemotherapy.

Quality control and quality assurance

Ines Mader

Although the extravasation of cytotoxic agents is one of the rarer complications in the context of chemotherapy, it can lead to severe complications when vesicant drugs are involved. Prevention and appropriate treatment are therefore essential, so as to avoid serious sequelae. Quality control and quality assurance are making an appreciable contribution to optimising proceedings in the context of an extravasation event.
The following measures are components of quality control and assurance:

- **Information and education for patients**
- **Training and continuing professional education for doctors and nursing staff**
- **Appointment of an individual as the "first port of call"**
- **Interdisciplinary communication and cooperation**
- **Implementation of guidelines**
- **Documentation**
- **Knowledge management**

As with all other adverse effects, the probability of an extravasation occurring will need to be factored into the risk-benefit balance for patients when deciding on cytotoxic chemotherapy. The patients will need to be informed about possible side effects of this treatment as for any other. If patient information is delivered face to face, witnesses are required, but it can also be delivered in writing.
Regular training sessions help raise sensitivity and awareness in medical and nursing staff, but they also impart knowledge with regard to a qualified, appropriate intervention in an emergency.
As a support for the organisation, an individual should be appointed as the first port of call for extravasations within the department/hospital, whose responsibility should include training and standardised documentation per patient and providing and maintaining the extravasation kit. The contact person should be competent and as such should be contacted in case of an extravasation event, to coordinate further proceedings. In addition, plastic surgeons (for example) should be consulted.
To reduce variation in activities, it is recommended to set out, complement, and regularly update guidelines. These are scientifically based recommendations for action with a focus on clinical practice, and staff should deviate from these guidelines only in exceptional circumstances and for sounds reasons. This helps guarantee standardised procedures in emergency settings. A further advantage is the increasingly

important putting in place of safeguards against questions of legal liability and other legal affairs.
Standardised documentation relating to the patient (see chapter "Documentation") is crucial to follow and evaluate the measures taken in an event afterwards. The following should be documented:

- Description of event
- Symptoms
- Measures taken
- Further developments
- Aftercare

Knowledge management

There are hardly any prospective clinical studies on the subject of extravasation of cytotoxic drugs. Our current knowledge is based mostly on retrospective evaluations, individual case reports, and animal studies. This explains the wide range of recommended measures that in some cases are even contradictory. In addition to the critical debate on the subject of extravasation, clinical evidence is urgently required. This can come only from prospective studies that stringently apply standardised treatment guidelines in large patient cohorts, so as to overcome the current stagnation in our knowledge.

Open questions and outlook

Robert Mader

Because of the particular conditions in which extravasations occur, several relevant questions have not been answered satisfactorily or indeed at all. Even if no solution to outstanding questions may be expected in the near future, this chapter is aiming to raise awareness for one thing: we have an awful lot of work ahead of us!

For the subject of extravasation, the main attention must focus on preventive measures. This book contains a catalogue of the most important questions that should be asked before administering therapy, but these do not always assess the individual patient's situation in its totality. If the aim is to standardise prevention—for example, in the sense of a checklist—then the current state of knowledge will require much improvement. Questions about the state of a patient's veins, hyposensitivities or hypersensitivities, or about the compliance of an informed patient require reliable prospective assessment, which currently cannot be provided. Further, the risk factors—as the basis for preventive measures or a contribution towards early detection for individual patients—need to be balanced, which is incompatible with the often hectic daily activities in a hospital.

For a long time it was seen as a safe and confirmed approach to take recourse to central venous catheter in patients with difficult veins or complex therapeutic schemes with vesicant substances. This approach now seems questionable in the light of recent data: even in central venous application, extravasations have occurred repeatedly, which add to the astonishingly high proportion of 7.5% of all applications [6]. Further, in this type of administration, symptoms may occur with an enormous time delay and extravasations may be noticed only when necroses are already extensive. It is obvious in the light of this that positioning control of central venous catheters needs to be discussed somewhat more extensively. Radiological controls after placing the catheter of in moments of suspicion alone are not sufficient.

The type of damage associated with cytotoxic agents has been central to the discussion for a long time now and gains prominence whenever a new substance is licensed. It takes years for sufficient clinical information to accumulate to be able to classify with a degree of certainty a substance with regard to its tissue toxic potential. And even after years of clinical use, there are certain cytotoxic agents that we cannot conclusively classify—for example, busulfan and estramustine. If even a relatively simple classification into three types of damage is riven with uncertainties, further investigations are naturally made even more difficult. Further subclassifications are desirable, however, because the vesicant potential of paclitaxel is not comparable to that of the anthracyclines. The mechanisms that underlie the tissue damage associated with extravasation thus require independent consideration and cannot be derived just from a substances profile of effects and side effects.

In the event of an extravasation of a vesicant substance, there is no certainty in predicting the clinical course and the extent of the damage that is to be expected. Plastic surgeons are often confronted with this problem when they are asked during consultations to make predictions for the future. After extravasations of anthracyclines, necroses can develop completely unexpectedly and with a time delay, which should serve to underline the ubiquitous uncertainty. Plastic surgeons have often expressed a desire for definite answers with regard to the resection margins in the course of plastic reconstruction cover as transplants are still often rejected, which puts the patients under enormous psychological and physical strain. We cannot predict with certainty the state of the healthy tissue that enables successful surgical intervention. As a first measure, intraoperative frozen section and close cooperation with pathologists can be recommended.

The medical emergency extravasation is subject to many empirical variables. In spite of much pharmaceutical knowledge, it is not possible to extrapolate tissue toxicity on the basis of physical-chemical attributes. In the best-case scenario, similarities of reactions can be deduced—as for the vinca alkaloids and the anthracyclines—which in turn require empirical confirmation. A possible way out would be studies of the acute tissue toxicity including vesicant potential, which might provide important clues as information for the licensing process of the substance. A glance at the guidelines of the European Agency for the Evaluation of Medicinal Products (EMEA) shows that similar considerations have been entertained for several years ("Note for guidance on the pre-clinical evaluation of anticancer medicinal products" from 1998). The chapter "Evaluation of toxicity" provides for testing local tolerance, with a remark of the potentially high tissue toxicity of cytotoxic substances. From a clinical perspective, it would be helpful to define these requirements explicitly for extravasations also and conduct studies accordingly. This information should be included in the specialised information, in order to assess the tissue toxicity of newly licensed substances even before their use. This information is required from the manufacturers, as waiting is not a solution in this scenario.

In clinical practice, distinguishing hypersensitivity reactions or phlebitides from extravasations causes problems that cannot always be solved when time is short. This differential diagnosis causes fewer problems for experienced clinicians, which again emphasises the need for training and educating inexperienced colleagues as well as the need

for specialisation in extravasation within hospitals and institutions dealing with patients (see chapter "Forming clinical working groups"). Although the substance specific measures after extravasation have been well documented for some substances, some central issues remain. An extravasation is not always noticed immediately and causes symptoms days later in some cases. According to the literature this time delay is usually longer than 5 days [158]. How much time is allowed to lapse before the effectiveness of antidotes would be compromised? Antidotes have been set out and tested for the time immediately after the extravasation even. Even animal studies have not provided any new insights as the antidotes are always administered within an hour after the subcutaneous lesion was placed. Dexrazoxane has been studied in this regard. An animal study has shown that its efficacy against anthracyclines remained for at least 3 hours after the extravasation event but was clearly reduced for daunorubicin after 6 hours [165]. Even smaller time windows seem to apply to the antidote hyaluronidase [183]. If the patient presents again only on the day after treatment, the supportive effects of dexrazoxane and probably other antidotes cannot be assumed to be certain. For this reason, educating patients in addition to regular monitoring of the infusion is of such crucial importance: early detection provides us with a set of instruments whose effectiveness is time critical.
As dexrazoxane has been approved based on the data from two single-arm studies [221], it is not clear how its effectivity compares with that of the highly established clinical use of DMSO/topical cooling. This procedure has also been tested in a prospective clinical trial with very similar number of patients treated and a very similar rate of success [146]. This is a serious flaw in the study design of both prospective clinical studies using dexrazoxane as the Bertelli data clearly prove that DMSO/topical cooling is an effective procedure for the management of anthracycline extravasations. As a consequence, we have lost an opportunity to compare and to discuss the effectivity of both antidotes, but also the option to consider complementary strategies, which might have been even more helpful for our patients. The indication for dexrazoxane clearly requires the treatment to be initiated within 6 hours after extravasation. Overlooking the data of more than 70 extravsations with anthracyclines, the author's experience is that approximately half of these extravasations are diagnosed one or several days after the event itself. Alluding to the questions raised in the paragraph before, the question still remains: what is our strategy in these cases?
Another aspect that has not been given much attention in the discussion so far is the combination of antidotes. Only very few of the tested antidotes are used in clinical practice because many of them have not shown to have any benefits for the patients when used in isolation. This does

not mean that some of these antidotes cannot be used as supportive measures with other effective antidotes—in the context of clinical studies. The authors' own studies have shown that in many cases, all vessels in the environment of the extravasation are thrombosed. The resultant lack of movement in removing the cytotoxic substance may increase the damage. Low molecular heparins combined with other antidotes may be a rational option in this scenario. However, in the animal model, the efficacy of heparin for doxorubicin induced necroses was low, independent of which heparin was used [148].

The pathological changes to the tissue in the context of extravasation have been characterised only insufficiently. This explains the ongoing discussion about the use of corticosteroids. Although many authors know that inflammatory processes do not dominate in the event, the literature has many mentions of corticosteroid use. To clarify the state of affairs in this regard should be possible by cooperating with pathologists and using tissue samples from the operation, to gain certainty in this relatively simple question. It should be pointed out here that insights gained from animal studies—especially those using rodents—can be transferred to humans only to a very limited degree. The pig is the recommended animal to study cutaneous toxicity as its skin anatomically resembles human skin.

A real worry is the problem of documentation [6], which continues with the lack of minimum recommendations for scientific publications. Without standardised documentation with defined minimum standards we will learn very little from publications, which are mostly case reports. This means that in individual publications, not even the concentration of the infusion was known, and neither was the volume of the extravasation. Often, the allocation of patients to therapy is lacking and therefore information about the extravasation and its course, as well as the administration and dosage of antidotes. This is a challenge for the reviewers of specialist journals, who carry some responsibility for the fact that many manuscript have not benefited from critical review. The publication of case studies with regard to quality and usability shows clearly the oversight in setting out minimum standards for documentation and implement these internationally. It cannot be emphasised enough how important this is for the subject of extravasation, where knowledge is created by means of case reports and clinical studies are the exception.

New therapeutic developments will change the pharmacological landscape fundamentally over the ext 15 years. In addition to antihormonal substances that are mostly given p.o., molecular specific therapies will increasingly take over from the traditional cytotoxic agents. These will be targeted at growth receptors such as HER-2/neu, affect the proteasome, simultaneously inhibit COX-2, and intervene in the cellular cycle regulation and prevent neoangiogenesis. Differentiation factors such as retinoids and—even if not immediately—genetic drugs will be used that all have one thing in common: they hardly possess any vesicant potential, mostly probably not even irritant effects. Today's trend towards oral formulations will increase—for example, as in vinorelbine or temozolomide. Potentially locally toxic taxans—such as paclitaxel—will be used in polymer bound form with reduced local toxicity, similar to the liposomal formulations of daunorubicin, doxorubicin, and vincristine, whose local toxicity is clearly lower than that of their free original substances. Monoclonal humanised antibodies are increasingly used in oncology. These currently include:

- Rituximab (MabThera® which targets antigen CD20, in the treatment of B-cell lymphoma;
- Trastuzumab (Herceptin®), which targets the *HER-2/neu* receptor (also *erbB*-2), in the treatment of breast cancer;
- Bevacizumab (Avastin®), which targets the angiogenesis factor VEGF (vascular endothelial growth factor), in the treatment of colon cancer;
- Cetuximab (Erbitux®), which targets EGFR (endothelial growth factor receptor), in the treatment of colon cancer;
- Alemtuzumab (MabCampath®), which targets antigen CD52, in the treatment of chronic lymphatic leukaemia.

All antibodies bind to a defined epitope, which prompts their therapeutic effect. However, they are not side effect free because this epitope can be expressed on healthy cells too, which is presumably responsible for the cardiotoxicity of trastuzumab. Clinical experience to date has shown type 1 hypersensitivity reactions [111], which are usually controllable but in rare cases can result in side effects of WHO grades 3 or 4. Because of this mechanism of action, vesicant behaviour is highly unlikely. At least it may be assumed that the monoclonal antibodies after extravasation have only low grade irritant potential. To date, the few reported cases were free of appreciable side effects, which is consistent with our own experiences. Still, it should be pointed out that this optimistic assessment will be confirmed only by the clinical experience gained from large numbers of cases.

Thanks to the molecular specific therapeutic drugs, extravasation may become a finished chapter in the history of haemato-oncology even within 15 years. But we should not forget that cytotoxic drugs will certainly continue to be an important topic in less developed countries. Even for this time period, it is worth contributing to the highest principle of all treatments with regard to extravasation: primum nihil nocere!

References

[1] Laughlin RA, Landeen JM, Habal MB: The management of inadvertent subcutaneous adriamycin infiltration. Am J Surg 137: 408–412, 1979.

[2] Barlock AL, Howser DM, Hubbard SM: Nursing management of adriamycin extravasation. Am J Nurs 79: 94–96, 1979.

[3] Cox K, Stuart-Harris R, Abdini G, et al: The management of cytotoxicdrug extravasation: guide-lines drawn up by a working party for the Clinical Oncological Society of Australia. Med J Aust 148: 185–189, 1988.

[4] Brown AS, Hoelzer DJ, Piercy SA: Skin necrosis from extravasation of intravenous fluids in children. Plast Reconstr Surg 64: 145–150, 1979.

[5] Heckler FR: Current thoughts on extravasation injuries. Clin Plast Surg 16: 557–563, 1989.

[6] Krämer I: Zehn Jahre Dokumentation von Zytostatika-Paravasat-Ereignissen: Auswertung von 175 Paravasate-Dokumentationen. Krankenhauspharmazie 23: 269–274, 2002.

[7] Wang JJ, Cortes E, Sinks LF, et al: Therapeutic effect and toxicity of adriamycin in patients with neoplastic disease. Cancer 28: 837–843, 1971.

[8] Rudolph R, Stein RS, Pattillo RA: Skin ulcers due to adriamycin. Cancer 38: 1087–1094, 1976.

[9] Bowers DG, Lynch JB: Adriamycin extravasation. Plast Reconstr Surg 61: 86–92, 1978.

[10] Barth J: Paravasate und deren Behandlung. In: Barth J (ed) Zytostatika-Herstellung in der Apotheke. Deutscher Apotheker Verlag, Chapter VI-3: 1–9, 2000.

[11] Stanley A: Managing complications of chemotherapy administration. In: Allwood M, Stanley A, Wright P (eds) The Cytotoxics Handbook. Radcliffe Medical Press, 4th edition: 119–193, 2002.

[12] Upton J, Mulliken JB, Murray JE: Major intravenous extravasation injuries. Am J Surg 137: 497–506, 1979.

[13] Sonneveld P, Wassenaar HA, Nooter K: Long persistence of doxorubicin in human skin after extravasation. Cancer Treat Rep 68: 895–896, 1984.

[14] Dorr RT, Dordal MS, Koenig LM, et al: High levels of doxorubicin in the tissues of a patient experiencing extravasation during a 4-day infusion. Cancer 64: 2462–2464, 1989.

[15] Yosowitz P, Ekland DA, Shaw RC, et al: Peripheral intravenous infiltration necrosis. Ann Surg 182: 553–556, 1975.

[16] Lynch DJ, Key JC, White RR: Management and prevention of infiltration and extravasation injury. Surg Clin North Am 59: 939–949, 1979.
[17] Daniel RK, Williams HB: The free transfer of skin flaps by microvascular anastomoses. An experimental study and a reappraisal. Plast Reconstr Surg 52: 16–31, 1973.
[18] Berdel WE, Schmoll HJ, Büchele T, et al: Prävention und Therapie von Paravasaten/Extravasaten. In: Schmoll HJ, Höffken K, Possinger K (eds) Kompendium Internistische Onkologie. Standards in Diagnostik und Therapie. Springer, vol 1, 3rd edition: 1689–1701, 1999.
[19] Harwood KV: Treatment of anthracycline extravasation-recommendations for practice. J Clin Oncol 5: 1705, 1987.
[20] Schneider G: Paravasate von Zytostatika. Diagnostik und Therapie. Aina S. Schneider Verlag, 6th edition: 1–17, 1999.
[21] Köstering H, Nagel GA: Prophylaxe und Therapie von Zytostatika-Hautnekrosen. Onkologie 6: 317–320, 1980.
[22] Ignoffo RJ, Friedman MA: Therapy of local toxicities caused by extravasation of cancer chemotherapeutic drugs. Cancer Treat Rev 7: 17–27, 1980.
[23] Mullin S, Beckwith MC, Tyler LS: Prevention and management of antineoplastic extravasation injury. Hosp Pharm 35: 57–76, 2000.
[24] Linder RM, Upton J, Osteen R: Management of extensive doxorubicin hydrochloride extravasation injuries. J Hand Surg 8: 32–38, 1983.
[25] Montrose PA: Extravasation management. Semin Oncol Nurs 3: 128–132, 1987.
[26] Faehnrich J: Extravasation. NITA 7: 49–52, 1984.
[27] Wetmore N: Extravasation. The dreaded complication. NITA 8: 47–49, 1985.
[28] Larson DL: Treatment of tissue extravasation by antitumor agents. Cancer 49: 1796–1799, 1982.
[29] Jordan K, Grothe W, Schmoll HJ: Paravasation von Zytostatika: Prävention und Therapie. Dtsch Med Wochenschr 130: 33–37, 2005.
[30] Beason R: Antineoplastic vesicant extravasation. J Intraven Nurs 13: 111–114, 1990.
[31] San Angel F: Current controversies in chemotherapy administration. J Intraven Nurs 18: 16–23, 1995.
[32] Krämer I: Zytostatika-Paravasate-Set. Krankenhauspharmazie 13: 154–160, 1992.
[33] Krämer I, Stützle M: Zytostatika-Paravasation – Wie ist vorzugehen? Krankenhauspharmazie 23: 261–268, 2002.

[34] Reilly JJ, Neifeld JP, Rosenberg SA: Clinical course and management of accidental adriamycin extravasation. Cancer 40: 2053–2056, 1977.
[35] MacCara ME: Extravasation: a hazard of intravenous therapy. Drug Intell Clin Pharm 17: 713–717, 1983.
[36] Anderson JM, Walters RS, Hortobagyi GN: Mediastinitis related to probable central vinblastine extravasation in a woman undergoing adjuvant chemotherapy for early breast cancer. Am J Cin Oncol 19: 566–568, 1996.
[37] Preuss P, Partoft S: Cytostatic extravasations. Ann Plast Surg 19: 323–327, 1987.
[38] Ener RA, Meglathery SB, Styler M: Extravasation of systemic hematooncological therapies. Ann Oncol 15: 858–862, 2004.
[39] Langstein HN, Duman H, Seelig D, et al: Retrospective study of the management of chemotherapeutic extravasation injury. Ann Plast Surg 49: 369–374, 2002.
[40] Hofer S, Schnabel K, Vogelbach P, et al: Das "Pinch-off"-Syndrom: eine Komplikation bei implantierbaren Kathetersystemen in die Vena subclavia. Schweiz Med Wochenschr 127: 1247–1250, 1997.
[41] Aitken DR, Minton JP: The "pinch off sign" a warning of impending problems with permanent subclavian catheters. Am J Surg: 633–636, 1984.
[42] Hinke DH, Zandt-Stastny DA, Goodman LR, et al: Pinch off syndrome: a complication of implantable subclavian venous access devices. Radiology 177: 353–356, 1990.
[43] Krutchen AE, Bjarnason H, Stackhouse DJ, et al: The mechanism of positional dysfunction of subclavian venous catheters. Radiology 200: 159–163, 1996.
[44] Nostdahl T, Waagsbo NA: Costoclavicular pinching: a complication of long-term central venous catheters. a report of three cases. Acta Anaesthesiol Scand 42: 872–875, 1998.
[45] Spiegel RJ: The acute toxicities of chemotherapy. Cancer Treat Rep 8: 197–207, 1981.
[46] Chait LA, Dinner MI: Ulceration caused by cytotoxic drugs. S Afr Med J 49: 1935–1936, 1975.
[47] Rudolph R, Larson DL: Etiology and treatment of chemotherapeutic agent extravasation injuries: a review. J Clin Oncol 5: 1116–1126, 1987.
[48] Schummer W, Schummer C, Müller A, et al: Extravasation – eine seltene Komplikation zentralvenöser Katheter? Fallbericht einer drohenden Arrosion der A. carotis. Anästhesist 8: 711–717, 2003.
[49] Dragon LH, Braine HG: Necrosis of the hand after daunorubicin infusion distal to an arteriovenous fistula. Ann Intern Med 91: 58–59, 1979.

[50] Levey RH, Sallen S, Weinstein H, et al: Surgical techniques for vascular access for chemotherapy in infants and children. J Pediatr Surg 13: 724–729, 1978.
[51] Tully JL, Friedland GH, Baldini LM, et al: Complications of intravenous therapy with steel needles and teflon® catheters. Am J Med 70: 702–706, 1981.
[52] Powell LL: Oncology Nursing Society cancer chemotherapy guidelines recommendations for practice. Pittsburgh: Oncology Nursing Press, 1996.
[53] Kassner E: Evaluation and treatment of chemotherapy extravasation injuries. J Pediatr Oncol Nurs 17: 135–148, 2000.
[54] Meranze SG, Burke DR, Feurer ID, et al: Spontaneous retraction of indwelling catheters: previously unreported complications. J Parenter Enteral Nutr 12: 310–312, 1988.
[55] Kurul S, Saip P, Aydin T: Totally implantable venous-access ports: local problems and extravasation injury. Lancet Oncol 3: 684–692, 2002.
[56] Davies AG, Russell WC, Thompson JP: Extravasation and tissue necrosis secondary to central line infusions. Anaesthesia 58: 820–821, 2003.
[57] Klotz HP, Schopke W, Kohler A, et al: Catheter fracture: a rare complication of totally implantable subclavian venous access devices. J Surg Oncol 62: 222–225, 1996.
[58] Kraft A, Weinig S, Edinger M, et al: Anthrazyklin-Extravasate. Der Onkologe 6: 674–686, 2000.
[59] Lauvin R, Miglianico L, Hellegouarc HR: Skin cancer occurring 10 years after the extravasation of doxorubicin. N Engl J Med 332: 754, 1995.
[60] Kellner O, Dempke W, Schmoll HJ, et al: Zentralvenöse Katheter in der Hämatologie und Onkologie. In: Schmoll HJ, Höffken K, Possinger K (eds) Kompendium Internistische Onkologie. Standards in Diagnostik und Therapie. Springer, vol 1, 3rd edition: 1739–1753, 1999.
[61] Kock HJ, Pietsch M, Krause U, et al: Implantable vascular access systems: experience in 1,500 patients with totally implanted central venous port systems. World J Surg 22: 12–16, 1998.
[62] Schulmeister L, Camp-Sorrell D: Chemotherapy extravasation from implanted ports. Oncol Nurs Forum 27: 531–538, 2000.
[63] Freytes CO, Reid P, Smith KL: Long-term experience with a totally implanted catheter system in cancer patients. J Surg Oncol 45: 99–102, 1990.
[64] Stein M, Wagner RH: Komplikationen zentralvenöser Portsysteme: Erfahrungsbericht über 2359 Implantationen. Dtsch Med Wochenschr 130: 1129–1132, 2005.

[65] Rauthe G, Altmann C: Venous port systems in the field of gynaecological oncology. Eur J Gynaecol Oncol 19: 173–78, 1998.
[66] Lemmers NW, Gels ME, Sleijfer DT, et al: Complications of venous access ports in 132 patients with disseminated testicular cancer treated with polychemotherapy. J Clin Oncol 14: 2916–2922, 1996.
[67] Lokich JL, Bothe A, Benotti P, et al: Complications and management of implanted venous access catheters. J Clin Oncol 3: 710–717, 1985.
[68] Biffi R, Pozzi S, Agazzi A, et al: Use of totally implantable central venous access ports for high-dose chemotherapy and peripheral blood stem cell transplantation: results of a monocentre series of 376 patients. Ann Oncol 15: 296–300, 2004.
[69] Strum SB, McDermed JE, Korn AR, et al: Improved methods for venous access: the port-a-cath, a totally implanted catheter system. J Clin Oncol 4: 596–603, 1986.
[70] Mueller BU, Skelton J, Callender DDP, et al: A prospective randomized trial comparing the infectious and noninfectious complications of an externalized catheter versus a subcutaneously implanted device in cancer patients. J Clin Oncol 10: 1943–1948, 1992.
[71] Shetty PC, Mody MK, Kastan DJ, et al: Outcome of 350 implanted chest ports placed by interventional radiologists. J Vasc Intervent Radiol 8: 991–995, 1997.
[72] Poorter RL, Lauw FN, Bemelmann WA, et al: Complications of an implantable venous access device (Port-a-Cath) during intermittent continuous infusion of chemotherapy. Eur J Cancer 32A: 2262–2266, 1996.
[73] Brothers TE, Moll LK, Miederhuber JE, et al: Experience with subcutaneous infusion ports in three hundred patients. Surg Gynecol Obstet 166: 295–301, 1988.
[74] Bothe A, Piccione W, Ambrosino JJ, et al: Implantable central venous access system. Am J Surg 147: 565–569, 1984.
[75] Reed WP, Newman KA, Applefeld MM, et al: Drug extravasation as a complication of venous access ports. Ann Intern Med 102: 788–789, 1985.
[76] Rodier JM, Malbec L, Lauraine EP, et al: Mediastinal infusion of epirubicin and 5-fluorouracil. A complication of totally implantable central venous systems. Report of a case. J Cancer Res Clin Oncol 122: 566–567, 1996.
[77] Cathcart-Rake WF, Mowery WE: Intrapericardial infusion of 5-fluorouracil. An unusual complication of a Hickman catheter. Cancer 67: 735–737, 1991.
[78] Manheimer F, Aranda CP, Smith RL: Necrotizing pneumonitis caused by 5-fluorouracil infusion. A complication of a Hickman catheter. Cancer 70: 554–556, 1992.

[79] Duhrsen U, Heinrichs V, Beecken WD, et al: Local and systemic sequelae of mediastinal daunorubicin extravasation in a patient with acute myelomonocytic leukemia. Ann Oncol 8: 1167–1168, 1997.

[80] Bozkurt AK, Uzel B, Akman C, et al: Intrathoracic extravasation of antineoplastic agents. Case report and systematic review. Am J Clin Oncol 26: 121–123, 2003.

[81] Watterson J, Heisel M, Cich JA, et al: Intrathoracic extravasation of sclerosing agents associated with central venous catheters. Am J Pediatr Hematol Oncol 10: 240–251, 1988.

[82] Barutca S, Kadikoylu G, Bolaman Z, et al: Extravasation of paclitaxel into breast tissue from central catheter port. Support Cancer Care 10: 563–565, 2002.

[83] El Saghir NS, Otrock ZK: Docetaxel extravasation into the normal breast during breast cancer treatment. Anti-Cancer Drugs 15: 401–404, 2004.

[84] Webster PJ, D'Souza D: Extravasation of epirubicin/vincristine and ifosfamide/mesna from a central venous catheter. J Oncol Pharm Practice 1: 41–44, 1995.

[85] Kretzschmar A, Pink D, Thuss-Patience P, et al: Extravasations of oxaliplatin. J Clin Oncol 21: 4068–4069, 2003.

[86] Eckert R, Maier KP: Necrotizing panniculitis after extravasation of oxaliplatin. Ann Oncol 13 (Suppl 5): 29, 2002.

[87] Wong C, Joshi N, Nachimuthu S, et al: Cough in a patient with an infusion port. Chest 120: 1031–1033, 2001.

[88] Germain BS, Houlihan N, D'Amato S: Dimethyl sulfoxide therapy in the treatment of vesicant extravasation. J Intrav Nurs 17: 261–266, 1994.

[89] Clark KR, Higgs MJ: Breast abscess following central venous catheterization. Intensive Care Med 17: 123–124, 1991.

[90] Pacelli CM, Eitzman DT: Tracheal ostruction secondary to extravasation of intravenous fluids from central catheter port. Am J Med 92: 701–702, 1992.

[91] Bach F, Videbaek C, Holst-Christensen J, et al: Cytostatic extravasation. A serious complication of long-term venous access devices. Cancer 68: 538–539, 1991.

[92] Johnson JC: Complications of vascular access devices. Emerg Med Clin N Am 12: 691–705, 1994.

[93] Pronzato P, Queirolo P, Vidili MG, et al: Continuous venous infusion of vinblastine in metastatic breast cancer. Chemother 37: 146–149, 1991.

[94] Rudolph R, Suzuki M, Luce JK: Experimental skin necrosis produced by adriamycin. Cancer Treat Rep 63: 529–537, 1979.

[95] Luedke DW, Kennedy PS, Rietschel RL: Histopathogenesis of skin and subcutaneous injury induced by adriamycin. Plast Reconstr Surg 63: 463–465, 1979.
[96] Petro JA, Graham WP, Miller SH, et al: Experimental and clinical studies of ulcers induced with adriamycin. Surg Forum 30: 535–537, 1979.
[97] Dorr RT, Alberts DS, Chen HS: The limited role of corticosteroids in ameliorating experimental doxorubicin skin toxicity in the mouse. Cancer Chemother Pharmacol 5: 17–20, 1980.
[98] Coleman JJ, Walker AP, Didolkar MS: Treatment of adriamycin-induced skin ulcers: a prospective controlled study. J Surg Oncol 22: 129–135, 1983.
[99] Loth TS, Eversmann WW: Treatment methods for extravasationd of chemotherapeutic agents: a comparative study. J Hand Surg 11A: 388–396, 1986.
[100] Yoo MS, Ahn SK, Cho EH et al: Experimental study of gross and histopathological changes after extravasation of adriamycin and efficacy of intralesional injection of steroid. Kor J Dermatol 34: 732–738, 1996.
[101] Bhawan J, Petry J, Rybak ME: Histologic changes induced in skin by extravasation of doxorubicin (adriamycin). J Cutan Pathol 16: 158–163, 1989.
[102] Whang SW, Lee SH, Elias PM, et al: Intralesional steroids reduce inflammation from extravasated chemotherapeutic agents. Br J Dermatol 145: 680–682, 2001.
[103] Dorr RT, Alberts DS: Vinca alkaloid skin toxicity: antidote and drug disposition studies in the mouse. J Natl Cancer Inst 74: 113–120, 1985.
[104] Moreno de Vega MJ, Dauden E, Abajo P, et al: Skin necrosis from ectravasation of vinorelbine. J Eur Acad Dermatol Venereol 16: 488–490, 2002.
[105] Haskell CM, Canellos GP, Leventhal BG, et al: L-asparaginase: therapeutic and toxic effects in patients with neoplastic disease. N Engl J Med 281: 1028–1034, 1969.
[106] Weiss RB, Bruno S: Hypersensitivity reactions to cancer chemotherapeutic agents. Ann Int Med 94: 66–72, 1981.
[107] Cornwell GG, Pajak TF, McIntyre OR: Hypersensitivity reactions to i.v. melphalan during treatment of multiple myeloma: cancer and leukemia group B experience. Cancer Treat Rep 63: 399–403, 1979.
[108] Grem JL, King SA, Costanza ME, et al: Hypersensitivity reactions to trimetrexate. Invest New Drugs 8: 211–214, 1990.
[109] Bokemeyer C: Dermatotoxizität antineoplastischer Substanzen. In: Schmoll HJ, Höffken K, Possinger K (eds) Kompendium

Internistische Onkologie. Standards in Diagnostik und Therapie. Springer, vol 1, 3rd edition: 1411–1420, 1999.
[110] Vogelzang NJ: "Adriamycin flare": a skin reaction resembling extravasation. Cancer Treat Rep 63: 2067–2069, 1979.
[111] Alley E, Green R, Schuchter L: Cutaneous toxicities of cancer therapy. Curr Opin Oncol 14: 212–216, 2002.
[112] Bokemeyer C: Allergische Reaktionen. In: Schmoll HJ, Höffken K, Possinger K (eds) Kompendium Internistische Onkologie. Standards in Diagnostik und Therapie. Springer, vol 1, 3rd edition: 1421–1426, 1999.
[113] Cohen SC, DiBella NJ, Michalak JC: Recall injury from adriamycin. Ann Intern Med 83: 232, 1975.
[114] Wilson J, Carder P, Gooi J, et al: Recall phenomenon following epirubicin. Clin Oncol (R Coll Radiol) 11: 424–425, 1999.
[115] Meehan JL, Sporn JR: Case report of taxol administration via central vein producing a recall reaction at a site of prior taxol extravasation. J Natl Cancer Inst 86: 1250–1251, 1994.
[116] Shapiro J, Richardson GE: Paclitaxel-induced "recall" soft tissue injury occuring at the site of previous extravasation with subsequent intravenous treatment in a different limb. J Clin Oncol 12: 2237–2238, 1994.
[117] Hidalgo M, Benito J, Colomer R, et al: Recall reaction of a severe local peripheral neuropathy after paclitaxel extravasation. J Natl Cancer Inst 88: 1320, 1996.
[118] Koppel RA, Boh EE: Cutaneous reactions to chemotherapeutic agents. Am J Med Sci 321: 327–335, 2001.
[119] D'Angio GJ, Farber S, Maddock CL: Potentiation of x-ray effects by Actinomycin D. Radiology 73: 175–177, 1959.
[120] Stelzer KJ, Griffin TW, Koh WJ: Radiation recall skin toxicity with bleomycin in a patient with Kaposi sarcoma related to acquired immune deficiency syndrome. Cancer 71: 1322–1325, 1993.
[121] Zulian GB, Aapro MS: Docetaxel and radiation recall severe mucositis. Ann Oncol 5: 964, 1994.
[122] Yeo W, Leung SF, Johnson PJ: Radiation recall dermatitis with docetaxel: establishment of a requisite radiation threshold. Eur J Cancer 33: 699–700, 1997.
[123] Morkas M, Fleming D, Hahl M: Diagnosis in oncology. case 2. radiation recall associated with docetaxel. J Clin Oncol 20: 867–869, 2002.
[124] Hill AB, Tattersall SF: Recall of radiation pneumonitis after intrapleural administration of doxorubicin. Med J Aust 1: 39–40, 1983.

[125] Donaldson SS, Glick JM, Wilbur JR: Adriamycin activating a recall phenomenon after radiation therapy. Ann Intern Med 81: 407–408, 1974.

[126] Fontana JA: Radiation recall associated with VP-16–213 therapy. Cancer Treat Rep 63: 224–225, 1979.

[127] Perez EA, Campbell DL, Ryu JK: Radiation recall dermatitis induced by edatrexate in a patient with breast cancer. Cancer Invest 13: 604–607, 1995.

[128] Castellano D, Hitt R, Cortes-Funes H, et al: Radiation recall reaction induced by gemcitabine. J Clin Oncol 18: 695–696, 2000.

[129] Gabel C, Eifel PJ, Tornos C, et al: Radiation recall reaction to idarubicin resulting in vaginal necrosis. Gynecol Oncol 57: 266–269, 1995.

[130] Dabaja MAK, Morgensztern D, Markoe AM, et al: Radiation recall dermatitis induced by methotrexate in a patient with Hodgkin's disease. Am J Clin Oncol 23: 531–533, 2000.

[131] McCarty MJ, Peake MF, Lillis P, et al: Paclitaxel induced radiation recall dermatitis. Med Pediatr Oncol 27: 185–186, 1996.

[132] Nemechek PM, Corder MC: Radiation recall associated with vinblastine in a patient treated for Kaposi sarcoma related to acquired immune deficiency syndrome. Cancer 70: 1605–1606, 1992.

[133] Kitani H, Kosaka T, Fujihara T, et al: The "recall effect" in radiotherapy: is subeffective, reparable damage involved? Int J Radiat Oncol Biol Phys 18: 689–695, 1990.

[134] Camidge R, Price, A: Characterizing the phenomenon of radiation recall dermatitis. Radiother Oncol 59: 237–246, 2001.

[135] Burdon J, Bell R, Sullivan J, et al: Adriamycin induced recall phenomenon 15 years after radiotherapy. JAMA 239: 931, 1978.

[136] Khan MS, Holmes JD: Reducing the morbidity from extravasation injuries. Ann Plast Surg 48: 628–632, 2002.

[137] Hankin FM, Louis DS: Extravasation of chemotherapeutic agents. Am Fam Physician 31: 147–150, 1985.

[138] Hessen JA: Protocol for treatment of vesicant antineoplastic extravasation. Hosp Pharm 24: 705–709, 1989.

[139] Hirsh JD, Conlon PF: Implementing guidelines for managing extravasation of antineoplastics. Am J Hosp Pharm 40: 1516–1519, 1983.

[140] Dorr RT: Antidotes to vesicant chemotherapy extravasations. Blood Rev 4: 41–60, 1990.

[141] Harwood KV, Aisner J: Treatment of chemotherapy extravasation: current status. Cancer Treat Rep 68: 939–945, 1984.

[142] Scuderi N, Onesti MG: Antitumor agents: extravasation, management, and surgical treatment. Ann Plast Surg 32: 39–44, 1994.
[143] Gault DT: Extravasation injuries. Br J Plast Surg 46: 91–96, 1993.
[144] Cicchetti S, Jemec B, Gault DT: Two case reports of vinorelbine extravasation: management and review of the literature. Tumori 86: 289–292, 2000.
[145] Giunta R, Akpaloo J, Kovacs L, et al: Technik der subkutanen Spülung bei hochtoxischen Paravasaten – ein Kurzbeitrag. Handchir Mikrochir Plast Chir 34: 399–402, 2002.
[146] Bertelli G, Gozza A, Forno GB, et al: Topical dimethylsulfoxide for the prevention of soft tissue injury after extravasation of vesicant cytotoxic drugs: a prospective clinical study. J Clin Oncol 13: 2851–2855, 1995.
[147] Owen OE, Dellatorre DL, van Scott EJ, et al: Accidental intramuscular injection of mechlorethamine. Cancer 45: 2225–2226, 1980.
[148] Askar I, Erbas MK, Gurlek A: Effects of heparin fractions on the prevention of skin necrosis resulting from adriamycin extravasation: an experimental study. Ann Plast Surg 49: 297–301, 2002.
[149] Hajarizadeh H, Lebredo L, Barrie R, et al: Protective effect of doxorubicin in vitamin C or dimethylsulfoxide against skin ulceration in the pig. Ann Surg Oncol 1: 411–414, 1994.
[150] Schwartsmann G, Sander EB, Vinholes J, et al: N-acetylcysteine protects skin lesion induced by local extravasation of doxorubicin in a rat model. Am J Pediatr Hematol Oncol 14: 280–281, 1992.
[151] Nobbs P, Barr RD: Soft-tissue injury caused by antineoplastic drugs is inhibited by topical dimethyl sulphoxide and alpha tocopherol. Br J Cancer 48: 873–876, 1983.
[152] Ludwig CU, Stoll HR, Obrist R, et al: Prevention of cytotoxic drug induced skin ulcers with dimethyl sulfoxide (DMSO) and α-tocopherole. Eur J Cancer Clin Oncol 23: 327–329, 1987.
[153] Averbuch SD, Gaudiano G, Koch TH, et al: Doxorubicin-induced skin necrosis in the swine model: protection with a novel radical dimer. J Clin Oncol 4: 88–94, 1986.
[154] Averbuch SD, Boldt M, Gaudiano G, et al: Experimental chemotherapyinduced skin necrosis in swine. J Clin Invest 81: 142–148, 1988.
[155] Comas D, Mateu J: Treatment of extravasation of both doxorubicin and vincristine administration in a y-site infusion. Ann Pharmacother 30: 244–246, 1996.
[156] Spugnini EP: Use of hyaluronidase for the treatment of extravasation of chemotherapeutic agents in six dogs. JAMA 221: 1437–1440, 2002.

[157] Modena T, Conti B, Genta I, et al: Hyaluronidase-injectable microparticles intended for the treatment of extravasation. J Microencapsulation 15: 85–92, 1998.
[158] Parikh PM, Pai VP, Ranjan S, et al: Phlogenzym® is safe and effective in reducing morbidity of vesicant chemotherapy extravasation – a prospective study. Int J Immunotherapy 17: 163–170, 2001.
[159] Kolarić K, Zupanc D, Stahl KW, et al: Verhinderung von Extravasatnekrosen als Komplikation nach intravenöser Zytostatikatherapie. Onkologie 11: 238–240, 1988.
[160] Abbes M, Picard JL, Bourgeon Y, et al: A propos de quarante et une complications locales de chimiothèrapie. Ann Chir Plast Esthèt 31: 149–156, 1986.
[161] Tsavaris NB, Karagiaouris P, Tzannou I, et al: Conservative approach to the treatment of chemotherapy-induced extravasation. J Dermatol Surg Oncol 16: 519–522, 1990.
[162] Andoh T, Ishida R: Catalytic inhibitors of DNA topoisomerase II. Biochim Biophys Acta 1400: 155–171, 1998.
[163] Langer Sw, Sehested M, Jensen PB: Dexrazoxane is a potent and specific inhibitor of anthracycline induced subcutaneous lesions in mice. Ann Oncol 12: 405–410, 2001.
[164] Sehested M, Jensen PB, Sorensen BS, et al: Antagonistoc effect of the cardioprotector (+)–1,2-bis(3,5-dioxopiperazinyl-1-yl)propane (ICRF-187) in DNA breaks and cytotoxicity induced by the topoisomerase II directed drugs daunorubicin and etoposide (VP-16). Biochem Pharmacol 46: 389–393, 1993.
[165] Langer SW, Sehested M, Jensen PB: Treatment of anthracycline extravasation with dexrazoxane. Clin Cancer Res 6: 3680–3686, 2000.
[166] Lane P, Vichi P, Bain DL, et al: Temperature dependence studies of adriamycin uptake and cytotoxicity. Cancer Res 47: 4038–4042, 1987.
[167] Dorr RT, Alberts DS, Stone A: Cold protection and heat enhancement of doxorubicin skin toxicity in the mouse. Cancer Treat Rep 69: 431–437, 1985.
[168] Herman TS: Temperature dependence of adriamycin, cis-diamminedichlo-roplatinum, bleomycin, and 1,3-bis(2-chloroethyl)-1 -nitrosourea cytotoxicity in vitro. Cancer Res 43: 517–520, 1983.
[169] Harwood KV, Gonin R: Short term vs. long term local cooling after doxorubicin (DOX) extravasation: an eastern cooperative oncology group (ECOG) study. Proc ASCO 13: 447, 1994.
[170] Goodman M, Stewart I, Lydon J, et al: Use caution when managing paclitaxel and taxotere infiltrations. Oncol Nurs Forum 23: 541–542, 1996.

[171] David NA: The pharmacology of dimethyl sulfoxide 6544. Ann Rev Pharmacol 12: 353–374, 1972.

[172] Kligman AM: Topical pharmacology and toxicology of dimethyl sulfoxide – part I. JAMA 193: 796–804, 1965.

[173] Görög P, Kovàcs IB: Effect of dimethyl sulfoxide (DMSO) on various experimental cutaneous reactions. Pharmacology 2: 313–319, 1969.

[174] Desai MH, Teres D: Prevention of doxorubicin-induced skin ulcers in the rat and pig with dimethyl sulfoxide (DMSO). Cancer Treat Rep 66: 1371–1374, 1982.

[175] Massart C, Le Tellier C, Gibassier J, et al: Modulation by dimethyl sulphoxide of the toxicity induced by cis-diamminedichloroplatinum in cultured thyrocytes. Toxicol in vitro 7: 87–94, 1993.

[176] Jones MM, Basinger MA, Field L, et al: Coadministration of dimethyl sulfoxide reduces cisplatin nephrotoxicity. Anticancer Res 11: 1939–1942, 1991.

[177] de Lemos ML: Role of dimethylsulfoxide for management of chemotherapy extravasation. J Oncol Pharm Practice 10: 197–200, 2004.

[178] Barth J, Bildat E: Empfehlungen zur Behandlung von Paravasaten mit Vinorelbin. Krankenhauspharmazie 21: 622–624, 2000.

[179] Olver IN, Aisner J, Hament A, et al: A prospective study of topical dimethyl sulfoxide for treating anthracycline extravasation. J Clin Oncol 6: 1732–1735, 1988.

[180] Creus N, Mateu J, Masso J, et al: Toxicity to topical dimethylsulfoxide (DMSO) when used as an extravasation agent. Pharm World Sci 24: 175–176, 2002.

[181] Bertelli G, Dini D, Forno GB, et al: Hyaluronidase as an antidote to extravasation of vinca alkaloids: clinical results. J Cancer Res Clin Oncol 120: 505–506, 1994.

[182] Cohen MH: Amelioration of adriamycin skin necrosis: an experimental study. Cancer Treat Rep 63: 1003–1004, 1979.

[183] Laurie SW, Wilson KL, Kernahan DA, et al: Intravenous extravasation injuries: the effectiveness of hyaluronidase in their treatment. Ann Plast Surg 13: 191–194, 1984.

[184] Disa JJ, Chang RR, Mucci SJ, et al: Prevention of adriamycin-induced fullthickness skin loss using hyaluronidase infiltration. Plast Reconstr Surg 101: 370–374, 1998.

[185] Stanley A: Managing complications of chemotherapy. In: Allwood M, Stanley A, Wright P (eds) The Cytotoxics Handbook. Radcliffe Medical Press, 3rd edition: 105–124, 1997.

[186] Schwartzman J, Henderson AT, King WE: Hyaluronidase in fluid administration. J Pediatr 33: 267–273, 1948.

[187] Sehested M, Jensen PB: Mapping of DNA topoisomerase II poisons (etoposide, clerocidin) and catalytic inhibitors (aclarubicin, ICRF-187) to four distinct steps on the toposisomerase II catalytic cycle. Biochem Pharmacol 51: 879–886, 1996.
[188] Bos AM, van der Graaf WT, Willemse PH: A new conservative approach to extravasation of anthracyclines with dimethylsulfoxide and dexrazoxane. Acta Oncol 40: 541–541, 2001.
[189] Langer SW, Sehested M, Jensen PB: Dexrazoxane in anthracycline extravasation. J Clin Oncol 18: 3063, 2000.
[190] Jensen JN, Lock-Andersen J, Langer SW, et al: Dexrazoxane – a promising antidote in the treatment of accidental extravasation of anthracyclines. Scand J Plast Reconstr Hand Surg 37: 174–175, 2003.
[191] El Saghir N, Otrock Z, Mufarrij A, et al: Dexrazoxane for anthracycline extravasation and GM-CSF for skin ulceration and wound healing. Lancet Oncol 5: 320–321, 2004.
[192] Wilson DW, Grier D, Reimer R, et al: Structure-activity relationship of daunorubicin and its peptide derivatives. J Med Chem 19: 381–384, 1976.
[193] Bartkowski-Dodds L, Daniels JR: Use of sodium bicarbonate as a means of ameliorating doxorubicin-induced dermal necrosis in rats. Cancer Chemother Pharmacol 4: 179–181, 1980.
[194] Barr RD, Sertic J: Soft-tissue necrosis induced by extravasated cancer chemotherapeutic agents: a study of active intervention. Br J Cancer 44: 267–269, 1981.
[195] Laskar PA, Ayres JW: Degradation of carmustine in aqueous media. J Pharm Sci 66: 1073–1076, 1977.
[196] Colvin M, Hartner J, Summerfield M: Stability of carmustine in the presence of sodium bicarbonate. Am J Hosp Pharm 37: 677–678, 1980.
[197] Schneider SM, Distelhorst CW: Chemotherapy-induced emergencies. Semin Oncol 16: 572–578, 1989.
[198] Jackson IT, Robinson DW: Severe tissue damage following accidental subcutaneous infusion of bicarbonate solution. Scot Med J 21: 200–201, 1976.
[199] Gaze NR: Tissue necrosis caused by commonly used intravenous infusions. Lancet 2: 417–419, 1978.
[200] Kappel B, Hindenburg AA, Taub RN: Treatment of anthracycline extravasation – a warning against the use of sodium bicarbonate. J Clin Oncol 5: 825–826, 1987.
[201] Groos E, Walker L, Masters JR: Intravesical chemotherapy: studies on the relationship between pH and cytotoxicity. Cancer 58: 1199–1203, 1986.

[202] Tsavaris NB, Komitsopoulou P, Karagiaouris P, et al: Prevention of tissue necrosis due to accidental extravasation of cytostatic drugs by a conservative approach. Cancer Chemother Pharmacol 30: 330–333, 1992.
[203] Howell SB, Taetle R: Effect of sodium thiosulfate on cis-dichloroammine-platinum (II) toxicity and antitumor activity in L1210 leukemia. Cancer Treat Rep 64: 611–616, 1980.
[204] Buchanan GR, Buchsbaum HJ, O'Banion K, et al: Extravasation of dactinomycin, vincristine, and cisplatin: studies in an animal model. Med Pediatr Oncol 13: 375–380, 1985.
[205] Dorr RT, Soble M, Alberts DS: Efficacy of sodium thiosulfate as a local antidote to mechlorethamine skin toxicity in the mouse. Cancer Chemother Pharmacol 22: 299–302, 1988.
[206] Baskin SI, Horowitz AM, Nealley EW: The antidotal action of sodium nitrite and sodium thiosulfate against cyanide poisoning. J Clin Pharmacol 32: 368–375, 1992.
[207] Rudolph R: Ulcers of the hand and wrist caused by doxorubicin hydrochloride. Orthop Rev 7: 93–95, 1978.
[208] Larson DL: What is the appropriate management of tissue extravasation by antitumor agents? Plast Reconstr Surg 75: 397–402, 1985.
[209] Pitkänen J, Asko-Seljavaara S, Gröhn P, et al: Adriamycin extravasation: surgical treatment and possible prevention of skin and soft-tissue injuries. J Surg Oncol 23: 259–262, 1983.
[210] Shenaq SM, Abbase EH, Friedman JD: Soft-tissue reconstruction following extravasation of chemotherapeutic agents. Surg Oncol Clin N Am 5: 825–845, 1996.
[211] Seyfer AE, Solimando DA: Toxic lesions of the hand associated with chemotherapy. J Hand Surg 8: 39–42, 1983.
[212] D'Andrea F, Onesti MG, Nicoletti GF, et al: Surgical treatment of ulcers caused by the extravasation of cytotoxic drugs. Scand J Plast Reconstr Surg Hand Surg 38: 288–292, 2004.
[213] Devereux DF, Thibault LE, Boretos J, et al: The quantitative and qualitative impairment of wound healing by adriamycin. Cancer 43: 932–938, 1979.
[214] Devereux DF, Kent H, Brennan MF: Time dependent effects of adriamycin and x-ray therapy on wound healing in the rat. Cancer 45: 2805–2810, 1980.
[215] Devereux DF, Triche TJ, Webber BL, et al: A study of adriamycin-reduced wound breaking strength in rats. Cancer 45: 2811–2815, 1980.
[216] Vandeweyer E, Heymans O, Deraemaecker R: Extravasation injuries and emergency suction as treatment. Plast Reconstra Surg 105: 109–110, 2000.

[217] Yilmaz M, Demirdover C, Mola Fahri: Treatment options in extravasation injury: an experimental study in rats. Plast Reconstr Surg 109: 2418–2423, 2002.

[218] Cohen FJ, Manganaro J, Bezozo RC: Identification of involved tissue during surgical treatment of doxorubicin-induced extravasation necrosis. J Hand Surg 8: 43–45, 1983.

[219] Nogler-Semenitz E, Mader I, Fürst-Weger P, et al: Paravasation von Zytostatika. Wien Klin Wochenschr 116: 289–295, 2004.

[220] Summary of product characteristics Savene® (Denmark), Topo Target, July 2006.

[221] Mouridsen HT, Langer SW, Buter J, et al: Treatment of anthracycline extravasation with Savene (dexrazoxane): results from two prospective cilinical multicentre studies. Ann Oncol 18: 546–550, 2007.

[222] Tebbi CK, London WB, Friedmann D, et al: Dexrazoxane-associated risk for acute myeloic leukemia/myelodysplastic syndrome and other secondary malignancies in pediatric Hodgkin's disease. J Clin Oncol 25: 493–500, 2007.

Substance-specific part

Remarks on the substance-specific part

Ines Mader

1. General remarks

In the following section, cytotoxic substances are listed in alphabetical order by their substance name, not their trade names, so that in the emergency setting, practitioners can access the relevant information speedily. The substance monographs are divided into two parts:

1. Instructions for what to do in an emergency
2. Synopsis of the relevant literatures

We included all cytotoxic agents that are licensed for use in Europe. This 2nd edition includes two substances that were not previously mentioned:

- Pemetrexed
- Bortezomib

2. Remarks about the substance monographs

We retained the tried and tested structure used in the 1st edition of this book.

CONSENSUS

This includes the authors' work on:

- Classification of the type of damage
- General measures to be initiated in an emergency
- Substance specific measures (if available)

and

- Warnings

Type of damage mentioned in the literature:

- As described in the primary and secondary literature, without including animal studies

Symptoms and progression as mentioned in the literature:

To describe the symptoms and clinical course, we included with very few exceptions exclusively information from original articles and the summary of product characteristics.

In contrast to the 1st edition, we structured the monographs by:

- Initial symptoms (within 24 hours after extravasation)
- Delayed-onset symptoms (first reaction occurring or initial symptoms deteriorating, days, weeks, or months after the event)
- Outcome with sequelae (permanent damage) and
- Single case reports of unusual developments

Measures mentioned in the literature:

To list and assess the described measures, we consulted original articles as well as secondary literature.
The evaluation of successful treatment relates only to conservative measures.

- **With successful treatment:**
  The success of the treatment was assessed in relation to the damage potential of the respective substance (for example, prevention of necrosis in vesicant substances)

- **Unsuccessful treatment:**
  In vesicant substances:

  - Development of necroses or ulceration
  - Recurrence of symptoms after initial therapy as well as asymptomatic intervals or intensification of initial symptoms
  - Late sequelae such as impaired sensitivity, impaired movement of the affected limb
  - Surgical intervention where conservative measures have failed

  In irritant substances:

  - Blistering
  - Eruptions
  - Persistent pain
  - Recurrence of symptoms after initial therapy as well as asymptomatic intervals or intensification of initial symptoms

- **Success of treatment not reported:**
  The literature does not provide details about successful (or otherwise) treatment.

Particular remarks:

For the special remarks, the authors conducted a comprehensive review of the literature and discussions of effective treatment measures.
We also list substance specific side effects that may aid differential diagnosis.

Conclusion:

The authors conducted a comprehensive review of the types of damage and substance specific measures.

Literature:

The literature search methods and explanations about primary and secondary literature, as well as about additionally read literature can be found in the introduction to this book.

Amsacrine

CONSENSUS

Type of damage: vesicant

Recommended treatment:

General measures:

1. Stop injection/infusion immediately
2. Get extravasation kit
3. Put on (sterile) gloves
4. Replace infusion lead or syringe with 5 ml disposable syringe and aspirate slowly as much as possible of the extravasated drug; **Cave**! do not exert pressure on extravasation area
5. Remove i.v. access while aspirating
6. If blisters occur: aspirate with 1 ml syringe and s.c. cannula, use new equipment for every new attempt at aspiration
7. Elevate limb and immobilise
8. Start **substance specific measures**
9. Ensure adequate analgesia
10. Complete extravasation documentation sheet (mention extent of extravasation)
11. Inform and instruct the patient and relatives
12. Regular control (aftercare)
13. Always consult a (plastic) surgeon within 24 hours

Substance specific measures:

DMSO:

1. Apply DMSO (99%) every 8 hours (e.g. with a sterile gauze pad) without pressure
2. Allow to air-dry – **Cave**! do not cover
3. Continue for a minimum of 7 days

Immediately afterwards topical cooling:

1. Apply cold, dry pack immediately for at least 1 hour (for example, using a cold-hot pack)
2. Continue several times daily for 15 minutes each time

Cave! after extravasation:

1. No flushing of i.v. access
2. No moist compresses
3. No alcohol compresses
4. No occlusive dressings

Type of damage reported in literature:

High risk of necrosis [4,5]

Vesicant [1,3,8–11,14]

Symptoms and clinical course reported in literature:

Initial symptoms: No data available

Delayed-onset symptoms: Necrosis and ulceration (1 patient) [1]

Residual findings: No data available

Measures reported in literature:

Successful treatment:
- Animal experiments: local application of DMSO [2,4]

Unsuccessful treatment:
- Animal experiments: enhanced ulceration after application of local heat, heparin, and N-acetylcysteine [2,4]
- Animal experiments: hyaluronidase, hydrocortisone, sodium bicarbonate, and topical cooling did not significantly improve local symptoms [2,4]

Outcome of treatment not reported:
- Ice packs over 1–3 days, topical application of DMSO (70–100%) every 3–4 hours for 3–14 days, consultation of plastic surgeon just in time [5]
- Cold compresses immediately applied for 30–60 minutes, then for 24 hours alternating every 15 minutes (with/without compresses), topical application of 1.5 ml DMSO (50–99%) every 6 hours for 14 days [6]

- On day 1, DMSO every 2 hours, hydrocortisone (1%) applied topically, cold compresses for 30 minutes, followed by alternating DMSO or hydrocortisone at 3 hourly intervals for the following 14 days [8]

- DMSO (99%) at least every 6 hours for 3-14 days, cold compresses immediately for 20 minutes, afterwards 4 × daily for 20 minutes for 3-4 days [9]

- Ice packs [16]

- Topical cooling for 1 hour initially, several times daily for 15 minutes thereafter; DMSO (99%) every 8 hours for 8 days; maintain therapy free interval between cooling and DMSO [18]

- No specific measures mentioned [10,11,13,14]

Particular remarks: Phlebitis up to 17% [1,4,6,7,15], pain, and erythema [4] are not associated with extravasation, these symptoms may be reduced by prolonging the duration of the infusion by several hours and dilution in at least 500 ml glucose 5% [4,12]

DMSO: Reports about a positive effect in preventing necrosis are available from animal experiments only [2,4,6,15,17]

Conclusion: Amsacrine is classified exclusively as vesicant in the literature; although the substance is rarely administered, one case report of necrosis after extravasation has been reported; the substance is therefore classified as vesicant

On the basis of positive results using DMSO and topical cooling after extravasation of other DNA-intercalating agents, these substance specific and non-invasive interventions are recommended

Original articles

[1] Legha SS, Gutterman JU, Hall SW, et al: Phase I clinical investigation of 4´-(9-acridinylamino)methanesulfon-m-anisidide (NSC 249992), a new acridine derivative. Cancer Res 38: 3712–3716, 1978.

[2] Soble MJ, Dorr RT, Plezia P, et al: Dose-dependent skin ulcers in mice treated with DNA binding antitumor antibiotics. Cancer Chemother Pharmacol 20: 33–36, 1987.

Secondary literature

[3] Dorr RT: Extravasation of vesicant antineoplastics: clinical and experimental findings. Ariz Med 38: 271–275, 1981.

[4] Dorr RT: Antidotes to vesicant chemotherapy extravasations. Blood Rev 4: 41–60, 1990.

[5] Schneider G: Paravasate von Zytostatika. Diagnostik und Therapie. Aina S. Schneider Verlag, 6th edition: 1–17, 1999.

[6] Dorr RT: Pharmacologic management of vesicant chemotherapy extravasations. In: Dorr RT, Von Hoff DD (eds) Cancer Chemotherapy Handbook. Appleton & Lange, 2nd edition: 109–118, 1994.

[7] Louie AC, Issell BF: Amsacrine (AMSA) – a clinical review. J Clin Oncol 3: 562–592, 1985.

[8] Stanley A: Managing complications of chemotherapy administration. In: Allwood M, Stanley A, Wright P (eds) The Cytotoxics Handbook. Radcliffe Medical Press, 4th edition: 119–193, 2002.

[9] Krämer I, Stützle M: Zytostatika-Paravasation – Wie ist vorzugehen? Krankenhauspharmazie 23: 261–268, 2002.

[10] Bertelli G: Prevention and management of extravasation of cytotoxic drugs. Drug Safety 12: 245–255, 1995.

[11] Gain M, Melzer S, Meyer-Jürshof A, et al: Allgemeiner Teil: Behandlung von Paravasaten. In: Gain M, et al (eds) ADKA-Zytostatika-Handbuch, Pharmazeutisch-wissenschaftliche Monographien. Verlag Heiner Biller, vol 1, 2nd edition: A42–44, 1997.

[12] Dorr RT, Von Hoff DD: Drug monographs: amsacrine. In: Dorr RT, Von Hoff DD (eds) Cancer Chemotherapy Handbook. Appleton & Lange, 2nd edition: 182–189, 1994.

[13] Mullin S, Beckwith MC, Tyler LS: Prevention and management of antineoplastic extravasation injury. Hosp Pharm 35: 57–76, 2000.

[14] Schneider SM, Distelhorst CW: Chemotherapy-induced emergencies. Semin Oncol 16: 572–578, 1989.

[15] Summary of product characteristics Amsidyl® (Switzerland), Pfizer, April 2003.

[16] Allwood M: Chemotherapeutic agents: amsacrine. In: Allwood M, Stanley A, Wright P (eds) The Cytotoxics Handbook. Radcliffe Medical Press, 4th edition: 268–270, 2002.
[17] Gain M, Melzer S, Meyer-Jürshof A, et al: Amsacrin: Behandlung von Paravasaten. In: Gain M, et al (eds) ADKA-Zytostatika-Handbuch, Pharmazeutisch-wissenschaftliche Monographien. Verlag Heiner Biller, vol 5: 20, 2001.
[18] Jordan K, Grothe W, Schmoll HJ: Paravasation von Zytostatika: Prävention und Therapie. Dtsch Med Wochenschr 130: 33–37, 2005.

Further reading:

- Ener RA, Meglathery SB, Styler M: Extravasation of systemic hemato-oncological therapies. Ann Oncol 15: 858–862, 2004.
- Fenchel K, Karthaus M: Zytostatika-Paravasate – gibt es neue Empfehlungen zum therapeutischen Vorgehen? Wien Med Wochenschr 151: 44–46, 2001.
- Henry MC, Port CD, Levine BS: Preclinical toxicologic evaluation of 4´-(9-acridinylamino)methanesulfon-m-anisidide (AMSA) in mice, dogs, and monkeys. Cancer Treat Rep 64: 855–860, 1980.
- Krämer I: Onkologische Pharmazie. In: Jaehde U, Radziwill R, Mühlebach S, et al (eds) Lehrbuch der Klinischen Pharmazie. Wissenschaftliche Verlagsgesellschaft mbH, 2nd edition: 307–336, 2003.
- Rauh J, Pluntke S, Müller C: Paravenöse Zytostatikainjektion: Prophylaxe und Sofortmaßnahmen im Notfall. MMW Fortschr Med 146: 682–686, 2004.

Revisions by Ines Mader

L-Asparaginase

CONSENSUS

Type of damage: non-vesicant

Recommended treatment:

General measures:

1. Stop injection/infusion immediately
2. Get extravasation kit
3. Put on (sterile) gloves
4. Replace infusion lead or syringe with 5 ml disposable syringe and aspirate slowly as much as possible of the extravasated drug; **Cave!** do not exert pressure on extravasation area
5. Remove i.v. access while aspirating
6. Elevate limb and immobilise
7. Complete extravasation documentation sheet (mention extent of extravasation)
8. Inform and instruct the patient and relatives
9. Regular control (aftercare)

Substance specific measures: none

Cave! after extravasation:

1. No flushing of i.v. access
2. No moist compresses
3. No alcohol compresses
4. No occlusive dressings

Type of damage reported in literature:

Non-vesicant [5,7–10,12,15,19]

No risk of necrosis [4,6]

Symptoms and clinical course reported in literature:

No data available

Measures reported in literature:

Successful treatment:
- No data available

Unsuccessful treatment:
- No data available

Outcome of treatment not reported:
- 1500 IU hyaluronidase s.c., application of heat and compression [5]
- Optional local infiltration of corticosteroids, warm to hot compresses for 1 hour [8]
- If local symptoms develop, hydrocortisone (1%) or heparin to be applied topically [10]
- Topical cooling 4 × daily for 20 minutes over 3–14 days [15]
- No specific measures mentioned [4,6,7,9,12,19]

Particular remarks:

Results of literature search: no clinical studies regarding extravasation have been published

Animal experiments: no local reactions reported after application of asparaginase s.c. and i.d. [3]

Very high immunogenic potential; incidence of hypersensitivity reactions: 6–70% described in the literature [1,2,5–7,11,13,16–18]

Conclusion: Since asparaginase is also administered i.m. [5,13,14,16], a tissue-damaging effect is unlikely; the substance is therefore classified as non-vesicant

No substance specific measures are required

Original articles

[1] Oettgen HF, Stephenson PA, Schwartz MK, et al: Toxicity of E. coli L- asparaginase in man. Cancer 25: 253–278, 1970.

[2] Haskell CM, Canellos GP, Leventhal BG, et al: L-asparaginase: therapeutic and toxic effects in patients with neoplastic disease. N Engl J Med 281: 1028–1034, 1969.

[3] Barr RD, Benton SG, Belbeck LW: Soft-tissue necrosis induced by extravasated cancer chemotherapeutic agents. J Natl Cancer Inst 66: 1129–1136, 1981.

Secondary literature

[4] Dorr RT: Antidotes to vesicant chemotherapy extravasations. Blood Rev 4: 41–60, 1990.

[5] Stanley A: Managing complications of chemotherapy administration. In: Allwood M, Stanley A, Wright P (eds) The Cytotoxics Handbook. Radcliffe Medical Press, 4th edition: 119–193, 2002.

[6] Schneider G: Paravasate von Zytostatika. Diagnostik und Therapie. Aina S. Schneider Verlag, 6th edition: 1–17, 1999.

[7] Schneider SM, Distelhorst CW: Chemotherapy-induced emergencies. Semin Oncol 16: 572–578, 1989.

[8] Ignoffo RJ, Friedman MA: Therapy of local toxicities caused by extravasation of cancer chemotherapeutic drugs. Cancer Treat Rev 7: 17–27, 1980.

[9] Dorr RT: Pharmacologic management of vesicant chemotherapy extravasations. In: Dorr RT, Von Hoff DD (eds) Cancer Chemotherapy Handbook. Appleton & Lange, 2nd edition: 109–118, 1994.

[10] Cox K, Stuart-Harris R, Abdini G, et al: The management of cytotoxic-drug extravasation: guide-lines drawn up by a working party for the Clinical Oncological Society of Australia. Med J Aust 148: 185–189, 1988.

[11] Fuxius S, Unger C: Pegaspargase. Arzneimitteltherapie 16: 170–173, 1998.

[12] Gain M, Melzer S, Meyer-Jürshof A, et al: Allgemeiner Teil: Behandlung von Paravasaten. In: Gain M, et al (eds) ADKA-Zytostatika-Handbuch, Pharmazeutisch-wissenschaftliche Monographien. Verlag Heiner Biller, vol 1, 2nd edition A42–44, 1997.
[13] Dorr RT, Von Hoff DD: Drug monographs: asparaginase. In: Dorr RT, Von Hoff DD (eds) Cancer Chemotherapy Handbook. Appleton & Lange, 2nd edition: 201–209, 1994.
[14] Summary of product characteristics Asparaginase medac (Germany), medac, March 2004.
[15] Krämer I, Stützle M: Zytostatika-Paravasation – Wie ist vorzugehen? Krankenhauspharmazie 23: 261–268, 2002.
[16] Albanell J, Baselga J: Systemic therapy emergencies. Semin Oncol 27: 347–361, 2000.
[17] Koppel RA, Boh EE: Cutaneous reactions to chemotherapeutic agents. Am J Med Sci 321: 327–335, 2001.
[18] Alley E, Green R, Schuchter L: Cutaneous toxicities of cancer therapy. Curr Opin Oncol 14: 212–216, 2002.
[19] Jordan K, Grothe W, Schmoll HJ: Paravasation von Zytostatika: Prävention und Therapie. Dtsch Med Wochenschr 130: 33–37, 2005.

Further reading:

- Fenchel K, Karthaus M: Zytostatika-Paravasate – gibt es neue Empfehlungen zum therapeutischen Vorgehen? Wien Med Wochenschr 151: 44–46, 2001.
- Rauh J, Pluntke S, Müller C: Paravenöse Zytostatikainjektion: Prophylaxe und Sofortmaßnahmen im Notfall. MMW Fortschr Med 146: 682–686, 2004.

Revisions by Patrizia Fürst-Weger

Bendamustine

CONSENSUS

Type of damage: irritant

Recommended treatment:

General measures:

1. Stop injection/infusion immediately
2. Get extravasation kit
3. Put on (sterile) gloves
4. Replace infusion lead or syringe with 5 ml disposable syringe and aspirate slowly as much as possible of the extravasated drug; **Cave!** do not exert pressure on extravasation area
5. Remove i.v. access while aspirating
6. If blisters occur: aspirate with 1 ml syringe and s.c. cannula, use new equipment for every new attempt at aspiration
7. Elevate limb and immobilise
8. Complete extravasation documentation sheet (mention extent of extravasation)
9. Inform and instruct the patient and relatives
10. Regular control (aftercare)

Substance specific measures: none

Cave! after extravasation:

1. No flushing of i.v. access
2. No moist compresses
3. No alcohol compresses
4. No occlusive dressings

Type of damage reported in literature:	Unknown tissue toxic potential [7] Irritant [8]
Symptoms and clinical course reported in literature:	**Initial symptoms:** No data available **Delayed-onset symptoms:** Skin alterations resembling those after extravasation of doxorubicin, but no skin necroses (2 patients) [2]; according to the summary of product characteristics necroses are very rare [5]—no further information available **Residual findings:** No data available
Measures reported in literature:	**Successful treatment:** - No data available **Unsuccessful treatment:** - No data available **Outcome of treatment not reported:** - Topical cooling of the extravasation site with ice-cold compresses, changed frequently [3] - Topical cooling 4 × daily for 20 minutes over 3–4 days [7] - No specific measure mentioned [8]
Particular remarks:	Results of literature search: no animal experiments and only two case studies regarding extravasation have been published Local irritations and phlebitis at the injection site [2,4,5], especially after i.v. bolus injection (35.4%[1]) are not associated with extravasation; these symptoms are likely to have been caused by the acidic pH of 3–4 [6] of the reconstituted drug

B

Conclusion:

The symptoms mentioned in the secondary literature such as necroses could not be verified in clinical case reports; bendamustine is classified as irritant because of the acidic pH of the reconstituted drug

Owing to little experience with extravasations of bendamustine, a final classification of the type of damage is not possible

Positive results of substance specific measures have not been described so far; until further data become available no substance specific measures can be ecommended

Original articles

[1] Ruffert K, Jahn H, Syrbe G, et al: Cytostasan® (Bendamustin) in der Alternativtherapie maligner Non-Hodgkin-Lymphome – Cytostasan (bendamustin) as an alternative therapeutic approach to treat malignant non-Hodgkin's lymphoma. Z Klin Med 44: 671–674, 1989.
[2] Brockmann B, Geschke E, Schmidt UM, et al: Therapieergebnisse und toxische Nebenwirkungen der Kombination Cytostasan, Adriamycin und Vincristin als "Second line"-Therapie beim metastasierten Mammakarzinom. In: Geburtshilfe und Frauenheilkunde. Georg Thieme Verlag 51: 383–386, 1991.

Secondary literature

[3] Gain M, Melzer S, Meyer-Jürshof A, et al: Bendamustin: Behandlung von Paravasaten. In: Gain M, et al (eds) ADKA-Zytostatika-Handbuch, Pharmazeutisch-wissenschaftliche Monographien. Verlag Heiner Biller, vol 4: 24, 2000.
[4] Sauer H: Substanzprofile, Zytostatika, Hormone, Zytokine: Bendamustin. In: Schmoll HJ, Höffken K, Possinger K (eds) Kompendium Internistische Onkologie. Standards in Diagnostik und Therapie. Springer, Vol 1, 3rd edition: 736–737, 1999.
[5] Summary of product characteristics Ribomustin® (Germany), ribosepharm, September 2003.
[6] Information for hospital pharmacists Ribomustin® (Germany), ribosepharm, October 1998.

[7] Krämer I, Stützle M: Zytostatika-Paravasation – Wie ist vorzugehen? Krankenhauspharmazie 23: 261–268, 2002.
[8] Jordan K, Grothe W, Schmoll HJ: Paravasation von Zytostatika: Prävention und Therapie. Dtsch Med Wochenschr 130: 33–37, 2005.

Further reading:

- Rauh J, Pluntke S, Müller C: Paravenöse Zytostatikainjektion: Prophylaxe und Sofortmaßnahmen im Notfall. MMW Fortschr Med 146: 682–686, 2004.

Revisions by Patrizia Fürst-Weger

Bleomycin

CONSENSUS

Type of damage: non-vesicant

Recommended treatment:

General measures:

1. Stop injection/infusion immediately
2. Get extravasation kit
3. Put on (sterile) gloves
4. Replace infusion lead or syringe with 5 ml disposable syringe and aspirate slowly as much as possible of the extravasated drug; **Cave!** do not exert pressure on extravasation area
5. Remove i.v. access while aspirating
6. Elevate limb and immobilise
7. Complete extravasation documentation sheet (mention extent of extravasation)
8. Inform and instruct the patient and relatives
9. Regular control (aftercare)

Substance specific measures: none

Cave! after extravasation:

1. No flushing of i.v. access
2. No moist compresses
3. No alcohol compresses
4. No occlusive dressings

Type of damage reported in literature:

Non-vesicant [2–7,11,14,16]

Weak irritant (not vesicant) [13]

Irritant [9,17]

Low risk of necrosis [8,12]

Vesicant [10]

Symptoms and clinical course reported in literature:

No data available

Measures reported in literature:

Successful treatment:
- No data available

Unsuccessful treatment:
- No data available

Outcome of treatment not reported:
- No special measures necessary, if in doubt perfuse with NaCl 0.9% [2]
- 100 mg hydrocortisone s.c. and i.v., respectively, ice or cold pack 4 × daily for 15–20 minutes, topical hydrocortisone [3,4]
- 1500 IU hyaluronidase s.c., application of heat and compression [5]
- Optional local infiltration of corticosteroids, warm to hot compresses for 1 hour [6]
- Topical cooling 4 × daily for 3-4 days [14]
- No specific measures mentioned [7–13,16,17]

Particular remarks:

Results of literature search: no animal experiments or clinical studies regarding extravasation have been published

B

Hypersensitivity reactions [11,18,19] or fever (incidence:20–25%) [11] are not related to extravasation

Enhanced radiosensitivity [18, 19] or recall phenomenon after radiotherapy reported [18,19]

Reports of erythema, swelling, fissures, hyperpigmentation of the palms after i.v. administration of bleomycin independent of administration site [1] are not associated with extravasation

Conclusion: Although bleomycin is classified as irritant/vesicant in some of the literature, no clinical case of tissue damage after extravasation has been documented

Since bleomycin can also be applied i.m. [2] and s.c. [15], a tissue-damaging effect is unlikely; the substance is therefore classified as non-vesicant

No substance specific measures are required

Original articles

[1] Seyfer AE, Solimando DA: Toxic lesions of the hand associated with chemotherapy. J Hand Surg 8: 39–42, 1983.

Secondary literature

[2] Summary of the product characteristics Bleomedac® (Germany), medac, September 2004.
[3] Gain M, Melzer S, Meyer-Jürshof A, et al: Allgemeiner Teil: Behandlung von Paravasaten. In: Gain M, et al (eds) ADKA-Zytostatika-Handbuch, Pharmazeutisch-wissenschaftliche Monographien. Verlag Heiner Biller, vol 1, 2nd edition: A42–44, 1997.
[4] Donislawski S, Gain M, Meyer-Jürshof A, et al: Bleomycin: Behandlung von Paravasaten. In: Donislawski S, et al (eds) ADKA-Zytostatika-Handbuch, Pharmazeutisch-wissenschaftliche Monographien. Verlag Heiner Biller, vol 2: 23, 1994.
[5] Stanley A: Managing complications of chemotherapy administration. In: Allwood M, Stanley A, Wright P (eds) The Cytotoxics Handbook. Radcliffe Medical Press, 4th edition: 119–193, 2002.

[6] Ignoffo RJ, Friedman MA: Therapy of local toxicities caused by extravasation of cancer chemotherapeutic drugs. Cancer Treat Rev 7: 17–27, 1980.
[7] Dorr RT: Pharmacologic management of vesicant chemotherapy extravasations. In: Dorr RT, Von Hoff DD (eds) Cancer Chemotherapy Handbook. Appleton & Lange, 2nd edition: 109–118, 1994.
[8] Schneider G: Paravasate von Zytostatika. Diagnostik und Therapie. Aina S. Schneider Verlag, 6th edition: 1–17, 1999.
[9] Mullin S, Beckwith MC, Tyler LS: Prevention and management of antineoplastic extravasation injury. Hosp Pharm 35: 57–76, 2000.
[10] Bertelli G: Prevention and management of extravasation of cytotoxic drugs. Drug Safety 12: 245–255, 1995.
[11] Schneider SM, Distelhorst CW: Chemotherapy-induced emergencies. Semin Oncol 16: 572–578, 1989.
[12] Dorr RT: Antidotes to vesicant chemotherapy extravasations. Blood Rev 4: 41–60, 1990.
[13] Barth J: Paravasate und deren Behandlung. In: Barth J (eds) Zytostatika-Herstellung in der Apotheke. Deutscher Apotheker Verlag, chapter VI-3: 1–9, 2000.
[14] Krämer I, Stützle M: Zytostatika-Paravasation – Wie ist vorzugehen? Krankenhauspharmazie 23: 261–268, 2002.
[15] Dorr RT, Von Hoff DD: Drug monographs: bleomycin sulfate. In: Dorr RT, Von Hoff DD (eds) Cancer Chemotherapy Handbook. Appleton & Lange, 2nd edition: 227–236, 1994.
[16] Jordan K, Grothe W, Schmoll HJ: Paravasation von Zytostatika: Prävention und Therapie. Dtsch Med Wochenschr 130: 33–37, 2005.
[17] Ener RA, Meglathery SB, Styler M: Extravasation of systemic hemato-oncological therapies. Ann Oncol 15: 858–862, 2004.
[18] Koppel RA, Boh EE: Cutaneous reactions to chemotherapeutic agents. Am J Med Sci 321: 327–335, 2001.
[19] Alley E, Green R, Schuchter L: Cutaneous toxicities of cancer therapy. Curr Opin Oncol 14: 212–216, 2002.

Further reading:

- Krämer I: Zehn Jahre Dokumentation von Zytostatika-Paravasat-Ereignissen: Auswertung von 175 Paravasate-Dokumentationen. Krankenhauspharmazie 23: 269–274, 2002.
- Krämer I: Onkologische Pharmazie. In: Jaehde U, Radziwill R, Mühlebach S, et al (eds) Lehrbuch der Klinischen Pharmazie. Wissenschaftliche Verlagsgesellschaft mbH, 2nd edition: 307–336, 2003.

B

- Preuss P, Partoft S: Cytostatic extravasations. Ann Plast Surg 19: 323–327, 1987.
- Rauh J, Pluntke S, Müller C: Paravenöse Zytostatikainjektion: Prophylaxe und Sofortmaßnahmen im Notfall. MMW Fortschr Med 146: 682–686, 2004.

Revisions by Elisabeth Nogler-Semenitz

Bortezomib

CONSENSUS

Type of damage: irritant

Recommended treatment:

General measures:

1. Stop injection/infusion immediately
2. Get extravasation kit
3. Put on (sterile) gloves
4. Replace infusion lead or syringe with 5 ml disposable syringe and aspirate slowly as much as possible of the extravasated drug; **Cave!** do not exert pressure on extravasation area
5. Remove i.v. access while aspirating
6. If blisters occur: aspirate with 1 ml syringe and s.c. cannula, use new equipment for every new attempt at aspiration
7. Elevate limb and immobilise
8. Complete extravasation documentation sheet (mention extent of extravasation)
9. Inform and instruct the patient and relatives
10. Regular control (aftercare)

Substance specific measures: none

Cave! after extravasation:

1. No flushing of i.v. access
2. No moist compresses
3. No alcohol compresses
4. No occlusive dressings

B

Type of damage reported in literature:	Irritant [3]
Symptoms and clinical course reported in literature:	**Initial symptoms:** Skin irritations [1] according to the summary of product characteristics from the US, but no further information available **Delayed-onset symptoms:** No tissue damage [1] **Residual findings:** No data available
Measures reported in literature:	No data available
Particular remarks:	Results of literature search: no animal experiments or clinical studies regarding extravasation have been published Clinical studies have shown local skin irritations in 5% of patients [1] Occasionally occurring erythema at the injection site is not associated with extravasation [2]
Conclusion:	Since the literature includes reports of skin irritations, bortezomib is classified as irritant Owing to little or no experience with extravasations of bortezomib, a final evaluation of the type of damage is not possible Positive results of substance specific measures have not been described so far; until further data become available, substance specific measures can therefore not be recommended

Original articles

–

Secondary literature

[1] Prescribing information Velcade® (USA), Millennium Pharmaceuticals Inc, März 2005.
[2] Summary of product characteristics Velcade® (Austria), Janssen-Cilag, April 2004.

[3] Cancer Care Ontario, Appendix 2 – Extravasation, June 2005.

Further reading:

– Krämer I: Bortezomib: a new approach to anticancer treatment. EJHP-S 11: 3–10, 2005.

Revisions by Sabine Wassertheurer

Busulfan

CONSENSUS

Type of damage: irritant

Recommended treatment:

General measures:

1. Stop injection/infusion immediately
2. Get extravasation kit
3. Put on (sterile) gloves
4. Replace infusion lead or syringe with 5 ml disposable syringe and aspirate slowly as much as possible of the extravasated drug; **Cave!** do not exert pressure on extravasation area
5. Remove i.v. access while aspirating
6. If blisters occur: aspirate with 1 ml syringe and s.c. cannula, use new equipment for every new attempt at aspiration
7. Elevate limb and immobilise
8. Complete extravasation documentation sheet (mention extent of extravasation)
9. Inform and instruct the patient and relatives
10. Regular control (aftercare)

Substance specific measures: none

Cave! after extravasation:

1. No flushing of i.v. access
2. No moist compresses
3. No alcohol compresses
4. No occlusive dressings

Type of damage reported in literature:	Irritant [2,6]
Symptoms and clinical course reported in literature:	No data available
Measures reported in literature:	**Successful treatment:** – No data available **Unsuccessful treatment:** – No data available **Outcome of treatment not reported:** – No specific measure mentioned [6]
Particular remarks:	Results of literature search: no animal experiments or clinical studies regarding extravasation have been published Inflammation (25%[1]) and pain (15%[1]) at the site of injection [1,5] are not associated with extravasation; these symptoms are likely to have been caused by the excipient polyethylenglycol 400 [3] and the acidic pH of 3.4–3.9 [1] of the infusion solution Hypersensitivity reactions have been described in the literature [1,4]; incidence: mild to moderate 24%, severe 2% [1]
Conclusion:	Although busulfan is classified as irritant in the literature, no clinical case of irritation of tissue after extravasation has been documented; the substance is classified as irritant because of the excipient and the acidic pH of the infusion solution Since busulfan is given rarely, there is lack of experience with extravasation; a final classification of the type of damage is not possible

B

Positive results of substance specific measures have not been described so far; until further data become available no substance specific measures can be recommended

Original articles

–

Secondary literature

[1] Prescribing Information Busulfex® (USA), Orphan Medical Inc, February 1999.
[2] Mullin S, Beckwith MC, Tyler LS: Prevention and management of antineoplastic extravasation injury. Hosp Pharm 35: 57–76, 2000.
[3] Price JC: Polyethylene glycol. In: Wade A, et al (eds) Handbook of Pharmaceutical Excipients, 2nd edition: 355–361, 1994.
[4] Koppel RA, Boh EE: Cutaneous reactions to chemotherapeutic agents. Am J Med Sci 321: 327–335, 2001.
[5] Summary of product characteristics Busilvex® (Germany), Pierre Fabre Médicament, October 2003.
[6] Jordan K, Grothe W, Schmoll HJ: Paravasation von Zytostatika: Prävention und Therapie. Dtsch Med Wochenschr 130: 33–37, 2005.

Revisions by Patrizia Fürst-Weger

Carboplatin

CONSENSUS

Type of damage: non-vesicant

Recommended treatment:

General measures:

1. Stop injection/infusion immediately
2. Get extravasation kit
3. Put on (sterile) gloves
4. Replace infusion lead or syringe with 5 ml disposable syringe and aspirate slowly as much as possible of the extravasated drug; **Cave!** do not exert pressure on extravasation area
5. Remove i.v. access while aspirating
6. Elevate limb and immobilise
7. Complete extravasation documentation sheet (mention extent of extravasation)
8. Inform and instruct the patient and relatives
9. Regular control (aftercare)

Substance specific measures: none

Cave! after extravasation:

1. No flushing of i.v. access
2. No moist compresses
3. No alcohol compresses
4. No occlusive dressings

Type of damage reported in literature:

No damage or moderate damage [5]

Weak irritant (not vesicant) [12]

Irritant [6,7,9,13,14]

No risk of necrosis [10]

Symptoms and clinical course reported in literature:

No data available

Measures reported in literature:

Successful treatment:

- 4 drops of DMSO (99%) per 10 cm^2 applied topically to an area twice the size of the affected area, repeat every 8 hours for 1 week or until symptoms have subsided; local cooling for 60 minutes, every 8 hours for 3 days (cold-hot pack) (5 patients) [2,8]
- Cold compresses for 24 hours (2 patients) [3]

Unsuccessful treatment:

- No data available

Outcome of treatment not reported:

- After extravasation in the context of combination chemotherapy with carboplatin and epirubicin (extravasated substance not identified): DMSO, topical cooling, glucocorticoid i.d. (1 patient) [4]
- After extravasation in the context of combination chemotherapy with carboplatin and etoposide or cyclophosphamide (extravasated substance not identified): no specific measure mentioned (1 patient, respectively) [4]
- Cold compresses for 24 hours [5]
- 100 mg hydrocortisone i.v. and s.c. respectively, additionally topical hydrocortisone, icepack; after initial reaction has subsided, warm compresses [6]

- Topical glucocorticoids [7]
- Hydrocortisone cream (1%) every 6 hours over 14 days, hydrocortisone and hyaluronidase s.c., warm compresses; sodium thiosulfate in particularly severe cases [8]
- No specific measure mentioned [4 (9 patients), 12–14]

Particular remarks: Animal experiments: blister formation after administration of concentrations ≥ 10 mg/ml; complete healing after 21 days [1]

Local reactions such as erythema, pain, and irritations of the intima at the application site [11] are not associated with extravasation

Incidence of hypersensitivity reactions is less than 2% [11]

Extravasations of solutions containing carboplatin progress without complications, since carboplatin is given only in diluted form [8]

DMSO and topical cooling: positive effects have been reported [2]

Conclusion: Although carboplatin is occasionally classified as irritant in the literature, no clinical case of irritation of tissue after extravasation has been documented; the substance is therefore classified as non-vesicant

No substance specific measures – such as DMSO and topical cooling – are required

Original articles

[1] Marnocha RS, Hutson PR: Intradermal carboplatin and ifosfamide extravasation in the mouse. Cancer 70: 850–853, 1992.
[2] Bertelli G, Gozza A, Forno GB, et al: Topical dimethylsulfoxide for the prevention of soft tissue injury after extravasation of vesicant cytotoxic drugs: a prospective clinical study. J Clin Oncol 13: 2851–2855, 1995.
[3] Langstein HN, Duman H, Seelig D, et al: Retrospective study of the management of chemotherapeutic extravasation injury. Ann Plast Surg 49: 369–374, 2002.

[4] Krämer I: Zehn Jahre Dokumentation von Zytostatika-Paravasat-Ereignissen: Auswertung von 175 Paravasate-Dokumentationen. Krankenhauspharmazie 23: 269–274, 2002.

C

Secondary literature

[5] Bristol Myers Squibb, personal communication, October 1998.
[6] Stanley A: Managing complications of chemotherapy administration. In: Allwood M, Stanley A, Wright P (eds) The Cytotoxics Handbook. Radcliffe Medical Press, 4th edition: 119–193, 2002.
[7] Krämer I, Stützle M: Zytostatika-Paravasation – Wie ist vorzugehen? Krankenhauspharmazie 23: 261–268, 2002.
[8] Gain M, Melzer S, Meyer-Jürshof A, et al: Carboplatin: Behandlung von Paravasaten. In: Gain M, et al (eds) ADKA-Zytostatika-Handbuch, Pharmazeutisch-wissenschaftliche Monographien. Verlag Heiner Biller, vol 3: 43, 1998.
[9] Gain M, Melzer S, Meyer-Jürshof A, et al: Allgemeiner Teil: Behandlung von Paravasaten. In: Gain M, et al (eds) ADKA-Zytostatika-Handbuch, Pharmazeutisch-wissenschaftliche Monographien. Verlag Heiner Biller, Vol 1, 2nd edition: A42–44, 1997.
[10] Dorr RT, Von Hoff DD: Drug monographs: carboplatin. In: Dorr RT, Von Hoff DD (eds) Cancer Chemotherapy Handbook. Appleton & Lange, 2nd edition: 259–267, 1994.
[11] Summary of product characteristics Carboplatin "Ebewe" (Austria), Ebewe, November 2002.
[12] Barth J: Paravasate und deren Behandlung. In: Barth J (ed) Zytostatika-Herstellung in der Apotheke. Deutscher Apotheker Verlag, chapter VI-3: 1–9, 2000.
[13] Ener RA, Meglathery SB, Styler M: Extravasation of systemic hemato-oncological therapies. Ann Oncol 15: 858–862, 2004.
[14] Jordan K, Grothe W, Schmoll HJ: Paravasation von Zytostatika: Prävention und Therapie. Dtsch Med Wochenschr 130: 33–37, 2005.

Further reading:

- Fenchel K, Karthaus M: Zytostatika-Paravasate – gibt es neue Empfehlungen zum therapeutischen Vorgehen? Wien Med Wochenschr 151: 44–46, 2001.
- Kassner E: Evaluation and treatment of chemotherapy extravasation injuries. J Pediatr Oncol Nurs 17: 135–148, 2000.

- Rauh J, Pluntke S, Müller C: Paravenöse Zytostatikainjektion: Prophylaxe und Sofortmaßnahmen im Notfall. MMW Fortschr Med 146: 682–686, 2004.
- Schrijvers DL: Extravasation: a dreaded complication of chemotherapy. Ann Oncol 14: iii26–iii30, 2003.

Revisions by Patrizia Fürst-Weger

Carmustine

CONSENSUS

Type of damage: irritant

Recommended treatment:

General measures:

1. Stop injection/infusion immediately
2. Get extravasation kit
3. Put on (sterile) gloves
4. Replace infusion lead or syringe with 5 ml disposable syringe and aspirate slowly as much as possible of the extravasated drug; **Cave!** do not exert pressure on extravasation area
5. Remove i.v. access while aspirating
6. If blisters occur: aspirate with 1 ml syringe and s.c. cannula, use new equipment for every new attempt at aspiration
7. Elevate limb and immobilise
8. Complete extravasation documentation sheet (mention extent of extravasation)
9. Inform and instruct the patient and relatives
10. Regular control (aftercare)

Substance specific measures: none

Cave! after extravasation:

1. No flushing of i.v. access
2. No moist compresses
3. No alcohol compresses
4. No occlusive dressings

Type of damage reported in literature:

No risk of necrosis [13,19]

Irritant [8,15–18,20,21,23–26] and/or weak vesicant in large amounts and high concentrations [11]

Vesicant [9,22]

Symptoms and clinical course reported in literature:

No data available

Measures reported in literature:

Successful treatment:
- No data available

Unsuccessful treatment:
- Animal experiments: topical treatment with DMSO and α-tocopherol [7]

Outcome of treatment not reported:
- Infiltration of 5 ml sodium bicarbonate (8.4%), optional local infiltration of corticosteroids, warm to hot compresses for 1 hour [8]
- Infiltration of 1–3 ml sodium bicarbonate (2.1% [9,23] or 8.4% [20]), aspiration after 2 minutes [9]
- If local symptoms develop, hydrocortisone (1%) or heparin to be applied topically [17]
- Topical cooling 4 × daily for 20 minutes over 3–4 days [24]
- No specific measure mentioned [11,13,15,16,18, 19,25,26]

Particular remarks:

Results of literature search: no clinical studies regarding extravasation have been published

Animal experiments: ulceration after i.d. administration [7]

C

Burning sensation at the infusion site [1,2,8,14,15,19], pain [14], and phlebitis [8,13,14,19] are not associated with extravasation; these symptoms are due to ethanol [1,2,8,13,15]

Sufficient dilution [2,8,15] in 250 ml [12,13] to 500 ml [14] of the infusion solution and decreasing of the flow rate [2,8,12] are recommended as prophylactic measures; the infusion should take at least 1–2 hours [14]

Sodium bicarbonate is recommended as an antidote by some authors [8,9,20]; this measure may be due to the fast inactivation of carmustine in an alkaline medium [5,6,8,10,12,13]; **Cave!** sodium bicarbonate may cause necrosis by itself [3,4]

Conclusion: Although carmustine is classified as irritant/vesicant in the literature, no clinical case of tissue damage after extravasation has been documented; the substance is classified as irritant, because of the excipient in the reconstituted solution (ethanol [14])

Positive results of substance specific measures have not been described so far; until further data become available no substance specific measures can be recommended

Original articles

[1] De Vita VT, Carbone PP, Owens AH, et al: Clinical trials with 1,3-bis (2-chloroethyl)-1-nitrosourea, NSC-409962. Cancer Res 25: 1876–1881, 1965.
[2] Marsh JC, DeConti RC, Hubbard SP: Treatment of Hodgkin's disease and other cancers with 1,3-bis(2-chloroethyl)-1-nitrosourea (BCNU; NSC-409962). Cancer Chemother Rep 55: 599–606, 1971.
[3] Gaze NR: Tissue necrosis caused by commonly used intravenous infusions. Lancet 2: 417–419, 1978.
[4] Jackson IT, Robinson DW: Severe tissue damage following accidental subcutaneous infusion of bicarbonate solution. Scot Med J 21: 200–201, 1976.

[5] Colvin M, Hartner J, Summerfield M: Stability of carmustine in the presence of sodium bicarbonate. Am J Hosp Pharm 37: 677–678, 1980.
[6] Laskar PA, Ayres JW: Degradation of carmustine in aqueous media. J Pharm Sci 66: 1073–1076, 1977.
[7] Loth TS, Eversmann WW: Treatment methods for extravasations of chemotherapeutic agents: a comparative study. J Hand Surg 11A: 388–396, 1986.

C

Secondary literature

[8] Ignoffo RJ, Friedman MA: Therapy of local toxicities caused by extravasation of cancer chemotherapeutic drugs. Cancer Treat Rev 7: 17–27, 1980.
[9] Stanley A: Managing complications of chemotherapy administration. In: Allwood M, Stanley A, Wright P (eds) The Cytotoxics Handbook. Radcliffe Medical Press, 4th edition: 119–193, 2002.
[10] Allwood M: Chemotherapeutic agents: carmustine. In: Allwood M, Stanley A, Wright P (eds) The Cytotoxics Handbook. Radcliffe Medical Press, 4th edition: 282–285, 2002.
[11] Dorr RT: Pharmacologic management of vesicant chemotherapy extravasations. In: Dorr RT, Von Hoff DD (eds) Cancer Chemotherapy Handbook. Appleton & Lange, 2nd edition: 109–118, 1994.
[12] Dorr RT, Von Hoff DD: Drug monographs: carmustine. In: Dorr RT, Von Hoff DD (eds) Cancer Chemotherapy Handbook. Appleton & Lange, 2nd edition: 267–275, 1994.
[13] Dorr RT: Antidotes to vesicant chemotherapy extravasations. Blood Rev 4: 41–60, 1990.
[14] Summary of product characteristics Carmubris® (Germany), Bristol-Myers Squibb, February 2005.
[15] Krämer I: Zytostatika-Paravasate-Set. Krankenhauspharmazie 13: 154–160, 1992.
[16] Schneider SM, Distelhorst CW: Chemotherapy-induced emergencies. Semin Oncol 16: 572–578, 1989.
[17] Cox K, Stuart-Harris R, Abdini G, et al: The management of cytotoxic-drug extravasation: guide-lines drawn up by a working party for the Clinical Oncological Society of Australia. Med J Aust 148: 185–189, 1988.
[18] Bertelli G: Prevention and management of extravasation of cytotoxic drugs. Drug Safety 12: 245–255, 1995.
[19] Schneider G: Paravasate von Zytostatika. Diagnostik und Therapie. Aina S. Schneider Verlag, 6th edition: 1–17, 1999.

C

[20] Donislawski S, Gain M, Meyer-Jürshof A, et al: Carmustin: Behandlung von Paravasaten. In: Donislawski S, et al (eds) ADKA-Zyto statika-Handbuch, Pharmazeutisch-wissenschaftliche Monographien. Verlag Heiner Biller, vol 2: 21, 1994.
[21] Holmes BC: Administration of cancer chemotherapy agents. In: Dorr RT, Von Hoff DD (eds) Cancer Chemotherapy Handbook. Appleton & Lange, 2nd edition: 57–94, 1994.
[22] Gain M, Melzer S, Meyer-Jürshof A, et al: Allgemeiner Teil: Behandlung von Paravasaten. In: Gain M, et al (eds) ADKA-Zytostatika-Handbuch, Pharmazeutisch-wissenschaftliche Monographien. Verlag Heiner Biller, vol 1, 2nd edition: A42–44, 1997.
[23] Barth J: Paravasate und deren Behandlung. In: Barth J (ed) Zytostatika-Herstellung in der Apotheke. Deutscher Apotheker Verlag, chapter VI-3: 1–9, 2000.
[24] Krämer I, Stützle M: Zytostatika-Paravasation – Wie ist vorzugehen? Krankenhauspharmazie 23: 261–268, 2002.
[25] Ener RA, Meglathery SB, Styler M: Extravasation of systemic hemato-oncological therapies. Ann Oncol 15: 858–862, 2004.
[26] Jordan K, Grothe W, Schmoll HJ: Paravasation von Zytostatika: Prävention und Therapie. Dtsch Med Wochenschr 130: 33–37, 2005.

Further reading:

- Fenchel K, Karthaus M: Zytostatika-Paravasate – gibt es neue Empfehlungen zum therapeutischen Vorgehen? Wien Med Wochenschr 151: 44–46, 2001.
- Koppel RA, Boh EE: Cutaneous reactions to chemotherapeutic agents. Am J Med Sci 321: 327–335, 2001.
- Rauh J, Pluntke S, Müller C: Paravenöse Zytostatikainjektion: Prophylaxe und Sofortmaßnahmen im Notfall. MMW Fortschr Med 146: 682–686, 2004.
- Schrijvers DL: Extravasation: a dreaded complication of chemotherapy. Ann Oncol 14: iii26–iii30, 2003.

Revisions by Patrizia Fürst-Weger

Cisplatin

CONSENSUS

Type of damage: irritant
vesicant at a concentration ≥ 0.4 mg/ml

Recommended treatment:

General measures:

1. Stop injection/infusion immediately
2. Get extravasation kit
3. Put on (sterile) gloves
4. Replace infusion lead or syringe with 5 ml disposable syringe and aspirate slowly as much as possible of the extravasated drug; **Cave!** do not exert pressure on extravasation area
5. Remove i.v. access while aspirating
6. If blisters occur: aspirate with 1 ml syringe and s.c. cannula, use new equipment for every new attempt at aspiration
7. Elevate limb and immobilise
8. Start **substance specific measures**
9. Ensure adequate analgesia
10. Complete extravasation documentation sheet (mention extent of extravasation)
11. Inform and instruct the patient and relatives
12. Regular control (aftercare)
13. Always consult a (plastic) surgeon within 24 hours

Substance specific measures:

DMSO:

1. Apply DMSO (99%) every 8 hours (e.g. with a sterile gauze pad) without pressure
2. Allow to air-dry – **Cave!** do not cover
3. Continue for a minimum of 7 days

Immediately afterwards topical cooling:

1. Apply cold, dry pack immediately for at least 1 hour (for example, using a cold-hot pack)
2. Continue several times daily for 15 minutes each time

C

Cave! after extravasation:

1. No flushing of i.v. access
2. No moist compresses
3. No alcohol compresses
4. No occlusive dressings

Type of damage reported in literature:

Non-vesicant [15,17,19]

Weak irritant (not vesicant) [24]

Irritant [1,8,14,23] and/or weak vesicant in large amounts and high concentrations [20,26]

Exfoliant [13]

Low risk of necrosis [16,21]

Vesicant [2–4,12,18,22,23,27]

Symptoms and clinical course reported in literature:

Initial symptoms: Pain, swelling, inflammation (1 patient) [2]; erythema (1 patient) [3]

Delayed-onset symptoms: Pain and erythema (1 patient) [4]

- Blistering : 48 hours after extravasation at concentrations of 0.78 mg/ml [8] and at concentrations of 1 mg/ml (1 patient) [3] after several days
- Cellulitis and fibrosis 2 weeks after extravasation at a concentration of 0.42 mg/ml (1 patient) [1]
- Necroses within 2 weeks at concentrations of 0.75 mg/ml (1 patient) [2], at concentrations of 1 mg/ml (1 patient) [3] and at concentrations of 0.16 mg/ml (1 patient) [4]

Residual findings: After 10 weeks: residual fibrosis (1 patient) [1]

Measures reported in literature:

Successful treatment:

- 4 drops of DMSO (99%) per 10 cm^2 applied topically to an area twice the size of the affected area, repeat every 8 hours for 1 week or until symptoms have subsided; local cooling for 60 minutes, every 8 hours for 3 days (cold-hot pack) (37 patients) [6] or (26 patients) [7,12]
- Cold compresses for 24 hours (3 patients) [9]
- After extravasation in the context of combination chemotherapy with cisplatin, vinorelbine, and ifosfamide (extravasated substance not identified): intralesional injections of steroids (5 patients) [10]

Unsuccessful treatment:

- Warm compresses over 24 hours (1 patient) [1]
- No immediate treatment; after 14 days: antibiotics given; 1 week afterwards: a surgical intervention became necessary (1 patient) [2]
- After aspiration s.c. infiltration of corticosteroids, antibiotic treatment and local application of corticosteroids after development of necrosis (1 patient) [3]
- No immediate measures; after several days removal of necrotic tissue and application of hydrocolloid dressing; surgical intervention became necessary afterwards (1 patient) [4]
- Immediate treatment: ice packs hourly for 15 minutes over 24 hours; after 48 hours silver sulfadiazine cream and antibiotic treatment of the superinfection and mupirocin cream applied locally (1 patient) [8]

C

Outcome of treatment not reported:

- After extravasation in the context of combination chemotherapy with cisplatin and etoposide (extravasated substance not identified): no specific measure mentioned (1 patient) [11]

- After extravasation in the context of combination chemotherapy with cisplatin, etoposide, and vindesine (extravasated substance not identified): local glucocorticoids (1 patient) [11]

- Sodium thiosulfate (4%) in high concentrations of cisplatin [12]

- Infiltration of 1–3 ml sodium thiosulfate (3%), aspiration, 1500 IU hyaluronidase s.c., application of heat and compression [13]

- Topical glucocorticoids [14]

- Optional local infiltration of corticosteroids, warm to hot compresses for 1 hour [15]

- Sodium thiosulfate (4–8%) after extravasation of highly concentrated and/or large amounts of cisplatin solutions [12,19–21]; otherwise: 100 mg hydrocortisone s.c. and i.v., respectively, ice or cold pack 4 x daily for 15–20 minutes, topical hydrocortisone [18]

- If local symptoms develop, hydrocortisone (1%) or heparin to be applied topically combined with cold compresses (either once for 45 minutes or 20 minutes per day for 3 days) or warm compresses [22]

- After extravasation of at least 20 ml and a concentration of at least 0.5 mg/ml: sodium thiosulfate (4%) within 1 hour via i.v. access at the extravasation site or s.c., 2 ml for each mg of cisplatin; cold compresses every 6 hours for 15 minutes for 48–72 hours [23]

- Dry cold initially administered for 1 hour, followed by several applications daily for 15 minutes; DMSO (99%) every 8 hours for 8 days, maintain therapy free interval between cold and DMSO [27]

- No specific measures mentioned [11 (4 patients),16,17,24,26]

Particular remarks: Incidence of hypersensitivity reactions up to 20% [16,17,25] and radiation enhancement [28] have been described

The necrotic effect of diluted cisplatin solution (0.16 mg/ml) after extravasation is due to a recall phenomenon [4]

Corticosteroids: positive effect is questionable, because extravasations are only rarely accompanied by inflammatory processes (see chapter "Histopathological investigations")

DMSO and topical cooling: positive effects in preventing necroses have been reported [6,7]

Sodium thiosulfate inactivates cisplatin; systemic application in mice reduced the nephrotoxicity of cisplatin [5]; a positive effect regarding extravasation has not sufficiently been clinically proved [12] – disadvantage: invasive measure

Conclusion: Cisplatin is controversially classified in the literature; severe necroses have been reported after extravasations that were not treated at all [2,4] or inadequately [3]

As necroses have been documented only for concentrated solutions, cisplatin at a concentration ≥0.4 mg is classified as vesicant and in lower concentrations as irritant

Independently of the concentration of the cisplatin solution, the well-established and non-invasive measures DMSO and topical cooling are recommended

C

Original articles

[1] Lewis KP, Medina WD: Cellulitis and fibrosis due to cis-diamminedichloroplatinum (II) (platinol) infiltration. Cancer Treat Rep 64: 1162–1163, 1980.

[2] Leyden M, Sullivan J: Full-thickness skin necrosis due to inadvertent interstitial infusion of cisplatin. Cancer Treat Rep 67: 199, 1983.

[3] Algarra SM, Dy C, Bilbao I, et al: Cutaneous necrosis after intra-arterial treatment with cisplatin. Cancer Treat Rep 70: 687–688, 1986.

[4] Bairey O, Bishara J, Stahl B, et al: Severe tissue necrosis after cisplatin extravasation at low concentration: possible "immediate recall phenomenon". J Natl Cancer Inst 89: 1233–1234, 1997.

[5] Howell SB, Taetle R: Effect of sodium thiosulfate on cis-dichlorodiammineplatinum (II) toxicity and antitumor activity in L1210 leukemia. Cancer Treat Rep 64: 611–616, 1980.

[6] Bertelli G, Gozza A, Forno GB, et al: Topical dimethylsulfoxide for the prevention of soft tissue injury after extravasation of vesicant cytotoxic drugs: a prospective clinical study. J Clin Oncol 13: 2851–2855, 1995.

[7] Bertelli G, Dini D, Forno G, et al: Dimethylsulphoxide and cooling after extravasation of antitumour agents. Lancet 341: 1098–1099, 1993.

[8] Fields S, Koeller J, Topper RL, et al: Local soft tissue toxicity following cisplatin extravasation. J Natl Cancer Inst 82: 1649–1650, 1990.

[9] Langstein HN, Duman H, Seelig D, et al: Retrospective study of the management of chemotherapeutic extravasation injury. Ann Plast Surg 49: 369–374, 2002.

[10] Whang SW, Lee SH, Elias PM, et al: Intralesional steroids reduce inflammation from extravasated chemotherapeutic agents. Br J Dermatol 145: 680–682, 2001.

[11] Krämer I: Zehn Jahre Dokumentation von Zytostatika-Paravasat-Ereignissen: Auswertung von 175 Paravasate-Dokumentationen. Krankenhauspharmazie 23: 269–274, 2002.

Secondary literature

[12] Bertelli G: Prevention and management of extravasation of cytotoxic drugs. Drug Safety 12: 245–255, 1995.

[13] Stanley A: Managing complications of chemotherapy administration. In: Allwood M, Stanley A, Wright P (eds) The Cytotoxics Handbook. Radcliffe Medical Press, 4th edition: 119–193, 2002.

C

[14] Krämer I, Stützle M: Zytostatika-Paravasation – Wie ist vorzugehen? Krankenhauspharmazie 23: 261–268, 2002.
[15] Ignoffo RJ, Friedman MA: Therapy of local toxicities caused by extravasation of cancer chemotherapeutic drugs. Cancer Treat Rev 7: 17–27, 1980.
[16] Schneider G: Paravasate von Zytostatika. Diagnostik und Therapie. Aina S. Schneider Verlag, 6th edition: 1–17, 1999.
[17] Schneider SM, Distelhorst CW: Chemotherapy-induced emergencies. Semin Oncol 16: 572–578, 1989.
[18] Gain M, Melzer S, Meyer-Jürshof A, et al: Allgemeiner Teil: Behandlung von Paravasaten. In: Gain M, et al (eds) ADKA-Zytostatika-Handbuch, Pharmazeutisch-wissenschaftliche Monographien. Verlag Heiner Biller, vol 1, 2nd edition: A42–44, 1997.
[19] Gain M, Melzer S, Meyer-Jürshof A, et al: Cisplatin: Behandlung von Paravasaten. In: Gain M, et al (eds) ADKA-Zytostatika-Handbuch, Pharmazeutisch-wissenschaftliche Monographien. Verlag Heiner Biller, vol 1, 2nd edition: 61, 1997.
[20] Dorr RT: Pharmacologic management of vesicant chemotherapy extravasations. In: Dorr RT, Von Hoff DD (eds) Cancer Chemotherapy Handbook. Appleton & Lange, 2nd edition: 109–118, 1994.
[21] Dorr RT: Antidotes to vesicant chemotherapy extravasations. Blood Rev 4: 41–60, 1990.
[22] Cox K, Stuart-Harris R, Abdini G, et al: The management of cytotoxic-drug extravasation: guide-lines drawn up by a working party for the Clinical Oncological Society of Australia. Med J Aust 148: 185–189, 1988.
[23] Mullin S, Beckwith MC, Tyler LS: Prevention and management of antineoplastic extravasation injury. Hosp Pharm 35: 57–76, 2000.
[24] Barth J: Paravasate und deren Behandlung. In: Barth J (ed) Zytostatika-Herstellung in der Apotheke. Deutscher Apotheker Verlag, chapter VI-3: 1–9, 2000.
[25] Alley E, Green R, Schuchter L: Cutaneous toxicities of cancer therapy. Curr Opin Oncol 14: 212–216, 2002.
[26] Ener RA, Meglathery SB, Styler M: Extravasation of systemic hemato-oncological therapies. Ann Oncol 15: 858–862, 2004.
[27] Jordan K, Grothe W, Schmoll HJ: Paravasation von Zytostatika: Prävention und Therapie. Dtsch Med Wochenschr 130: 33–37, 2005.
[28] Koppel RA, Boh EE: Cutaneous reactions to chemotherapeutic agents. Am J Med Sci 321: 327–335, 2001.

C

Further reading:

- Albanell J, Baselga J: Systemic therapy emergencies. Semin Oncol 27: 347–361, 2000.
- Buchanan GR, Buchsbaum HJ, O'Banion K, et al: Extravasation of dactinomycin, vincristine, and cisplatin: studies in an animal model. Med Pediatr Oncol 13: 375–380, 1985.
- Dorr RT, Alberts DS, Soble M: Lack of experimental vesicant activity for the anticancer agents cisplatin, melphalan, and mitoxantrone. Cancer Chemother Pharmacol 16: 91–94, 1986.
- Fenchel K, Karthaus M: Zytostatika-Paravasate – gibt es neue Empfehlungen zum therapeutischen Vorgehen? Wien Med Wochenschr 151: 44–46, 2001.
- Kassner E: Evaluation and treatment of chemotherapy extravasation injuries. J Pediatr Oncol Nurs 17: 135–148, 2000.
- Khan MS, Holmes JD: Reducing the morbidity from extravasation injuries. Ann Plast Surg 48: 628–632, 2002.
- Rauh J, Pluntke S, Müller C: Paravenöse Zytostatikainjektion: Prophylaxe und Sofortmaßnahmen im Notfall. MMW Fortschr Med 146: 682–686, 2004.
- Schrijvers DL: Extravasation: a dreaded complication of chemotherapy. Ann Oncol 14: iii26–iii30, 2003.

Revisions by Patrizia Fürst-Weger

Cladribine

CONSENSUS

Type of damage: non-vesicant

Recommended treatment:

General measures:

1. Stop injection/infusion immediately
2. Get extravasation kit
3. Put on (sterile) gloves
4. Replace infusion lead or syringe with 5 ml disposable syringe and aspirate slowly as much as possible of the extravasated drug; **Cave!** do not exert pressure on extravasation area
5. Remove i.v. access while aspirating
6. Elevate limb and immobilise
7. Complete extravasation documentation sheet (mention extent of extravasation)
8. Inform and instruct the patient and relatives
9. Regular control (aftercare)

Substance specific measures: none

Cave! after extravasation:

1. No flushing of i.v. access
2. No moist compresses
3. No alcohol compresses
4. No occlusive dressings

C

Type of damage reported in literature:

Non-vesicant [3–5,9]

No tissue toxic potential [10]

Weak irritant (not vesicant) [8]

Irritant [7]

Vesicant [6]

Symptoms and clinical course reported in literature:

Single case report: after extravasation of ca. 5–10 ml infusion solution (0.0116 mg/ml): slightly erythematous indurated area around the venous access point, no pain, only a small induration 16 hours later, almost completely gone after 3 days (1 patient) [2]

Measures reported in literature:

Successful treatment:
- No measure (1 patient) [2]

Unsuccessful treatment:
- No data available

Outcome of treatment not reported:
- 1500 IU hyaluronidase s.c., application of heat and compression [3]
- Ice pack [11] or cooling [4,6] 4 × daily for 20 minutes for 3–4 days [10]
- No specific measures mentioned [5,7–9]

Particular remarks:

Results of literature search: no animal experiments or clinical studies regarding extravasation have been published

No signs of toxicity around the injection site after s.c. administration [1]

One case of tissue reaction after extravasation has been described; no lasting damage even without specific measures [2]

Conclusion:

Although cladribine is classified as irritant/vesicant in some of the literature, no clinical case of lasting tissue damage after extravasation has been documented; since cladribine can also be administered s.c., a tissue-damaging effect is unlikely; the substance is therefore classified as non-vesicant

No substance specific measures are required

Original articles

[1] Juliusson G, Heldal D, Hippe E, et al: Subcutaneous injections of 2-chlorodeoxyadenosine for symptomatic hairy cell leukemia. J Clin Oncol 13: 989–995, 1995.
[2] Mateu-de Antonio J, Acuna-Reina L, Pans JC, et al: Lack of toxicity in a cladribine extravasation. Ann Pharmacother 33: 873, 1999.

Secondary literature

[3] Stanley A: Managing complications of chemotherapy administration. In: Allwood M, Stanley A, Wright P (eds) The Cytotoxics Handbook. Radcliffe Medical Press, 4th edition: 119–193, 2002.
[4] van Gemmern R: Gewebstoxizität und Paravasatbehandlung neuer Zytostatika. Krankenhauspharmazie 17: 471–473, 1996.
[5] Gain M, Melzer S, Meyer-Jürshof A, et al: Cladribin: Behandlung bei Paravasaten. In: Gain M, et al (eds) ADKA-Zytostatika-Handbuch, Pharmazeutisch-wissenschaftliche Monographien. Verlag Heiner Biller, vol 7: 39, 2003.
[6] Berdel WE, Schmoll HJ, Büchele T, et al: Prävention und Therapie von Paravasaten/Extravasaten. In: Schmoll HJ, Höffken K, Possinger K (eds) Kompendium Internistische Onkologie. Standards in Diagnostik und Therapie. Springer, Vol 1, 3rd edition: 1689–1701, 1999.
[7] Mullin S, Beckwith MC, Tyler LS: Prevention and management of antineoplastic extravasation injury. Hosp Pharm 35: 57–76, 2000.
[8] Barth J: Paravasate und deren Behandlung. In: Barth J (ed) Zytostatika-Herstellung in der Apotheke. Deutscher Apotheker Verlag, chapter vi-3: 1–9, 2000.
[9] Jordan K, Grothe W, Schmoll HJ: Paravasation von Zytostatika: Prävention und Therapie. Dtsch Med Wochenschr 130: 33–37, 2005.
[10] Krämer I, Stützle M: Zytostatika-Paravasation – Wie ist vorzugehen? Krankenhauspharmazie 23: 261–268, 2002.
[11] Summary of product characteristics Leustatin® (Germany), Janssen-Cilag, February 2004.

C

Further reading:

- Fenchel K, Karthaus M: Zytostatika-Paravasate – gibt es neue Empfehlungen zum therapeutischen Vorgehen? Wien Med Wochenschr 151: 44–46, 2001.
- Rauh J, Pluntke S, Müller C: Paravenöse Zytostatikainjektion: Prophylaxe und Sofortmaßnahmen im Notfall. MMW Fortschr Med 146: 682–686, 2004.

Revisions by Sabine Wassertheurer

Cyclophosphamide

CONSENSUS

Type of damage: non-vesicant

Recommended treatment:

General measures:

1. Stop injection/infusion immediately
2. Get extravasation kit
3. Put on (sterile) gloves
4. Replace infusion lead or syringe with 5 ml disposable syringe and aspirate slowly as much as possible of the extravasated drug; **Cave!** do not exert pressure on extravasation area
5. Remove i.v. access while aspirating
6. Elevate limb and immobilise
7. Complete extravasation documentation sheet (mention extent of extravasation)
8. Inform and instruct the patient and relatives
9. Regular control (aftercare)

Substance specific measures: none

Cave! after extravasation:

1. No flushing of i.v. access
2. No moist compresses
3. No alcohol compresses
4. No occlusive dressings

Type of damage reported in literature:

Non-vesicant [4–10,14,17]

Weak irritant (not vesicant) [13]

Irritant [12,16]

Symptoms and clinical course reported in literature:

No data available

Measures reported in literature:

Successful treatment:
- No data available

Unsuccessful treatment:
- No data available

Outcome of treatment not reported:
- After extravasation in the context of combination chemotherapy with cyclophosphamide and carboplatin (extravasated substance not identified): no specific measures mentioned (1 patient) [3]

- After extravasation in the context of combination chemotherapy with cyclophosphamide and epirubicin (extravasated substance not identified): no specific measures mentioned (1 patient); cooling, local glucocorticoids (1 patient); DMSO, cooling, glucocorticoids i.d., sodium hydrogen carbonate (1 patient); DMSO, glucocorticoids i.d., hyaluronidase (1 patient) [3]

- After extravasation in the context of combination chemotherapy with cyclophosphamide and vincristine (extravasated substance not identified): local glucocorticoids (1 patient) [3]

- Flushing with NaCl 0.9% [4]

- 1500 IU hyaluronidase s.c., application of heat and compression [5]

- Optional local infiltration of corticosteroids, warm to hot compresses for 1 hour [6]
- 100 mg hydrocortisone s.c and i.v., respectively, ice or cold pack 4 x daily for 15–20 minutes, topical hydrocortisone [8,9]
- If local symptoms develop, hydrocortisone (1%) or heparin to be applied topically [12]
- Topical cooling 4 x daily for 20 minutes over 3–4 days [14]
- No specific measures mentioned [3 (8 patients), 7,10,13,16,17]

Particular remarks: Results of literature search: no clinical studies regarding extravasation have been published

Animal experiments: no local reactions after s.c. application of cyclophosphamide; tissue damage after i.d. administration of high doses [2]

Phlebitis at injection site [11] is not associated with extravasation

Cyclophosphamide is an atoxic prodrug and is mostly activated in the liver [1,4,11,15]; cyclophosphamide can also be injected i.m. [15], no problems after extravasation are therefore to be expected

Conclusion: Although cyclophosphamide is classified as irritant in some of the literature, no clinical case of irritation of tissue after extravasation has been documented; the substance is therefore classified as non-vesicant

No substance specific measures are required

C

Original articles

[1] Brock N, Hilgard P, Peukert M, et al: Basis and new developments in the field of oxazaphosphorines. Cancer Invest 6: 513–532, 1988.
[2] Barr RD, Benton SG, Belbeck LW: Soft-tissue necrosis induced by extravasated cancer chemotherapeutic agents. J Natl Cancer Inst 66: 1129–1136, 1981.
[3] Krämer I: Zehn Jahre Dokumentation von Zytostatika-Paravasat-Ereignissen: Auswertung von 175 Paravasate-Dokumentationen. Krankenhauspharmazie 23: 269–274, 2002.

Secondary literature

[4] Summary of product characteristics Endoxan® (Germany), Baxter, January 2002.
[5] Stanley A: Managing complications of chemotherapy administration. In: Allwood M, Stanley A, Wright P (eds) The Cytotoxics Handbook. Radcliffe Medical Press, 4th edition: 119–193, 2002.
[6] Ignoffo RJ, Friedman MA: Therapy of local toxicities caused by extravasation of cancer chemotherapeutic drugs. Cancer Treat Rev 7: 17–27, 1980.
[7] Dorr RT: Pharmacologic management of vesicant chemotherapy extravasations. In: Dorr RT, Von Hoff DD (eds) Cancer Chemotherapy Handbook. Appleton & Lange, 2nd edition: 109–118, 1994.
[8] Donislawski S, Gain M, Meyer-Jürshof A, et al: Cyclophosphamid: Behandlung von Paravasaten. In: Donislawski S, et al (eds) ADKA-Zytostatika-Handbuch, Pharmazeutisch-wissenschaftliche Monographien. Verlag Heiner Biller, vol 2: 39, 1994.
[9] Gain M, Melzer S, Meyer-Jürshof A, et al: Allgemeiner Teil: Behandlung von Paravasaten. In: Gain M, et al (eds) ADKA-Zytostatika-Handbuch, Pharmazeutisch-wissenschaftliche Monographien. Verlag Heiner Biller, vol 1, 2nd edition: A42–44, 1997.
[10] Schneider SM, Distelhorst CW: Chemotherapy-induced emergencies. Semin Oncol 16: 572–578, 1989.
[11] Dorr RT, Von Hoff DD: Drug monographs: cyclophosphamide. In: Dorr RT, Von Hoff DD (eds) Cancer Chemotherapy Handbook. Appleton & Lange, 2nd edition: 319–332, 1994.
[12] Cox K, Stuart-Harris R, Abdini G, et al: The management of cytotoxic-drug extravasation: guide-lines drawn up by a working party for the Clinical Oncological Society of Australia. Med J Aust 148: 185–189, 1988.
[13] Barth J: Paravasate und deren Behandlung. In: Barth J (ed) Zytostatika-Herstellung in der Apotheke. Deutscher Apotheker Verlag, chapter VI-3: 1–9, 2000.

[14] Krämer I, Stützle M: Zytostatika-Paravasation – Wie ist vorzugehen? Krankenhauspharmazie 23: 261–268, 2002.
[15] Summary of product characteristics Endoxan "Baxter" (Austria), Baxter, January 2002.
[16] Ener RA, Meglathery SB, Styler M: Extravasation of systemic hemato-oncological therapies. Ann Oncol 15: 858–862, 2004.
[17] Jordan K, Grothe W, Schmoll HJ: Paravasation von Zytostatika: Prävention und Therapie. Dtsch Med Wochenschr 130: 33–37, 2005.

Further reading:

- Fenchel K, Karthaus M: Zytostatika-Paravasate – gibt es neue Empfehlungen zum therapeutischen Vorgehen? Wien Med Wochenschr 151: 44–46, 2001.
- Otto J, Goebell PJ, Otto T: Urologischer Notfall in der Onkologie. Der Onkologe 10: 351–357, 2004.
- Rauh J, Pluntke S, Müller C: Paravenöse Zytostatikainjektion: Prophylaxe und Sofortmaßnahmen im Notfall. MMW Fortschr Med 146: 682–686, 2004.
- Schrijvers DL: Extravasation: a dreaded complication of chemotherapy. Ann Oncol 14: iii26–iii30, 2003.

Revisions by Patrizia Fürst-Weger

Cytarabine

CONSENSUS

Type of damage: non-vesicant

Recommended treatment:

General measures:

1. Stop injection/infusion immediately
2. Get extravasation kit
3. Put on (sterile) gloves
4. Replace infusion lead or syringe with 5 ml disposable syringe and aspirate slowly as much as possible of the extravasated drug; **Cave!** do not exert pressure on extravasation area
5. Remove i.v. access while aspirating
6. Elevate limb and immobilise
7. Complete extravasation documentation sheet (mention extent of extravasation)
8. Inform and instruct the patient and relatives
9. Regular control (aftercare)

Substance specific measures: none

Cave! after extravasation:

1. No flushing of i.v. access
2. No moist compresses
3. No alcohol compresses
4. No occlusive dressings

Type of damage reported in literature:

Non-vesicant [3–8,10,12,16]

No tissue toxic potential [17]

Weak irritant (not vesicant) [15]

Irritant [11]

No risk of necrosis [9]

Symptoms and clinical course reported in literature:

No data available

Measures reported in literature:

Successful treatment:
- No data available

Unsuccessful treatment:
- No data available

Outcome of treatment not reported:
- Optional local infiltration of corticosteroids, warm to hot compresses for 1 hour [3]
- If local symptoms develop, hydrocortisone (1%) or heparin to be applied topically [4]
- 1500 IU hyaluronidase s.c., application of heat and compression [6]
- 100 mg hydrocortisone s.c. and i.v., respectively, ice or cold pack 4 × daily for 15–20 minutes, topical hydrocortisone [8,12]
- Topical cooling 4 × daily for 20 minutes over 3–4 days [17]
- No specific measures mentioned [5, 9–11,15,16]

Particular remarks:

Results of literature search: no clinical studies regarding extravasation have been published

C

Animal experiments: no local reactions after s.c. and i.d. administration of cytarabine [2]

No local discomfort and skin reactions after s.c. administration [1]

Hypersensitivity reactions [18,19] and recall phenomenon after radiotherapy [18] are not associated with the extravasation

Conclusion: Although cytarabine is classified as irritant in some of the literature, no clinical case of irritation of tissue after extravasation has been documented; since cytarabine can also be administered i.m. [14] and s.c. [13], a tissue-damaging effect is unlikely; the substance is therefore classified as non-vesicant

No substance specific measures are required

Original articles

[1] Slevin ML, Piall EM, Aherne GW, et al: Subcutaneous infusion of cytosine arabinoside: a practical alternative to intravenous infusion. Cancer Chemother Pharmacol 10: 112–114, 1983.

[2] Barr RD, Benton SG, Belbeck LW: Soft-tissue necrosis induced by extravasated cancer chemotherapeutic agents. J Natl Cancer Inst 66: 1129–1136, 1981.

Secondary literature

[3] Ignoffo RJ, Friedman MA: Therapy of local toxicities caused by extravasation of cancer chemotherapeutic drugs. Cancer Treat Rev 7: 17–27, 1980.

[4] Cox K, Stuart-Harris R, Abdini G, et al: The management of cytotoxic-drug extravasation: guidelines drawn up by a working party for the Clinical Oncological Society of Australia. Med J Aust 148: 185–189, 1988.

[5] Dorr RT: Pharmacologic management of vesicant chemotherapy extravasations. In: Dorr RT, Von Hoff DD (eds) Cancer Chemotherapy Handbook. Appleton & Lange, 2nd edition: 109–118, 1994.

[6] Stanley A: Managing complications of chemotherapy administration. In: Allwood M, Stanley A, Wright P (eds) The Cytotoxics Handbook. Radcliffe Medical Press, 4th edition: 119–193, 2002.
[7] Pharmacia & Upjohn, personal communication, November 1998.
[8] Gain M, Melzer S, Meyer-Jürshof A, et al: Cytarabin: Behandlung von Paravasaten. In: Gain M, et al (eds) ADKA-Zytostatika-Handbuch, Pharmazeutisch-wissenschaftliche Monographien. Verlag Heiner Biller, vol 3: 42, 1998.
[9] Schneider G: Paravasate von Zytostatika. Diagnostik und Therapie. Aina S. Schneider Verlag, 6th edition: 1–17, 1999.
[10] Schneider SM, Distelhorst CW: Chemotherapy-induced emergencies. Semin Oncol 16: 572–578, 1989.
[11] Mullin S, Beckwith MC, Tyler LS: Prevention and management of antineoplastic extravasation injury. Hosp Pharm 35: 57–76, 2000.
[12] Gain M, Melzer S, Meyer-Jürshof A, et al: Allgemeiner Teil: Behandlung von Paravasaten. In: Gain M, et al (eds) ADKA-Zytostatika-Handbuch, Pharmazeutisch-wissenschaftliche Monographien. Verlag Heiner Biller, vol 1, 2nd edition: A42–44, 1997.
[13] Summary of product characteristics Alexan® (Austria), Ebewe, June 2003.
[14] Dorr RT, Von Hoff DD: Drug monographs: cytarabine. In: Dorr RT, Von Hoff DD (eds) Cancer Chemotherapy Handbook. Appleton & Lange, 2nd edition: 332–340, 1994.
[15] Barth J: Paravasate und deren Behandlung. In: Barth J (ed) Zytostatika-Herstellung in der Apotheke. Deutscher Apotheker Verlag, chapter VI-3: 1–9, 2000.
[16] Jordan K, Grothe W, Schmoll HJ: Paravasation von Zytostatika: Prävention und Therapie. Dtsch Med Wochenschr 130: 33–37, 2005.
[17] Krämer I, Stützle M: Zytostatika-Paravasation – Wie ist vorzugehen? Krankenhauspharmazie 23: 261–268, 2002.
[18] Koppel RA, Boh EE: Cutaneous reactions to chemotherapeutic agents. Am J Med Sci 321: 327–335, 2001.
[19] Alley E, Green R, Schuchter L: Cutaneous toxicities of cancer therapy. Curr Opin Oncol 14: 212–216, 2002.

Further reading:

- Fenchel K, Karthaus M: Zytostatika-Paravasate – gibt es neue Empfehlungen zum therapeutischen Vorgehen? Wien Med Wochenschr 151: 44–46, 2001.
- Rauh J, Pluntke S, Müller C: Paravenöse Zytostatikainjektion: Prophylaxe und Sofortmaßnahmen im Notfall. MMW Fortschr Med 146: 682–686, 2004.
- Schrijvers DL: Extravasation: a dreaded complication of chemotherapy. Ann Oncol 14: iii26–iii30, 2003.

Revisions by Sabine Wassertheurer

Dacarbazine

CONSENSUS

D

Type of damage: irritant

Recommended treatment:

General measures:

1. Stop injection/infusion immediately
2. Get extravasation kit
3. Put on (sterile) gloves
4. Replace infusion lead or syringe with 5 ml disposable syringe and aspirate slowly as much as possible of the extravasated drug; Cave! do not exert pressure on extravasation area
5. Remove i.v. access while aspirating
6. If blisters occur: aspirate with 1 ml syringe and s.c. cannula, use new equipment for every new attempt at aspiration
7. Elevate limb and immobilise
8. Complete extravasation documentation sheet (mention extent of extravasation)
9. Inform and instruct the patient and relatives
10. Regular control (aftercare)

Substance specific measures: none

Cave! protect affected area from direct sunlight

Cave! after extravasation:

1. No flushing of i.v. access
2. No moist compresses
3. No alcohol compresses
4. No occlusive dressings

Type of damage reported in literature:

No risk of necrosis [8,15]

Irritant [1,7,11,12,14,19,22,23,27] and/or weak vesicant in large amounts and high concentrations [17]

Low vesicant potential [26]

Vesicant [9,13,16,18]

D

Symptoms and clinical course reported in literature:

Initial symptoms: No data available

Delayed-onset symptoms: Pain and necroses [13] according to the summary of product characteristics – no further information available

Residual findings: No data available

Individual case report: No local reactions (1 patient) [2]

Measures reported in literature:

Successful treatment:
- Animal experiments: Sodium thiosulfate (8%) after i.d. administration of dacarbazine [1,15]

Unsuccessful treatment:
- Animal experiments: L-cysteine, DMSO, hyaluronidase, hydrocortisone, NaCl 0.9%, sodium thiosulfate (4%), application of heat and cooling increase ulceration [1,15]

Outcome of treatment not reported:
- After extravasation in the context of combination chemotherapy with dacarbazine and doxorubicin (extravasated substance not identified): DMSO, glucocorticoids i.d., sodium hydrogen carbonate (1 patient) [6]

- Topical cooling 4 × daily for 20 minutes over 3–4 days [7]

D

- Sodium thiosulfate (4%) in high concentrations of dacarbazine [10,16], protection of extravasation area from sunlight [10,15]

- Optional local infiltration with corticosteroids, warm to hot compresses for 1 hour [11]

- If local symptoms develop, hydrocortisone (1%) or heparin to be applied topically [12]

- On the first day DMSO every 2 hours, hydrocortisone (1%) applied topically, cold compresses for 30 minutes; subsequently for 14 days alternating DMSO or hydrocortisone at 3 hourly intervals applied topically [18]

- No specific measures mentioned [6 (1 patient),8,14,17,19,22,23,26,27]

Particular remarks:

Results of literature search: no clinical studies regarding extravasation have been published

Necroses are unlikely to develop as dacarbazine is a cytotoxically ineffective prodrug [13]

Effect of light:
- Photosensitivity reaction after administration of dacarbazine [2,3,13,20,21,24,25]

- Animal experiments: exposure to light after i.d. administration of dacarbazine resulted in increased skin toxicity [1,16]

- Phlebitis [15,17], local irritations [17], pain along the vein [2,4], burning [2,3] and erythema [3] of areas exposed to sunlight (head, hands) are not associated with extravasation; these symptoms are due to the degradation products of dacarbazine under the influence of light [3,4]

Protection from light: infusion of dacarbazine [2,4,5] (during production and administration) and patient (for several days after infusion) should be protected from intense light (sunlight) [1,16]

Sodium thiosulfate: positive effect is clinically not sufficiently proved [16]; disadvantage: invasive measure

Conclusion:

Although dacarbazine is classified as irritant/vesicant in the literature, no clinical case of tissue damage after extravasation has been documented; the classification as irritant is due to the effect of the drug's degradation products under the influence of intense light

The symptoms mentioned in the secondary literature, such as necroses, could not be verified in clinical case reports

Positive results of substance specific measures have not been described so far; until further data become available no substance specific measures can be recommended

The affected area must be protected from exposure to direct sunlight

Original articles

[1] Dorr RT, Alberts DS, Einspahr J, et al: Experimental dacarbazine antitumor activity and skin toxicity in relation to light exposure and pharmacologic antidotes. Cancer Treat Rep 71: 267–272, 1987.
[2] Buesa JM, Gracia M, Valle M, et al: Phase I trial of intermittent high-dose dacarbazine. Cancer Treat Rep 68: 499–504, 1984.
[3] Beck TM, Hart NE, Smith CE: Photosensitivity reaction following DTIC administration: report of two cases. Cancer Treat Rep 64: 725–726, 1980.
[4] Baird GM, Willoughby ML: Photodegradation of dacarbazine. The Lancet 2: 681, 1978.
[5] Koriech O, Shukla V: Reduced toxicity of DTIC with administration in the dark. Proc AACR-ASCO 21: 168, 1980.
[6] Krämer I: Zehn Jahre Dokumentation von Zytostatika-Paravasat-Ereignissen: Auswertung von 175 Paravasate-Dokumentationen. Krankenhauspharmazie 23: 269–274, 2002.

Secondary literature

[7] Krämer I, Stützle M: Zytostatika-Paravasation – Wie ist vorzugehen? Krankenhauspharmazie 23: 261–268, 2002.
[8] Schneider G: Paravasate von Zytostatika. Diagnostik und Therapie. Aina S. Schneider Verlag, 6th edition: 1–17, 1999.

D

[9] Gain M, Melzer S, Meyer-Jürshof A, et al: Allgemeiner Teil: Behandlung von Paravasaten. In: Gain M, et al (eds) ADKA-Zytostatika-Handbuch, Pharmazeutisch-wissenschaftliche Monographien. Verlag Heiner Biller, vol 1, 2nd edition: A42–44, 1997.
[10] Gain M, Melzer S, Meyer-Jürshof A, et al: Dacarbazin: Behandlung von Paravasaten. In: Gain M, et al (eds) ADKA-Zytostatika-Handbuch, Pharmazeutisch-wissenschaftliche Monographien. Verlag Heiner Biller, vol 1, 2nd edition: 30–31, 1997.
[11] Ignoffo RJ, Friedman MA: Therapy of local toxicities caused by extravasation of cancer chemotherapeutic drugs. Cancer Treat Rev 7: 17–27, 1980.
[12] Cox K, Stuart-Harris R, Abdini G, et al: The management of cytotoxic-drug extravasation: guide-lines drawn up by a working party for the Clinical Oncological Society of Australia. Med J Aust 148: 185–189, 1988.
[13] Summary of product characteristics Dacarbazine medac (Austria), medac, May 2001.
[14] Mullin S, Beckwith MC, Tyler LS: Prevention and management of antineoplastic extravasation injury. Hosp Pharm 35: 57–76, 2000.
[15] Dorr RT: Antidotes to vesicant chemotherapy extravasations. Blood Rev 4: 41–60, 1990.
[16] Bertelli G: Prevention and management of extravasation of cytotoxic drugs. Drug Safety 12: 245–255, 1995.
[17] Dorr RT: Pharmacologic management of vesicant chemotherapy extravasations. In: Dorr RT, Von Hoff DD (eds) Cancer Chemotherapy Handbook. Appleton & Lange, 2nd edition: 109–118, 1994.
[18] Stanley A: Managing complications of chemotherapy administration. In: Allwood M, Stanley A, Wright P (eds) The Cytotoxics Handbook. Radcliffe Medical Press, 4th edition: 119–193, 2002.
[19] Holmes BC: Administration of cancer chemotherapy agents. In: Dorr RT, Von Hoff DD (eds) Cancer Chemotherapy Handbook. Appleton & Lange, 2nd edition: 57–94, 1994.
[20] Dorr RT, Von Hoff DD: Drug monographs: dacarbazine. In: Dorr RT, Von Hoff DD (eds) Cancer Chemotherapy Handbook. Appleton & Lange, 2nd edition: 343–349, 1994.
[21] Material safety data sheet of the European Union, Version 94/11, Medac.
[22] Schneider SM, Distelhorst CW: Chemotherapy-induced emergencies. Semin Oncol 16: 572–578, 1989.
[23] Barth J: Paravasate und deren Behandlung. In: Barth J (ed) Zytostatika-Herstellung in der Apotheke. Deutscher Apotheker Verlag, chapter VI-3: 1–9, 2000.
[24] Koppel RA, Boh EE: Cutaneous reactions to chemotherapeutic agents. Am J Med Sci 321: 327–335, 2001.

[25] Alley E, Green R, Schuchter L: Cutaneous toxicities of cancer therapy. Curr Opin Oncol 14: 212–216, 2002.
[26] Ener RA, Meglathery SB, Styler M: Extravasation of systemic hemato-oncological therapies. Ann Oncol 15: 858–862, 2004.
[27] Jordan K, Grothe W, Schmoll HJ: Paravasation von Zytostatika: Prävention und Therapie. Dtsch Med Wochenschr 130: 33–37, 2005.

Further reading:

- Barr RD, Benton SG, Belbeck LW: Soft-tissue necrosis induced by extravasated cancer chemotherapeutic agents. J Natl Cancer Inst 66: 1129–1136, 1981.
- Fenchel K, Karthaus M: Zytostatika-Paravasate – gibt es neue Empfehlungen zum therapeutischen Vorgehen? Wien Med Wochenschr 151: 44–46, 2001.
- Khan MS, Holmes JD: Reducing the morbidity from extravasation injuries. Ann Plast Surg 48: 628–632, 2002.
- Rauh J, Pluntke S, Müller C: Paravenöse Zytostatikainjektion: Prophylaxe und Sofortmaßnahmen im Notfall. MMW Fortschr Med 146: 682–686, 2004.
- Schrijvers DL: Extravasation: a dreaded complication of chemotherapy. Ann Oncol 14: iii26–iii30, 2003.

Revisions by Patrizia Fürst-Weger

Dactinomycin

CONSENSUS

Type of damage: vesicant

Recommended treatment:

General measures:

1. Stop injection/infusion immediately
2. Get extravasation kit
3. Put on (sterile) gloves
4. Replace infusion lead or syringe with 5 ml disposable syringe and aspirate slowly as much as possible of the extravasated drug; **Cave!** do not exert pressure on extravasation area
5. Remove i.v. access while aspirating
6. If blisters occur: aspirate with 1 ml syringe and s.c. cannula, use new equipment for every new attempt at aspiration
7. Elevate limb and immobilise
8. Start **substance specific measures**
9. Ensure adequate analgesia
10. Complete extravasation documentation sheet (mention extent of extravasation)
11. Inform and instruct the patient and relatives
12. Regular control (aftercare)
13. Always consult a (plastic) surgeon within 24 hours

Substance specific measures:

DMSO:

1. Apply DMSO (99%) every 8 hours (e.g. with a sterile gauze pad) without pressure
2. Allow to air-dry – **Cave!** do not cover
3. Continue for a minimum of 7 days

Immediately afterwards topical cooling:

1. Apply cold, dry pack immediately for at least 1 hour (for example, using a cold-hot pack)
2. Continue several times daily for 15 minutes each time

Cave! after extravasation:

1. No flushing of i.v. access
2. No moist compresses
3. No alcohol compresses
4. No occlusive dressings

Type of damage reported in literature: Vesicant [1,2,4–19]

Symptoms and clinical course reported in literature:

Initial symptoms: Burning or stabbing sensation [16]

Delayed-onset symptoms: Deep, severe ulceration in several patients [1]

Residual findings: No data available

Measures reported in literature:

Successful treatment:
- Topical cooling (ice) 4 × daily for 15 minutes over 3 days [2]

- Animal experiments: local cooling [3]

Unsuccessful treatment:
- Animal experiments: application of heat, i.d. administration of ascorbic acid, sodium thiosulfate, NaCl 0.9%, steroids, ß-adrenergic drugs [3]

Outcome of treatment not reported:
- Infiltration of 4 ml sodium thiosulfate (4%) or 1 ml ascorbic acid (5%), optional local infiltration of corticosteroids, warm compresses for 1 hour [4]

- Ice pack for 1–3 days, 4 ml sodium thiosulfate (4%) s.c. [5]

- Immediate topical cooling for 20 minutes, then 4 × daily for 20 minutes over 3–4 days [6]

D

- On the first day DMSO every 2 hours, hydrocortisone (1%) applied topically, cold compresses for 30 minutes; subsequently alternate between DMSO and hydrocortisone at 3 hourly intervals over 7–10 days [8]
- Immediate topical cooling for 24 hours alternating with 1.5 ml topical DMSO (50%) every 6 hours; DMSO over 14 days [13]
- Intermittent application of ice over 3 days [16]
- Application of dry cold for 1 hour initially, followed by several times daily for 15 minutes; DMSO (99%) every 8 hours over 8 days; maintain therapy free interval between applying cold and DMSO [17]
- Immediate local cooling [18]
- No specific measures mentioned [5,7,9,11,12,14,15]

Particular remarks: Increased radiosensitivity and recall phenomenon after radiotherapy [20,21]

Cooling: a positive effect in preventing necrosis has been reported [2], also proved in animal experiments [3]

Conclusion: Dactinomycin is classified exclusively as vesicant in the literature

Positive results using DMSO and topical cooling after extravasation with other DNA-intercalating agents are reported; therefore these non-invasive interventions are recommended

Original articles

[1] Moore GE, DiPaolo JA, Kondo T: The chemotherapeutic effects and complications of actinomycin D in patients with advanced cancer. Cancer 11: 1204–1214, 1958.

[2] Larson DL: What is the appropriate management of tissue extravasation by antitumor agents? Plast Reconstr Surg 75: 397–402, 1985.
[3] Buchanan GR, Buchsbaum HJ, O'Banion K, et al: Extravasation of dactinomycin, vincristine, and cisplatin: studies in an animal model. Med Pediatr Oncol 13: 375–380, 1985.

D

Secondary literature

[4] Ignoffo RJ, Friedman MA: Therapy of local toxicities caused by extravasation of cancer chemotherapeutic drugs. Cancer Treat Rev 7: 17–27, 1980.
[5] Schneider G: Paravasate von Zytostatika. Diagnostik und Therapie. Aina S. Schneider Verlag, 6th edition: 1–17, 1999.
[6] Krämer J, Stützle M: Zytostatika-Paravasation – Wie ist vorzugehen? Krankenhauspharmazie 23: 261–268, 2002.
[7] Dorr RT: Pharmacologic management of vesicant chemotherapy extravasations. In: Dorr RT, Von Hoff DD (eds) Cancer Chemotherapy Handbook. Appleton & Lange, 2nd edition: 109–118, 1994.
[8] Stanley A: Managing complications of chemotherapy administration. In: Allwood M, Stanley A, Wright P (eds) The Cytotoxics Handbook. Radcliffe Medical Press, 4th edition: 119–193, 2002.
[9] Gain M, Melzer S, Meyer-Jürshof A, et al: Allgemeiner Teil: Behandlung von Paravasaten. In: Gain M, et al (eds) ADKA-Zytostatika-Handbuch, Pharmazeutisch-wissenschaftliche Monographien. Verlag Heiner Biller, vol 1, 2nd edition: A42–44, 1997.
[10] Bertelli G: Prevention and management of extravasation of cytotoxic drugs. Drug Safety 12: 245–255, 1995.
[11] Frei E: The clinical use of actinomycin. Cancer Chemother Rep 58: 49–54, 1974.
[12] Mullin S, Beckwith MC, Tyler LS: Prevention and management of antineoplastic extravasation injury. Hosp Pharm 35: 57–76, 2000.
[13] Dorr RT: Antidotes to vesicant chemotherapy extravasations. Blood Rev 4: 41–60, 1990.
[14] Schneider SM, Distelhorst CW: Chemotherapy-induced emergencies. Semin Oncol 16: 572–578, 1989.
[15] Barth J: Paravasate und deren Behandlung. In: Barth J (ed) Zytostatika-Herstellung in der Apotheke. Deutscher Apotheker Verlag, chapter. VI-3: 1–9, 2000.
[16] Summary of product characteristics Lyovac-Cosmegen® (Germany), MSD Sharp & Dohme, April 2003.

[17] Jordan K, Grothe W, Schmoll HJ: Paravasation von Zytostatika: Prävention und Therapie. Dtsch Med Wochenschr 130: 33–37, 2005.
[18] Fenchel K, Karthaus M: Zytostatika-Paravasate – gibt es neue Empfehlungen zum therapeutischen Vorgehen? Wien Med Wochenschr 151: 44–46, 2001.
[19] Ener RA, Meglathery SB, Styler M: Extravasation of systemic hemato-oncological therapies. Ann Oncol 15: 858–862, 2004.
[20] Koppel RA, Boh EE: Cutaneous reactions to chemotherapeutic agents. Am J Med Sci 321: 327–335, 2001.
[21] Alley E, Green R, Schuchter L: Cutaneous toxicities of cancer therapy. Curr Opin Oncol 14: 212–216, 2002.

Further reading:

- Albanell J, Baselga J: Systemic therapy emergencies. Semin Oncol 27: 347–361, 2000.
- Krämer I: Onkologische Pharmazie. In: Jaehde U, Radziwill R, Mühlebach S, et al (eds) Lehrbuch der Klinischen Pharmazie. Wissenschaftliche Verlagsgesellschaft mbH, 2nd edition: 307–336, 2003.
- Kurul S, Saip P, Aydin T: Totally implantable venous-access ports: local problems and extravasation injury. Lancet Oncol 3: 684–692, 2002.
- Loth TS, Eversmann WW: Treatment methods for extravasations of chemotherapeutic agents: a comparative study. J Hand Surg 11A: 388–396, 1986.
- Otto J, Goebell PJ, Otto T: Urologischer Notfall in der Onkologie. Der Onkologe 10: 351–357, 2004.
- Rauh J, Pluntke S, Müller C: Paravenöse Zytostatikainjektion: Prophylaxe und Sofortmaßnahmen im Notfall. MMW Fortschr Med 146: 682–686, 2004.
- Schrijvers DL: Extravasation: a dreaded complication of chemotherapy. Ann Oncol 14: iii26–iii30, 2003.
- Soble MJ, Dorr RT, Plezia P, et al: Dose-dependent skin ulcers in mice treated with DNA binding antitumor antibiotics. Cancer Chemother Pharmacol 20: 33–36, 1987.

Revisions by Elisabeth Nogler-Semenitz

D

Daunorubicin

D

CONSENSUS

Type of damage: vesicant

Recommended treatment:

General measures:

1. Stop injection/infusion immediately
2. Get extravasation kit
3. Put on (sterile) gloves
4. Replace infusion lead or syringe with 5 ml disposable syringe and aspirate slowly as much as possible of the extravasated drug; **Cave!** do not exert pressure on extravasation area
5. Remove i.v. access while aspirating
6. If blisters occur: aspirate with 1 ml syringe and s.c. cannula, use new equipment for every new attempt at aspiration
7. Elevate limb and immobilise
8. Start **substance specific measures**
9. Ensure adequate analgesia
10. Complete extravasation documentation sheet (mention extent of extravasation)
11. Inform and instruct the patient and relatives
12. Regular control (aftercare)
13. Always consult a (plastic) surgeon within 24 hours

Substance specific measures:

DMSO:

1. Apply DMSO (99%) every 8 hours (e.g. with a sterile gauze pad) without pressure
2. Allow to air-dry – **Cave!** do not cover
3. Continue for a minimum of 7 days

Immediately afterwards topical cooling:

1. Apply cold, dry pack immediately for at least 1 hour (for example, using a cold-hot pack)
2. Continue several times daily for 15 minutes each time

or as alternative intervention to DMSO/cooling

D

Dexrazoxane:

1. Administer 1000 mg dexrazoxane /m² i.v. within six hours after extravasation
2. Repeat the i.v. treatment on day 2 (1000 mg dexrazoxane /m²) and on day 3 (500 mg dexrazoxane /m²)

Cave! after extravasation:

1. No flushing of i.v. access
2. No moist compresses
3. No alcohol compresses
4. No occlusive dressings

Type of damage reported in literature:

Vesicant [1–3,7–18,21–27]

Symptoms and clinical course reported in literature:

Initial symptoms: Swelling, pain, erythema (3 patients) [1,2]

Delayed-onset symptoms: Induration [1]

Residual findings: Necrosis (1 patient each [3,7])[23]

Individual case report: Extravasation in a patient whose central venous catheter was placed incorrectly: initially retrosternal pain, within a few hours development of oedema with reddish discolouration of the skin, during 12 weeks: chest pain, cough, pleural and pericardial effusions, dysphagia, thyrotoxicosis, recall effect after daunorubicin containing treatment 18 and 35 days after extravasation (1 patient) [8]

Measures reported in literature:

Successful treatment:

- Infiltration of sodium bicarbonate and 4 mg dexamethasone, ice pack, application of 15 ml DMSO (70%) every 3–4 hours for 10 days (1 patient) [1,11]
- DMSO (99%) every 6 hours for 14 days (2 patients) [2]

- Extravasation in the mediastinum owing to incorrectly placed central venous catheter—mediastinal aspiration and infusion of 1500 ml NaCl 0.9% through the catheter, systemically administered prednisolone (1 patient) [8]

Unsuccessful treatment:

- Topical cooling (ice pack) 4 × daily for 15 minutes over 3 days; surgical intervention was necessary (1 patient) [3]

Outcome of treatment not reported:

- Infiltration of 5 ml sodium bicarbonate (8.4%), 4 mg dexamethasone, optional local infiltration of corticosteroids, warm to hot compresses for 1 hour [12]

- Ice packs over 1–3 days, topical application of DMSO (70–100%) every 3–4 hours for 3–14 days, early consultation of a plastic surgeon [13]

- Cold compresses immediately applied for 30–60 minutes, then for 24 hours alternating every 15 minutes (with/without compresses); DMSO (50–99%) every 6 hours for 3–14 days [15]

- On the first day DMSO every 2 hours, topical hydrocortisone (1%) and cold compresses for 30 minutes, over the next 7–10 days every 3 hours alternating DMSO and topical hydrocortisone [17]

- DMSO (99%) applied topically to an area twice the size of the affected area, every 6 hours over 14 days, optional ice pack for 15 minutes every 6 hours over 2 days [18]

D

- 4 drops DMSO (99%) per 10 cm^2 skin surface (treatment area: twice the size of the extravasation area), every 8 hours for at least 14 days, optional topical cooling with ice packs sequentially to DMSO treatment; in cases of persistent pain or development of skin necrosis or ulceration consider surgical débridement [16,19,24]

- Dry cold applied immediately for 1 hour, subsequently several times daily for 15 minutes; DMSO (99%) every 8 hours over 8 days; maintain therapy free interval between cold and DMSO [25]

- DMSO applied topically every 6 hours over 3–14 days, followed by cooling for 20 minutes 4 × daily for 3–4 days [26]

- 1–2 ml DMSO (50–99%) topically applied to an area twice the size of the extravasation, every 6–8 hours over 7–14 days, ice pack [27]

- Optional 100 mg hydrocortisone or 4 mg dexamethasone via i.v. access at the extravasation site and/or s.c., ice packs for 24–72 hours, optional topical hydrocortisone (1%), 4 × daily DMSO for several days; if pain persists after 72 hours: consult plastic surgeon [20]

- Immediate topical cooling for 24 hours alternating with 1.5 ml topical DMSO (50%) every 6 hours; DMSO over 14 days [21]

- Topical cooling over 24 hours [22]

Particular remarks: Concerning the risk of necrosis and the treatment after extravasation daunorubicin is often compared with doxorubicin [12–14]; but only few cases of extravasation of daunorubicin have been described

1 case report about the development of a necrosis of the distal digits after administration of daunorubicin through an intravenous shunt, which had been inserted for therapeutic reasons [7]

Local phlebitis, thrombophlebitis, phlebosclerosis [23], hypersensitivity reactions [28] are not associated with extravasation

Increased radiosensitivity and recall phenomenon after radiotherapy [29]

Corticosteroids: positive effect is questionable, because extravasations are only rarely accompanied by inflammatory processes [11,13,19] (see chapter "Histopathological investigations")

Dexrazoxane: in animal studies, systemic administration of dexrazoxane reduced the size of the skin lesion and accelerated healing. Three concsecutive applications were more efficacious than a single application only [9]. Intralesional administration was also efficacious in animal studies [10]

DMSO: positive effects in preventing necroses have been reported [1,2]

Sodium bicarbonate: can cause necroses by itself [4–6]

Conclusion:

In analogy to the chemically related substance doxorubicin, daunorubicin is classified as vesicant

The non-invasive measures DMSO and topical cooling are well established after extravasation of doxorubicin; therefore they are also recommended for daunorubicin

Although the efficacy of dexrazoxane has not been proven after extravasation of daunorubicin in terms of clinical evidence, the administration schedule of dexrazoxane established after extravasation of doxorubicin and epirubicin is applied to all anthracyclines

D

Original articles

[1] Lawrence HJ, Goodnight SH: Dimethyl sulfoxide and extravasation of anthracycline agents. Ann Intern Med 98: 1025, 1983.

[2] Olver IN, Aisner J, Hament A, et al: A prospective study of topical dimethyl sulfoxide for treating anthracycline extravasation. J Clin Oncol 6: 1732–1735, 1988.

[3] Larson DL: What is the appropriate management of tissue extravasation by antitumor agents? Plast Reconstr Surg 75: 397–402, 1985.

[4] Kappel B, Hindenburg AA, Taub RN: Treatment of anthracycline extravasation – a warning against the use of sodium bicarbonate. J Clin Oncol 5: 825–826, 1987.

[5] Jackson IT, Robinson DW: Severe tissue damage following accidental subcutaneous infusion of bicarbonate solution. Scot Med J 21: 200–201, 1976.

[6] Gaze NR: Tissue necrosis caused by commonly used intravenous infusions. Lancet 2: 417–419, 1978.

[7] Dragon LH, Braine HG: Necrosis of the hand after daunorubicin infusion distal to an arteriovenous fistula. Ann Intern Med 91: 58–59, 1979.

[8] Dührsen U, Heinrichs V, Beecken WD, et al: Local and systemic sequale of mediastinal daunorubicin extravasation in a patient with acute myelomonocytic leukemia. Ann Oncol 8: 1167–1169, 1997.

[9] Langer SW, Sehested M, Jensen PB: Treatment of anthracycline extravasation with dexrazoxane. Clin Cancer Res 6: 3680–3686, 2000.

[10] Langer SW, Sehested M, Jensen PB: Dexrazoxane is a potent and specific inhibitor of anthracycline induced subcutaneous lesions in mice. Ann Oncol 123: 405–410, 2001.

Secondary literature

[11] Bertelli G: Prevention and management of extravasation of cytotoxic drugs. Drug Safety 12: 245–255, 1995.

[12] Ignoffo RJ, Friedman MA: Therapy of local toxicities caused by extravasation of cancer chemotherapeutic drugs. Cancer Treat Rev 7: 17–27, 1980.

[13] Schneider G: Paravasate von Zytostatika. Diagnostik und Therapie. Aina S. Schneider Verlag, 6th edition 1–17, 1999.

[14] Krämer I: Onkologische Pharmazie. In: Jaehde U, Radziwill R, Mühlebach S, et al (eds) Lehrbuch der Klinischen Pharmazie. Wissenschaftliche Verlagsgesellschaft mbH, 2nd edition: 307–336, 2003.

[15] Dorr RT: Pharmacologic management of vesicant chemotherapy extravasations. In: Dorr RT, Von Hoff DD (eds) Cancer Chemotherapy Handbook. Appleton & Lange, 2nd edition: 109–118, 1994.
[16] Gain M, Melzer S, Meyer-Jürshof A, et al: Daunorubicin: Behandlung von Paravasaten. In: Gain M, et al (eds) ADKA-Zytostatika-Handbuch, Pharmazeutisch-wissenschaftliche Monographien. Verlag Heiner Biller, vol 5: 27–28, 2001.
[17] Stanley A: Managing complications of chemotherapy administration. In: Allwood M, Stanley A, Wright P (eds) The Cytotoxics Handbook. Radcliffe Medical Press, 4th edition: 119–193, 2002.
[18] Mullin S, Beckwith MC, Tyler LS: Prevention and management of antineoplastic extravasation injury. Hosp Pharm 35: 57–76, 2000.
[19] Kraft A, Weinig S, Edinger M, et al: Anthrazyklin-Extravasate. Der Onkologe 6: 674–686, 2000.
[20] Cox RF: Managing skin damage induced by doxorubicin hydrochloride and daunorubicin hydrochloride. Am J Hosp Pharm 41: 2410–2414, 1984.
[21] Dorr RT: Antidotes to vesicant chemotherapy extravasations. Blood Rev 4: 41–60, 1990.
[22] Schneider SM, Distelhorst CW: Chemotherapy-induced emergencies. Semin Oncol 16: 572–578, 1989.
[23] Gain M, Melzer S, Meyer-Jürshof A, et al: Daunorubicin: Nebenwirkungen. In: Gain M, et al (eds) ADKA-Zytostatika-Handbuch, Pharmazeutisch-wissenschaftliche Monographien. Verlag Heiner Biller, vol 5: 14, 2001.
[24] Summary of product characteristics Daunoblastin® (Germany), Pharmacia, March 2004.
[25] Jordan K, Grothe W, Schmoll HJ: Paravasation von Zytostatika: Prävention und Therapie. Dtsch Med Wochenschr 130: 33–37, 2005.
[26] Krämer I, Stützle M: Zytostatika-Paravasation – Wie ist vorzugehen? Krankenhauspharmazie 23: 261–268, 2002.
[27] Ener RA, Meglathery SB, Styler M: Extravasation of systemic hemato-oncological therapies. Ann Oncol 15: 858–862, 2004.
[28] Koppel RA, Boh EE: Cutaneous reactions to chemotherapeutic agents. Am J Med Sci 321: 327–335, 2001.
[29] Alley E, Green R, Schuchter L: Cutaneous toxicities of cancer therapy. Curr Opin Oncol 14: 212–216, 2002.

Further reading:

- Albanell J, Baselga J: Systemic therapy emergencies. Semin Oncol 27: 347–361, 2000.

D

- Fenchel K, Karthaus M: Zytostatika-Paravasate – gibt es neue Empfehlungen zum therapeutischen Vorgehen? Wien Med Wochenschr 151: 44–46, 2001.
- Gault DT: Extravasation injuries. Br J Plast Surg 46: 91–96, 1993.
- Kassner E: Evaluation and treatment of chemotherapy extravasation injuries. J Pediatr Oncol Nurs 17: 135–148, 2000.
- Krämer I: Zehn Jahre Dokumentation von Zytostatika-Paravasat-Ereignissen: Auswertung von 175 Paravasate-Dokumentationen. Krankenhauspharmazie 23: 269–274, 2002.
- Kurul S, Saip P, Aydin T: Totally implantable venous-access ports: local problems and extravasation injury. Lancet Oncol 3: 684–692, 2002.
- Rauh J, Pluntke S, Müller C: Paravenöse Zytostatikainjektion: Prophylaxe und Sofortmaßnahmen im Notfall. MMW Fortschr Med 146: 682–686, 2004.
- Rospond RM: Utilization of dimethyl sulfoxide for treating anthracycline extravasation. J Oncol Pharm Practice 1: 33–39, 1995.
- Schrijvers DL: Extravasation: a dreaded complication of chemotherapy. Ann Oncol 14: iii26–iii30, 2003.
- Soble MJ, Dorr RT, Plezia P, et al: Dose-dependent skin ulcers in mice treated with DNA binding antitumor antibiotics. Cancer Chemother Pharmacol 20: 33–36, 1987.

Revisions by Elisabeth Nogler-Semenitz

Daunorubicin liposomal

CONSENSUS

Type of damage: irritant

Recommended treatment:

General measures:

1. Stop injection/infusion immediately
2. Get extravasation kit
3. Put on (sterile) gloves
4. Replace infusion lead or syringe with 5 ml disposable syringe and aspirate slowly as much as possible of the extravasated drug; **Cave!** do not exert pressure on extravasation area
5. Remove i.v. access while aspirating
6. If blisters occur: aspirate with 1 ml syringe and s.c. cannula, use new equipment for every new attempt at aspiration
7. Elevate limb and immobilise
8. Start **substance specific measures**
9. Complete extravasation documentation sheet (mention extent of extravasation)
10. Inform and instruct the patient and relatives
11. Regular control (aftercare)

Substance specific measures:

Topical cooling:

1. Apply cold, dry pack immediately for at least 1 hour (for example, using a cold-hot pack)
2. Continue several times daily for 15 minutes each time

Cave! after extravasation:

1. No flushing of i.v. access
2. No moist compresses
3. No alcohol compresses
4. No occlusive dressings

D

Type of damage reported in literature:

Irritant [4,5,12]

Exfoliant [4]

Low risk of necrosis [9]

Potentially vesicant [6,10]

Vesicant [7]

Symptoms and clinical course reported in literature:

Initial symptoms: Pain free oedema (4 patients) [1]

Delayed-onset symptoms: Erythema (2 patients), increasingly severe pain (1 patient), hyperpigmentation or skin discolouration, leathery hardening of the skin (2 patients), induration (1 patient) [1], transient erythema, pain, swelling, symptoms subside within 6 months [10]

Residual findings: Reduced sensitivity (1 patient) [1]

Case report: Extravasation remained without sequelae [2], no necroses, [3] (no numbers of cases given)

Measures reported in literature:

Successful treatment:
- Infiltration of hydrocortisone or dexamethasone (in 1 patient hydrocortisone topically applied first), repeated ice packs over 1 day (3 patients) [1]
- Ice packs, 250 mg dicloxacillin 4 × daily p.o. for prophylaxis of cellulitis (1 patient) [1]

Unsuccessful treatment:
- No data available

Outcome of treatment not reported:
- 100 mg hydrocortisone s.c. and i.v., respectively, hydrocortisone applied topically, ice packs. There are indications that daunorubicin is released from the liposomes within 2–3 weeks, hence 8–12 hours after extravasation DMSO every 2 hours over 24 hours, then 4 × daily over 10–14 days [4]
- Topical cooling [12] for 30 minutes [5]

- Topical cooling 4 × daily for 20 minutes over 3–4 days [11]
- Immediate treatment: infiltration of 2–5 ml sodium bicarbonate (8.4%), infiltration with 4–8 mg dexamethasone, DMSO every 3–4 hours for 3–14 days [6]
- Immediate topical cooling for 24 hours alternating with 1.5 ml topical DMSO (50%) every 6 hours; DMSO over 14 days [9]

Particular remarks: Corticosteroids: positive effect is questionable, because extravasations are only rarely accompanied by inflammatory processes [7,8] (See chapter "Histopathological investigations")

Dicloxacillin: only for prophylaxis of secondary infection, no causal treatment of extravasation

Cooling: positive effects have been reported [1]

Avoid measures that might result in daunorubicin release from the liposomes, such as local instillation of an antidote, local compression etc [10]

Conclusion: Although daunorubicin liposomal is classified as vesicant in some of the literature, no clinical case of necroses after extravasation has been documented

The liposomal formulation seems to be less damaging than conventional daunorubicin [5]; daunorubicin liposomal is therefore classified as irritant

Owing to little experience with extravasations of daunorubicin liposomal, a final classification of the type of damage is not possible

The exclusive application of topical cooling is recommended; the lipid solving attribute of DMSO may cause a release of daunorubicin from the liposomes and may result in greater damage [5]

D

Original articles

[1] Cabriales S, Bresnahan J, Testa D, et al: Extravasation of liposomal daunorubicin in patients with AIDS-associated Kaposi s sarcoma: a report of four cases. Oncol Nurs Forum 25: 67–70, 1998.
[2] Guaglianone P, Chan K, Hanisch R, et al: Phase I clinical trial of liposomal daunorubicin (Daunoxome) in advanced malignancies. Proc ASCO 11: 135, 1992.
[3] Sharma D, Muggia F, Lucci L, et al: Liposomal daunorubicin (VS103): tolerance and clinical effects in AIDS-related Kaposi's sarcoma (KS) during a phase I study. Proc ASCO 9: 4, 1990.

Secondary literature

[4] Stanley A: Managing complications of chemotherapy administration. In: Allwood M, Stanley A, Wright P (eds) The Cytotoxics Handbook. Radcliffe Medical Press, 4th edition: 119–193, 2002.
[5] Mullin S, Beckwith MC, Tyler LS: Prevention and management of antineoplastic extravasation injury. Hosp Pharm 35: 57–76, 2000.
[6] van Gemmern R: Gewebstoxizität und Paravasatbehandlung neuer Zytostatika. Krankenhauspharmazie 17: 471–473, 1996.
[7] Bertelli G: Prevention and management of extravasation of cytotoxic drugs. Drug Safety 12: 245–255, 1995.
[8] Schneider G: Paravasate von Zytostatika. Diagnostik und Therapie. Aina S. Schneider Verlag, 6th edition: 1–17, 1999.
[9] Dorr RT: Antidotes to vesicant chemotherapy extravasations. Blood Rev 4: 41–60, 1990.
[10] Summary of product characteristics Daunoxome® (Germany), Gilead Sciences, March 2003.
[11] Krämer I, Stützle M: Zytostatika-Paravasation – Wie ist vorzugehen? Krankenhauspharmazie 23: 261–268, 2002.
[12] Jordan K, Grothe W, Schmoll HJ: Paravasation von Zytostatika: Prävention und Therapie. Dtsch Med Wochenschr 130: 33–37, 2005.

Further reading:

- Krämer I: Onkologische Pharmazie. In: Jaehde U, Radziwill R, Mühlebach S, et al (eds) Lehrbuch der Klinischen Pharmazie. Wissenschaftliche Verlagsgesellschaft mbH, 2nd edition: 307–336, 2003.
- Rauh J, Pluntke S, Müller C: Paravenöse Zytostatikainjektion: Prophylaxe und Sofortmaßnahmen im Notfall. MMW Fortschr Med 146: 682–686, 2004.

Revisions by Elisabeth Nogler-Semenitz

Docetaxel

CONSENSUS

Type of damage: irritant

Recommended treatment:

General measures:

1. Stop injection/infusion immediately
2. Get extravasation kit
3. Put on (sterile) gloves
4. Replace infusion lead or syringe with 5 ml disposable syringe and aspirate slowly as much as possible of the extravasated drug; **Cave!** do not exert pressure on extravasation area
5. Remove i.v. access while aspirating
6. If blisters occur: aspirate with 1 ml syringe and s.c. cannula, use new equipment for every new attempt at aspiration
7. Elevate limb and immobilise
8. Complete extravasation documentation sheet (mention extent of extravasation)
9. Inform and instruct the patient and relatives
10. Regular control (aftercare)

Substance specific measures: none

Cave! after extravasation:

1. No flushing of i.v. access
2. No moist compresses
3. No alcohol compresses
4. No occlusive dressings

D

Type of damage reported in literature:

Irritant [1,6,19,20]

Exfoliant [15]

Possibly vesicant [5,11]

Vesicant [9,17,23] in case of extravasation of large amounts and high concentrations [14,16]

Symptoms and clinical course reported in literature:

Peripheral venous application:
Initial symptoms: Pain, erythema, swelling (5 patients) [4]

Delayed-onset symptoms: Erythema, blistering, dysesthesia (11 patients) [1,4–6], severe pain with impaired movement of affected limb and skin discolouration (1 patient) [5], pruritus (3 patients, 4 extravasations) [6], recall reaction (1 patient) [10]

Residual findings: Hypoaesthesia (3 patients, 4 extravasations) [6]

Single case reports: Swelling around the cannula; after 4 hours, red swelling within the infiltrated area on the left forearm and pain; both subsided after 12 hours; after 24 hours only minimal residual swelling, redness completely disappeared; after 8 days: tissue damage affecting an area measuring 4.5 cm × 2.5 cm; itching and erythema; day 9: area of redness diminished, minimal itching, skin discolouration (hyperpigmentation) continued to expand until it covered an area of 4 cm × 8 cm; it then remained unchanged for 3 months, after which it disappeared slowly (1 patient) [8]

D

After the first administration on day 1 a mild painful swelling of the left hand was observed, 1 week later - a few hours after the second doxetacel application - erythematous swelling with tenderness and bulla formation at the original extravasation site on the left hand (recall reaction); skin lesion continued to progress and extended to the whole left hand, one palm-sized, well-demarcated, erythematous and slightly violaceous patch with flacid bulla formation was noted on the dorsum of the left hand, the range of motion of the left wrist was limited by tenderness and severe oedema; Day 29: only mild hyperpigmentation and desquamation; residual finding: change in sensations (1 patient) [9]

Central venous application:
Initial symptoms: Erythema and hyperthermia of affected region (1 patient) [11]

Delayed-onset symptoms: Blistering, skin desquamation, and bloody-serous secretion from small skin fissures (1 patient) [11]

Residual findings: Brown pigmentation of skin (1 patient) [11]

Measures reported in literature:

Successful treatment:
- 250 IU hyaluronidase in 6 ml NaCl 0.9% s.c. without local cooling or application of heat (2 patients) [1,14]
- Topical heat, no hyaluronidase (5 patients) [4]
- No specific measures (3 patients with 4 extravasations) [6]
- Oral antihistamines 2 × daily, hydrocortisone (1%) applied topically, topical heat (1 patient) [11]

D

Unsuccessful treatment:
- Local application of moist heat resulted in blistering and eruptions (1 patient) [2]

- Primary topical heat, later antibiotic and analgesic therapy (1 patient) [5]

- 10 ml NaCl (0.9%) perilesionally s.c., analgesia, local cooling for 8 minutes, then DMSO applied topically 3× for 45 minutes; repeated application of DMSO after recurrence of symptoms did not result in improvement of outcome compared with untreated area (1 patient) [8]

- Primary infiltration of hydrocortisone, local application of cold pack, later i.v. antibiotics, analgesia (1 patient) [9]

Outcome of treatment not reported:
- Topical corticosteroids and cooling [12]

- Ice packs for 15–20 minutes every 4–6 hours for 72 hours and treatment with DMSO or hyaluronidase [13]

- S.c. infiltration of 1–3 ml of a mixture of 100 mg hydrocortisone and 4 mg chloropheniramine in 10 ml, 1500 IU hyaluronidase, warm compresses; subsequently alternating between warm compresses and topically applied mepyramine or another antihistamine (for 3 days); in severe cases administration of 1 g sodium cromoglycate p.o., followed by 200 mg 4 × daily for the following 3 days [15]

- 250–300 IU hyaluronidase in 6 ml NaCl 0.9% s.c. neither local cooling nor application of heat [16]

- Topical cooling [22] once, for 3 hours [23]

- No specific measures mentioned [19,20]

Particular remarks:

Phlebitis and hypersensitivity reactions [3,4,18,25] are not associated with extravasation; these symptoms are likely to be due to the excipients in the formulation (polysorbate 80, ethanol [21])

Delayed onset of symptoms has often been described [5,6,9,11,23]

Reddish discolouration of skin above venous access without signs of extravasation or phlebitis in weekly administration of docetaxel [7]

The occurrence of a radiation recall phenomenon has been described [18,25]. A recall phenomenon with exacerbation of the symptoms of extravasation has also been described after repeated application of docetaxel at a different site (2 patients [7,10,23,24]

Local ulceration is likely to occur only in case of extravasation of large amounts and high concentration of infusion solution [14]

Antihistamines: only secondary prophylaxis, no causal treatment of extravasation

Glucocorticoids: positive effect is questionable, because extravasations are only rarely accompanied by inflammatory processes (See chapter "Histopathological investigations")

Hyaluronidase: insufficient clinical evidence for administration of hyaluronidase; disadvantage: invasive measure

Topical heat: positive as well as negative effects have been observed [4,5,11]

Watchful waiting is a possible strategy [8]

Conclusion:

Although docetaxel is classified as vesicant in some of the literature, no clinical case of necrosis after extravasation has been documented; the substance is classified as irritant due to the excipients in the formulation

Positive results of substance specific measures have not been described so far; until further data become available no substance specific measures can be recommended

D

Original articles

[1] Bertelli G, Cafferata MA, Ardizzoni A, et al: Skin ulceration potential of paclitaxel in a mouse skin model in vivo. Cancer 79: 2266–2268, 1997.

[2] Goodman M, Stewart I, Lydon J, et al: Use caution when managing paclitaxel and taxotere infiltrations. Oncol Nurs Forum 23: 541–542, 1996.

[3] Panday VR, Huizing MT, Huinink WW, et al: Hypersensitivity reactions to the taxanes paclitaxel and docetaxel. Clin Drug Invest 14: 418–427, 1997.

[4] Ascherman JA, Knowles SL, Attkiss K: Docetaxel (Taxotere) extravasation: a report of five cases with treatment recommendations. Ann Plast Surg 45: 438–441, 2000.

[5] Raley J, Geisler JP, Buekrs TE, et al: Docetaxel extravasation causing significant delayed tissue injury. Gyn Oncol 78: 259–260, 2000.

[6] Harrison BR, Ketts JR, Schultz MZ, et al: Docetaxel-induced extravasation injury: a report of three cases. J Oncol Pharm Practice 6: 122–125, 2000.

[7] Schrijvers DL, Van den Brande J, Vermorken JB: Supravenous discoloration of the skin due to docetaxel treatment. Br J Dermatol 142: 1069–1070, 2000.

[8] Berghammer P, Pöhnl R, Baur M, et al: Docetaxel extravasation. Support Cancer Care 9: 131–143, 2001.

[9] Ho CH, Yang CH, Chu CJ: Vesicant-type reaction due to docetaxel extravasation. Acta Derm Venereol 83: 467–468, 2003.

[10] Yae T, Tanaka Y, Yea E, et al: A case report of docetaxel-induced recall reaction. Jpn J Hosp Pharm 26: 642–646, 2000.

[11] El Saghir NS, Otrock ZK: Docetaxel extravasation into the normal breast during breast cancer treatment. Anti-Cancer Drugs 15: 401–404, 2004.

Secondary literature

[12] van Gemmern R: Gewebstoxizität und Paravasatbehandlung neuer Zytostatika. Krankenhauspharmazie 17: 471–473, 1996.
[13] Rhone-Poulenc Rorer, personal communication, August 1998.
[14] Dorr RT: Author reply to Bertelli G et al: Skin ulceration potential of paclitaxel in a mouse skin model in vivo. Cancer 79: 2268–2269, 1997.
[15] Stanley A: Managing complications of chemotherapy administration. In: Allwood M, Stanley A, Wright P (eds) The Cytotoxics Handbook. Radcliffe Medical Press, 4th edition: 119–193, 2002.
[16] Schneider G: Paravasate von Zytostatika. Diagnostik und Therapie. Aina S. Schneider Verlag, 6th edition: 1–17, 1999.
[17] Berdel WE, Schmoll HJ, Büchele T, et al: Prävention und Therapie von Paravasaten/Extravasaten. In: Schmoll HJ, Höffken K, Possinger K (eds) Kompendium Internistische Onkologie. Standards in Diagnostik und Therapie. Springer, vol 1, 3rd edition: 1689–1701, 1999.
[18] Bokemeyer C: Dermatoxizität antineoplastischer Substanzen. In: Schmoll HJ, Höffken K, Possinger K (eds) Kompendium Internistische Onkologie. Standards in Diagnostik und Therapie. Springer, Vol 1, 3rd edition: 1411–1426, 1999.
[19] Gain M, Melzer S, Meyer-Jürshof A, et al: Allgemeiner Teil: Behandlung von Paravasaten. In: Gain M, et al (eds) ADKA-Zytostatika-Handbuch, Pharmazeutisch-wissenschaftliche Monographien. Verlag Heiner Biller, vol 1, 2nd edition: A42–44, 1997.
[20] Mullin S, Beckwith MC, Tyler LS: Prevention and management of antineoplastic extravasation injury. Hosp Pharm 35: 57–76, 2000.
[21] Summary of product characteristics Taxotere® (Austria), Aventis, January 2005.
[22] Gain M, Melzer S, Meyer-Jürshof A, et al: Docetaxel: Behandlung von Paravasaten. In: Gain M, et al (eds) ADKA-Zytostatika-Handbuch, Pharmazeutisch-wissenschaftliche Monographien. Verlag Heiner Biller, vol 6: 30, 2002.
[23] Krämer I, Stützle M: Zytostatika-Paravasation – Wie ist vorzugehen? Krankenhauspharmazie 23: 261–268, 2002.
[24] Koppel RA, Boh EE: Cutaneous reactions to chemotherapeutic agents. Am J Med Sci 321: 327–335, 2001.
[25] Alley E, Green R, Schuchter L: Cutaneous toxicities of cancer therapy. Curr Opin Oncol 14: 212–216, 2002.

D

Further reading:

- Albanell J, Baselga J: Systemic therapy emergencies. Semin Oncol 27: 347–361, 2000.
- Ener RA, Meglathery SB, Styler M: Extravasation of systemic hemato-oncological therapies. Ann Oncol 15: 858–862, 2004.
- Fenchel K, Karthaus M: Zytostatika-Paravasate – gibt es neue Empfehlungen zum therapeutischen Vorgehen? Wien Med Wochenschr 151: 44–46, 2001.
- Jordan K, Grothe W, Schmoll HJ: Paravasation von Zytostatika: Prävention und Therapie. Dtsch Med Wochenschr 130: 33–37, 2005.
- Khan MS, Holmes JD: Reducing the morbidity from extravasation injuries. Ann Plast Surg 48: 628–632, 2002.
- Krämer I: Onkologische Pharmazie. In: Jaehde U, Radziwill R, Mühlebach S, et al (eds) Lehrbuch der Klinischen Pharmazie. Wissenschaftliche Verlagsgesellschaft mbH, 2nd edition: 307–336, 2003.
- Leonard GD, Zujewski JA: Docetaxel-related skin, nail and vascular toxicity. Ann Pharmacother 37: 148, 2003.
- Rauh J, Pluntke S, Müller C: Paravenöse Zytostatikainjektion: Prophylaxe und Sofortmaßnahmen im Notfall. MMW Fortschr Med 146: 682–686, 2004.
- Schrijvers DL: Extravasation: a dreaded complication of chemotherapy. Ann Oncol 14: iii26–iii30, 2003.

Revisions by Ines Mader

Doxorubicin

CONSENSUS

Type of damage: vesicant

Recommended treatment:

General measures:

1. Stop injection/infusion immediately
2. Get extravasation kit
3. Put on (sterile) gloves
4. Replace infusion lead or syringe with 5 ml disposable syringe and aspirate slowly as much as possible of the extravasated drug; **Cave**! do not exert pressure on extravasation area
5. Remove i.v. access while aspirating
6. If blisters occur: aspirate with 1 ml syringe and s.c. cannula, use new equipment for every new attempt at aspiration
7. Elevate limb and immobilise
8. Start **substance specific measures**
9. Ensure adequate analgesia
10. Complete extravasation documentation sheet (mention extent of extravasation)
11. Inform and instruct the patient and relatives
12. Regular control (aftercare)
13. Always consult a (plastic) surgeon within 24 hours

Substance specific measures:

DMSO:

1. Apply DMSO (99%) every 8 hours (e.g. with a sterile gauze pad) without pressure
2. Allow to air-dry – Cave! do not cover
3. Continue for a minimum of 7 days

Immediately afterwards topical cooling:

1. Apply cold, dry pack immediately for at least 1 hour (for example, using a cold-hot pack)
2. Continue several times daily for 15 minutes each time

or as alternative intervention to DMSO/cooling

D

Dexrazoxane:

1. Administer 1000 mg dexrazoxane /m^2 i.v. within six hours after extravasation
2. Repeat the i.v. treatment on day 2 (1000 mg dexrazoxane /m^2) and on day 3 (500 mg dexrazoxane /m^2)

Substance specific measures after simultaneous extravasation of vincristine and anthracyclines (for example, in the context of a VAD protocol):

Hyaluronidase:

Inject up to 1500 IU hyaluronidase around affected area depending on the size of the extravasation. **Cave!** local analgesia is recommended

Apply DMSO immediately afterwards:

1. Apply DMSO (99%) every 8 hours (e.g. with a sterile gauze pad) without pressure
2. Allow to air-dry – **Cave!** do not cover
3. Continue for a minimum of 7 days

Cave! no heat or cold must be applied

Cave! after extravasation:

1. No flushing of i.v. access
2. No moist compresses
3. No alcohol compresses
4. No occlusive dressings

Type of damage reported in literature:	Vesicant [1–7,62–76]
Symptoms and clinical course reported in literature:	**Initial symptoms:** Pain, erythema, swelling **Delayed-onset symptoms:** Increasing pain, desquamation of the horny layer of the epidermis, eschar formation, induration, hyperpigmentation, necroses, sometimes months after the event **Residual findings:** Pain on movement, contractures, scarring of skin, impaired joint movement including functional loss (many patients) [3,6–9,50] **Individual case report:** Necrosis after extravasation; surgical intervention was repeatedly rejected by patient, hence conservative treatment was given. Within 2 years, no complete healing, 10 years later squamous cell carcinoma at extravasation site (1 patient) [9]
Measures reported in literature:	**Successful treatment:** – Early surgical treatment (8 and 40 patients) [2,7] – 8 mg dexamethasone or hydrocortisone i.d., ice packs, 15 ml DMSO (50–99%) every 2–4 hours over at least 3 days (3 patients) [10] – 5–90 minutes after extravasation: infiltration of 500 mg hydrocortisone, application of betamethasone-gentamicin ointment every 12 hours for 2 days, then every 24 hours until healing is complete (8 and 10 patients) [11,12]; more than 5 days after extravasation: application of keratolytic ointment containing salicylic acid for 5 hours (1 patient) [11]; additionally infiltration of sodium thiosulfate solution (2%) followed by massage reduced the time of healing from 21 to 5 days (10 patients) [12]

D

- Infiltration of 150 TRU chondroitin sulfatase s.c, repeat after 24 hours, DMSO (90%) 4 × daily over 2 weeks (1 patient: VAD-protocol) [13]
- DMSO (90%), a-tocopherol acetate (10%) given topically every 12 hours over 48 hours (5 patients) [14]
- 4 drops DMSO (99%) per 10 cm^2 applied topically to an area twice the size of the affected area, repeat every 8 hours for 1 week or until symptoms have subsided; local cooling over 60 minutes, every 8 hours for 3 days (cold-hot pack) (8 patients [15] and 11 patients [16])
- Immediate infiltration of 2–5 ml sodium bicarbonate (8.4%), topical DMSO (99%) for 14 days, ice pack (3 patients) [17]
- DMSO (99%) every 6 hours over 14 days (18 patients) [18]
- Immediate infiltration of 5 ml sodium bicarbonate (8.4%) followed by 4 mg dexamethasone (1 patient) [19]
- S.c. injection of 20–90 ml NaCl 0.9%, to be repeated 3–6 times over the following days; topical corticosteroids under occlusion (26 patients) [20]
- If treatment within an hour after the event is possible: infiltration of 12–38 ml hyaluronidase (150 IU/l NaCl 0.9%) (about 120 patients) [21]
- 50–200 mg hydrocortisone s.c./i.d., topical hydrocortisone (1%) and ice packs (4 patients) [37]
- DMSO (99%) every 6 hours over 17 days (1 patient, VAD-protocol) [38]
- 4 ml sodium bicarbonate (6 patients) [39]

- Topical cooling, injection of 1500 IU hyaluronidase with 5 ml lidocaine 1% into extravasation area, flushout with 200 ml NaCl 0.9%, if possible elevation of limb, ice pack over 24 hours, hydrocortisone cream 2 × daily as long as erythema persists (6 patients) [46]

- Twice intralesional application of triamcinolone acetonide 7–8 ml (10 mg/l) at a week's distance. Healing in 4 and 5 weeks (2 patients) [47]

- Administration of dexrazoxane within 6 hours after extravasation, 1000 mg dexrazoxane /m^2 i.v. on day 1 to be repeated on day 2 (1000 mg/m^2) and on day 3 (500 mg/m^2) (23 patients) [48]

Unsuccessful treatment:

- 4 and 20 days after extravasation: infiltration of 5000 IU heparin, 4 mg dexamethasone or 100 mg hydrocortisone, ice pack for about 24 hours, 2 × daily topical hydrocortisone (1%) (2 patients) [3]

- Cooling with ice 15 minutes 4 × daily over 3 days (89 patients); in 25 patients surgical intervention became necessary [4]

- Cold compresses (4 patients) [5]

- 100 mg hydrocortisone i.v. or s.c. (3 patients); in 2 patients surgical intervention was necessary [5]

- Infiltration of 200 mg hydrocortisone, repeated surgical intervention (1 patient) [35]

- Local cooling with ice, topical cortisone, in 5 patients surgical intervention was necessary, occasional permanent functional impairment (16 patients) [36]

- 100 mg hydrocortisone i.v., ice packs (5 patients) [37]

D

- Anti-inflammatory ointment, DMSO applied topically 3 × daily, surgical intervention required [51]

- Extravasation in patient with Port-a-cath: 1 hours and 5 hours after the event, i.v. infusion of 1500 mg dexrazoxane, after 24 hours 750 mg dexrazoxane. 3 × DMSO application every 6 hours. Healing, only occasional pain and mild hyperpigmentation. 3 months after extravasation necrosis, after 4 months surgical intervention, healing achieved by using GM-CSF (300 µg) (1 patient) [50]

Outcome of treatment not reported:

- Bromelin, trypsin, and rutin combination: 1 tablet 3 × daily p.o. over 1 month. At the start of treatment within 24 hours warm compresses and hyaluronidase after extravasation of vinca alkaloid, cold compresses and hydrocortisone after anthracycline extravasation (6 patients with vinca alkaloid/anthracycline extravasation) [49]

- Infiltration of 5 ml sodium bicarbonate (8.4%), 4 mg dexamethasone, optional local infiltration of corticosteroids, warm to hot compresses for 1 hour [62]

- Topical DMSO every 6–8 hours for several days, local cooling [64,68,77]

- Ice packs over 1–3 days, topical application of DMSO (70–100%) every 3–4 hours for 3–14 days, early consultation of plastic surgeon [65]

- On the first day DMSO every 2 hours, topical hydrocortisone (1%) and cold compresses for 30 minutes, over 7–10 days every 3 hours alternating DMSO and topical hydrocortisone [66]

- DMSO (99%) at least every 6 hours over 3–14 days, followed by cold compresses immediately for 20 minutes, 4 × daily for 20 minutes over 3–4 days [67]

- DMSO (99%) to be applied to an area twice the size of the extravasation area, every 6 hours over 14 days; optional ice pack for 15 minutes every 6 hours over 2 days [69]

- Cold compresses immediately applied for 30–60 minutes, then for 24 hours alternating every 15 minutes (with/without compresses); DMSO (50–99%) every 6 hours for 3–14 days [70]

- Optional 100 mg hydrocortisone or 4 mg dexamethasone via i.v. access at the extravasation site or s.c., ice packs for 24–72 hours, optional topical hydrocortisone (1%), 4 × daily DMSO over several days, if pain persists after 72 hours: consultation of a plastic surgeon [71]

- Ice-packs [73]

- Immediate topical cooling for 24 hours alternating with 1.5 ml topical DMSO (50%) every 6 hours; DMSO for 14 days [74]

- 4 drops DMSO (99%) per 10 cm^2 skin surface (treatment area: twice the size of the extravasation area), every 8 hours for at least 14 days, optional topical cooling with ice packs sequentially to DMSO treatment; in cases of persistent pain or development of skin necrosis or ulceration consider surgical débridement [75]

- 100 mg hydrocortisone s.c. and i.v., respectively, DMSO (70–100%) every 3–4 hours for 14 days (minimum 3 days) locally applied, ice or cold pack 4 × daily for 15–20 minutes, topical hydrocortisone [76]

- Dry cold pack initially for 1 hour, followed by several times daily for 15 minutes; DMSO (99%) every 8 hours over 8 days; maintain therapy free interval between cold pack and DMSO [77]

- Application of 1–2 ml DMSO (50–99%) to an area twice the size of the extravasation area, every 6–8 hours over 7–14 days, ice packs [78]

Particular remarks: Ulcers may occur for a prolonged period of time [3,50]

Recall phenomena [79]: progression of a necrosis of an extravasation after repeated administration (2 months later) at another site [30]

Local reactions have been reported (erythema, urticaria) at the injection area (rarely generalised) that may be associated with preceding radiation treatment [31–33]

Hyperpigmentation of nails, mucosa, generalised hyperpigmentation, and hand-foot syndrome are not associated with extravasation [80]

Hypersensitivity reactions [79,80], enhanced radiosensitivity reactions, and recall after radiotherapy [79] are not associated with extravasation

Corticosteroids: positive effect is questionable, because extravasations are rarely accompanied by inflammatory processes [1,26,75]—in animal experiments the effect of corticosteroids has been described as inconsistent [25,27–29] (See chapter "Histopathological investigations")

DMSO and topical cooling: positive effects in preventing necroses have been reported [15,16,72]; repeated application of cold for 2–7 days did not yield advantage compared with 24 hours of cooling [40] Cave! Topical cooling alone is not sufficient [4,74,75]

Dexrazoxane: in animal studies, systemic administration of dexrazoxane reduced the size of the skin lesions and shortened the healing time. Threefold application was more efficacious than once only [52]. Intralesional administration was also efficacious in animal studies [53].

Gentamicin: only for prophylaxis of secondary infection, no causal treatment of extravasation

G-CSF and GM-CSF: 1 of 2 necroses healed 4 weeks after weekly administration of GM-CSF 400 µg s.c. over 3 weeks, the other necrosis was treated with G-CSF but did not improve [57]. Animal studies found a positive effect on the healing process of doxorubicin induced necroses [58,59]; positive effects not sufficiently proved

Heparin: unfractionated heparin, nadroparin, dalteparin, applied s.c., in animal studies significantly lowered the rate of ulceration and the size of the ulcer [54]; positive effect not sufficiently proved in human studies, invasive measure

Hyaluronidase: administration justified only in extravasation of vinca alkaloids and paclitaxel, positive effect in doxorubicin not sufficiently proved. Animal studies have shown a positive effect of hyaluronidase in dogs [56], of NaCl 0.9%, hyaluronidase, or heparin in rats if treatment was given within 15 minutes after the extravasation event [55]. The positive effects have not been proved in humans and treatment can therefore not be recommended.

NaCl 0.9% and hyaluronidase/NaCl 0.9%: showed a positive effect in s.c. injection, especially when treatment was administered within 1 hour after the extravasation event. Mechanism of action under discussion: dilution of the tissue toxic substance [21]. Disadvantage: invasive measure

Sodium bicarbonate: may itself cause necroses [22,23], also increases local cellular absorption of doxorubicin through raised pH from 5 to 8 and thus furthers tissue necroses [24]

Sodium thiosulfate: positive effect not sufficiently proved; disadvantage: invasive measure [12]

Propranolol and isoproterenol: positive effects described in animal experiments only [34]

D

α-tocopherol acetate: positive effect not sufficiently proved [14], report of positive effect of α-tocopherol succinate in animal experiments available [41]

Radical scavenger DHM3 (Bis (3,5-dimethyl-5-hydroxymethyl-2-oxomorpholine-3-yl) [44] and basic fibroblast growth factor (bFGF) [45]: positive effects observed in animal experiments only

Hyperbaric oxygen (HBO): results from animal studies were contradictory: positive effects with regard to healing [60], increase of cytotoxicity in early HBO treatment after extravasation [61], positive effects in humans not proved

In simultaneous extravasation of vincristine und anthracyclines: combination therapy of hyaluronidase and DMSO without heat or cold pack is recommended [67]

Surgical intervention:

- If adequate conservative treatment measures were started immediately after extravasation surgical intervention was necessary only in a small number of patients affected [10,14,16,18]
- Because of the damage mechanism – investigated in the animal model – surgical intervention before day 14 after extravasation is not indicated [42]
- Débridement only in symptomatic extravasations (pain and/or necroses or development of extensive ulcers) [75]
- Doxorubicin shows fluorescence in ultraviolet light; during débridement, tissue containing doxorubicin, which is to be removed, is made visible by UV light; in subsequent i.v. injection of fluorescein (10 mg/kg) vital tissue shows green fluorescence after 15 minutes and non-fluorescent necrotic tissue can be excised [43]

Conclusion: Owing to many reports of necroses doxorubicin is classified as vesicant

The well-established and non-invasive measures DMSO and topical cooling are recommended after extravasation of doxorubicin; as an alternative intervention, the i.v. administration of dexrazoxane has proven to be effective, if started within 6 hours after the extravasation event

Original articles

[1] Bhawan J, Petry J, Rybak ME: Histologic changes induced in skin by extravasation of doxorubicin (adriamycin). J Cutan Pathol 16: 158–163, 1989.
[2] Bowers DG, Lynch JB: Adriamycin extravasation. Plast Reconstr Surg 61: 86–92, 1978.
[3] Köstering H, Kasten U, Ruskowski H, et al: Lokale Toxizität des Adriamycins. In: Füllenbach D, et al (eds) Beiträge zur Onkologie. S. Karger 9: 76–93, 1981.
[4] Larson DL: What is the appropriate management of tissue extravasation by antitumor agents? Plast Reconstr Surg 75: 397–402, 1985.
[5] Reilly JJ, Neifeld JP, Rosenberg SA: Clinical course and management of accidental adriamycin extravasation. Cancer 40: 2053–2056, 1977.
[6] Rudolph R, Stein RS, Pattillo RA: Skin ulcers due to adriamycin. Cancer 38: 1087–1094, 1976.
[7] Linder RM, Upton J, Osteen R: Management of extensive doxorubicin hydrochloride extravasation injuries. J Hand Surg 8: 32–38, 1983.
[8] Rudolph R: Ulcers of the hand and wrist caused by doxorubicin hydrochloride. Orthop Rev 7: 93–95, 1978.
[9] Lauvin R, Miglianico L, Hellegouarc'h R: Skin cancer occurring 10 years after the extravasation of doxorubicin. N Engl J Med 332: 754, 1995.
[10] Lawrence HJ, Walsh D, Zapotowski KA, et al: Topical dimethylsulfoxide may prevent tissue damage from anthracycline extravasation. Cancer Chemother Pharmacol 23: 316–318, 1989.
[11] Tsavaris NB, Karagiaouris P, Tzannou I, et al: Conservative approach to the treatment of chemotherapy-induced extravasation. J Dermatol Surg Oncol 16: 519–522, 1990.
[12] Tsavaris NB, Komitsopoulou P, Karagiaouris P, et al: Prevention of tissue necrosis due to accidental extravasation of cytostatic drugs by a conservative approach. Cancer Chemother Pharmacol 30: 330–333, 1992.

D

[13] Comas D, Mateu J: Treatment of extravasation of both doxorubicin and vincristine administration in a y-site infusion. Ann Pharmacother 30: 244–246, 1996.
[14] Ludwig CU, Stoll HR, Obrist R, et al: Prevention of cytotoxic drug induced skin ulcers with dimethyl sulfoxide (DMSO) and a-tocopherole. Eur J Cancer Clin Oncol 23: 327–329, 1987.
[15] Bertelli G, Dini D, Forno G, et al: Dimethylsulphoxide and cooling after extravasation of antitumour agents. Lancet 341: 1098–1099, 1993.
[16] Bertelli G, Gozza A, Forno GB, et al: Topical dimethylsulfoxide for the prevention of soft tissue injury after extravasation of vesicant cytotoxic drugs: a prospective clinical study. J Clin Oncol 13: 2851–2855, 1995.
[17] Olver IN, Schwarz MA: Use of dimethyl sulfoxide in limiting tissue damage caused by extravasation of doxorubicin. Cancer Treat Rep 67: 407–408, 1983.
[18] Olver IN, Aisner J, Hament A, et al: A prospective study of topical dimethyl sulfoxide for treating anthracycline extravasation. J Clin Oncol 6: 1732–1735, 1988.
[19] Zweig JI, Kabakow B: An apparently effective countermeasure for doxorubicin extravasation. JAMA 239: 2116, 1978.
[20] Scuderi N, Onesti MG: Antitumor agents: extravasation, management, and surgical treatment. Ann Plast Surg 32: 39–44, 1994.
[21] Heckler FR: Current thoughts of extravasation injuries. Clin Plast Surg 16: 557–563, 1989.
[22] Jackson IT, Robinson DW: Severe tissue damage following accidental subcutaneous infusion of bicarbonate solution. Scot Med J 21: 200–201, 1976.
[23] Gaze NR: Tissue necrosis caused by commonly used intravenous infusions. Lancet 2: 417–419, 1978.
[24] Kappel B, Hindenburg AA, Taub RN: Treatment of anthracycline extravasation – a warning against the use of sodium bicarbonate. J Clin Oncol 5: 825–826, 1987.
[25] Cohen MH: Amelioration of adriamycin skin necrosis: an experimental study. Cancer Treat Rep 63: 1003–1004, 1979.
[26] Luedke DW, Kennedy PS, Rietschel RL: Histopathogenesis of skin and subcutaneous injury induced by adriamycin. Plast Reconstr Surg 63: 463–465, 1979.
[27] Dorr RT, Alberts DS, Chen HS: The limited role of corticosteroids in ameliorating experimental doxorubicin skin toxicity in the mouse. Cancer Chemother Pharmacol 5: 17–20, 1980.
[28] Coleman JJ, Walker AP, Didolkar MS: Treatment of adriamycin-induced skin ulcers: a prospective controlled study. J Surg Oncol 22: 129–135, 1983.

[29] Petro JA, Graham WP, Miller SH, et al: Experimental and clinical studies of ulcers induced with adriamycin. Surg Forum 30: 535–537, 1979.
[30] Cohen SC, DiBella NJ, Michalak JC: Recall injury from adriamycin. Ann Intern Med 83: 232, 1975.
[31] Etcubanas E, Wilbur JR: Uncommon side effects of adriamycin (NSC-123127). Cancer Chemother Rep 58: 757–758, 1974.
[32] Ostrowski MJ: An unusual allergic reaction in a vein following intravenous adriamycin. Clin Oncol 2: 179–180, 1976.
[33] Souhami L, Feld R: Urticaria following intravenous doxorubicin administration. JAMA 240: 1624–1626, 1978.
[34] Dorr RT, Alberts DS: Pharmacologic antidotes to experimental doxorubicin skin toxicity: a suggested role for beta-adrenergic compounds. Cancer Treat Rep 65: 1001–1006, 1981.
[35] Sonneveld P, Wassenaar HA, Nooter K: Long persistence of doxorubicin in human skin after extravasation. Cancer Treat Rep 68: 895–896, 1984.
[36] Pitkänen J, Asko-Seljavaara S, Gröhn P, et al: Adriamycin extravasation: surgical treatment and possible prevention of skin and soft-tissue injuries. J Surg Oncol 23: 259–262, 1983.
[37] Barlock AL, Howser DM, Hubbard SM: Nursing management of adriamycin extravasation. Am J Nurs 79: 94–96, 1979.
[38] Germain BS, Houlihan N, D´Amato S: Dimethyl sulfoxide therapy in the treatment of vesicant extravasation. J Intrav Nurs 17: 261–266, 1994.
[39] Bartkowski-Dodds L, Daniels JR: Use of sodium bicarbonate as a means of ameliorating doxorubicin-induced dermal necrosis in rats. Cancer Chemother Pharmacol 4: 179–181, 1980.
[40] Harwood K, Gonin R: Short term vs. long term local cooling after doxorubicin (DOX) extravasation: an eastern cooperative oncology group (ECOG) study. Proc ASCO 13: 447 (abstract 1544), 1994.
[41] Nobbs P, Barr RD: Soft-tissue injury caused by antineoplastic drugs is inhibited by topical dimethyl sulphoxide and alpha tocopherol. Br J Cancer 48: 873–876, 1983.
[42] Emiroglu M, Ercöcen AR, Demirseren ME, et al: Histopathological changes in adriamycin extravasation injury. Ann Plast Surg 41: 103–104, 1998.
[43] Cohen FJ, Manganaro J, Bezozo RC: Identification of involved tissue during surgical treatment of doxorubicin-induced extravasation necrosis. J Hand Surg 8: 43–45, 1983.
[44] Averbuch SD, Gaudiano G, Koch TH, et al: Doxorubicin-induced skin necrosis in the swine model: protection with a novel radical dimer. J Clin Oncol 4: 88–94, 1986.

D

[45] Vasilev SA, Morrow C, Morrow CP: Basic fibroblast growth factor in retardation of doxorubicin extravasation injury. Gynecol Oncol 44: 178–181, 1992.
[46] Kahn MS, Holmes JD: Reducing the morbidity from extravasation injuries. Ann Plast Surg 48: 628–632, 2002.
[47] Whang SW, Lee SH, Elias PM, et al: Intralesional steroids reduce inflammation from extravasated chemotherapeutic agents. Br J Dermatol 145: 680–682, 2001.
[48] Mouridsen HT, Langer SW, Buter J, et al: Treatment of anthracycline extravasation with Savene (dexrazoxane): results from two prospective cilinical multicentre studies. Ann Oncol 18: 546–550, 2007.
[49] Parikh PM, Ranjan S, Swami A, et al: Phlogenzym® is safe and effective in reducing morbidity of vesicant chemotherapy extravasation. A prospective study. Int J Immunother 17: 163–170, 2001.
[50] El Shagir N, Otrock Z, Mufarrij A, et al: Dexrazoxane for anthracycline extravasation and GM-CSF for skin ulceration and wound healing. Lancet Oncol 5: 320–321, 2004.
[51] Schrijvers DL: Extravasation: a dreaded complication of chemotherapy. Ann Oncol 14: iii26–iii30, 2003.
[52] Langer SW, Sehested M, Jensen PB: Treatment of anthracycline extravasation with dexrazoxane. Clin Cancer Res 6: 3680–3686, 2000.
[53] Langer SW, Sehested M, Jensen PB: Dexrazoxane is a potent and specific inhibitor of anthracycline induced subcutaneous lesions in mice. Ann Oncol 12: 405–410, 2001.
[54] Askar I, Erbas MK, Gurlek A: Effects of heparin fractions on the prevention of skin necrosis resulting from adriamycin extravasation: an experimental study. Ann Plast Surg 49: 297–301, 2002.
[55] Disa JJ, Chang RR, Mucci SJ, et al: Prevention of adriamycin-induced fullthickness skin loss using hyaluronidase infiltration. Plast Reconstr Surg 101: 370–374, 1998.
[56] Spugnini EP: Use of hyaluronidase for the treatment of extravasation of chemotherapeutic agents in six dogs. JAVMA 221: 1437–1440, 2002.
[57] Eroglu E, Sari A, Altuntas I, et al: The effect of GM-CSF (granulocyte macrophage colony stimulating factor) on doxorubicin-induced tissue necrosis and wound healing. Indian J Cancer 37: 153–157, 2000.
[58] Vargel I, Erdem A, Ertoy D, et al: Effects of growth factors on doxorubicin induced skin necrosis: documentation of histomorphological alteration and early treatment by GM-CSF. Ann Plast Surg 49: 646–653, 2002.
[59] Ultin HC, Guden M, Dede M, et al: Comparison of granulocyte-colony stimulating factor and granulocyte macrophage-colony

stimulating factor in the treatment of chemnotherapy extravasation ulcers. Eur J Gynaecol Oncol 21: 613–615, 2000.
[60] Atkas S, Toklu AS, Olgyc V: Hyperbaric oxygen therapy in adriamycin extravasation: a experimental animal study. Ann Plast Surg 45: 167–171, 2000.
[61] Monstrey SJ, Mullick P, Naranyanan K, et al: Hyperbaric oxygen therapy and free radical production: a experimental study in doxorubicin (adriamycin) extravasation injuries. Ann Plast Surg 36: 163–168, 1997.]

D

Secondary literature

[62] Ignoffo RJ, Friedman MA: Therapy of local toxicities caused by extravasation of cancer chemotherapeutic drugs. Cancer Treat Rev 7: 17–27, 1980.
[63] Köstering H, Nagel GA: Prophylaxe und Therapie von Zytostatika-Hautnekrosen. Onkologie 6: 317–320, 1980.
[64] Bertelli G: Prevention and management of extravasation of cytotoxic drugs. Drug Safety 12: 245–255, 1995.
[65] Schneider G: Paravasate von Zytostatika. Diagnostik und Therapie. Aina S. Schneider Verlag, 6th edition: 1–17, 1999.
[66] Stanley A: Managing complications of chemotherapy administration. In: Allwood M, Stanley A, Wright P (eds) The Cytotoxics Handbook. Radcliffe Medical Press, 4th edition: 119–193, 2002.
[67] Krämer I, Stützle M: Zytostatika-Paravasation – Wie ist vorzugehen? Krankenhauspharmazie 23: 261–268, 2002.
[68] Gain M, Melzer S, Meyer-Jürshof A, et al: Doxorubicin: Behandlung von Paravasaten: In: Gain M, et al (eds) ADKA-Zytostatika-Handbuch, Pharmazeutisch-wissenschaftliche Monographien. Verlag Heiner Biller, vol 3: 68–69, 1998.
[69] Mullin S, Beckwith MC, Tyler LS: Prevention and management of antineoplastic extravasation injury. Hosp Pharm 35: 57–76, 2000.
[70] Dorr RT: Pharmacologic management of vesicant chemotherapy extravasations. In: Dorr RT, Von Hoff DD (eds) Cancer Chemotherapy Handbook. Appleton & Lange, 2nd edition: 109–118, 1994.
[71] Cox RF: Managing skin damage induced by doxorubicin hydrochloride and daunorubicin hydrochloride. Am J Hosp Pharm 41: 2410–2414, 1984.
[72] Rospond RM: Utilization of dimethyl sulfoxide for treating anthracycline extravasation. J Oncol Pharm Practice 1: 33–39, 1995.
[73] Rudolph R, Larson DL: Etiology and treatment of chemotherapeutic agent extravasation injuries: a review. J Clin Oncol 5: 1116–1126, 1987.
[74] Dorr RT: Antidotes to vesicant chemotherapy extravasations. Blood Rev 4: 41–60, 1990.

[75] Kraft A, Weinig S, Edinger M, et al: Anthrazyklin-Extravasate. Der Onkologe 6: 674–686, 2000.
[76] Gain M, Melzer S, Meyer-Jürshof A, et al: Allgemeiner Teil: Behandlung von Paravasaten. In: Gain M, et al (eds) ADKA-Zytostatika-Handbuch, Pharmazeutisch-wissenschaftliche Monographien. Verlag Heiner Biller, vol 1, 2nd edition: A42–44, 1997.
[77] Jordan K, Grothe W, Schmoll HJ: Paravasation von Zytostatika: Prävention und Therapie. Dtsch Med Wochenschr 130: 33–37, 2005.
[78] Ener RA, Meglathery SB, Styler M: Extravasation of systemic hemato-oncological therapies. Ann Oncol 15: 858–862, 2004.
[79] Koppel RA, Boh EE: Cutaneous reactions to chemotherapeutic agents. Am J Med Sci 321: 327–335, 2001.
[80] Alley E, Green R, Schuchter L: Cutaneous toxicities of cancer therapy. Curr Opin Oncol 14: 212–216, 2002.

Further reading:

- Albanell J, Baselga J: Systemic therapy emergencies. Semin Oncol 27: 347–361, 2000.
- Andersson AP, Dahlstrøm KK: Clinical results after doxorubicin extravasation treated with excision guided by fluorescence microscopy. Eur J Cancer 29A: 1712–1714, 1993.
- Barr RD, Benton SG, Belbeck LW: Soft-tissue necrosis induced by extravasated cancer chemotherapeutic agents. J Natl Cancer Inst 66: 1129–1136, 1981.
- Barr RD, Sertic J: Soft-tissue necrosis induced by extravasated cancer chemotherapeutic agents: a study of active intervention. Br J Cancer 44: 267–269, 1981.
- Desai MH, Teres D: Prevention of doxorubicin-induced skin ulcers in the rat and pig with dimethyl sulfoxide (DMSO). Cancer Treat Rep 66: 1371–1374, 1982.
- Diekmann J, Ransom J: Extravasation of doxorubicin from a hickman catheter: a case presentation. Oncol Nurs Forum 12: 50–52, 1985.
- Disa JJ, Chang RR, Mucci SJ, et al: Prevention of adriamycin-induced fullthickness skin loss using hyaluronidase infiltration. Plast Reconstr Surg 101: 370–374, 1998.
- Donaldson SS, Glick JM, Wilbur JR: Adriamycin activating a recall phenomenon after radiation therapy. Ann Intern Med 81: 407–408, 1974.
- Dorr RT, Alberts DS: Failure of DMSO and vitamin E to prevent doxorubicin skin ulceration in the mouse. Cancer Treat Rep 67: 499–501, 1983.

- Dorr RT, Alberts DS, Stone A: Cold protection and heat enhancement of doxorubicin skin toxicity in the mouse. Cancer Treat Rep 69: 431–437, 1985.
- Fenchel K, Karthaus M: Zytostatika-Paravasate – gibt es neue Empfehlungen zum therapeutischen Vorgehen? Wien Med Wochenschr 151: 44–46, 2001.
- Harwood KV: Treatment of anthracycline extravasation – recommendations for practice. J Clin Oncol 5: 1705, 1987.
- Harwood KV, Bachur N: Evaluation of dimethyl sulfoxide and local cooling as antidotes for doxorubicin extravasation in a pig model. Oncol Nurs Forum 14: 39–44, 1987.
- Ignoffo RJ, Tomlin W, Rubinstein E, et al: A model for skin toxicity of antineoplastic drugs: doxorubicin (DOX), mitomycin-C (MMC), and vincristine (VCR). Clin Res 29: 437A, 1981.
- Kassner E: Evaluation and treatment of chemotherapy extravasation injuries. J Pediatr Oncol Nurs 17: 135–148, 2000.
- Krämer I: Zehn Jahre Dokumentation von Zytostatika-Paravasat-Ereignissen: Auswertung von 175 Paravasate-Dokumentationen. Krankenhauspharmazie 23: 269–274, 2002.
- Krämer I: Onkologische Pharmazie. In: Jaehde U, Radziwill R, Mühlebach S, et al (eds) Lehrbuch der Klinischen Pharmazie. Wissenschaftliche Verlagsgesellschaft mbH, 2nd edition: 307–336, 2003.
- Kurul S, Saip P, Aydin T: Totally implantable venous-access ports: local problems and extravasation injury. Lancet Oncol 3: 684–692, 2002.
- Langstein HN, Duman H, Seelig D, et al: Retrospective study of the management of chemotherapeutic extravasation injury. Ann Plast Surg 49: 369–374, 2002.
- Laughlin RA, Landeen JM, Habal MB: The management of inadvertent subcutaneous adriamycin infiltration. Am J Surg 137: 408–412, 1979.
- Loth TS, Eversmann WW: Treatment methods for extravasations of chemotherapeutic agents: a comparative study. J Hand Surg 11A: 388–396, 1986.
- Luedke D, Sunwoo Y, Luedke S, et al: Doxorubicin (D) induced soft tissue necrosis: occurrence despite pH manipulation. Proc AACR – ASCO 21: 330, 1980.
- Okano T, Ohnuma T, Efremidis A, et al: Doxorubicin-induced skin ulcer in the piglet. Cancer Treat Rep 67: 1075–1078, 1983.
- Preuss P, Partoft S: Cytostatic extravasations. Ann Plast Surg 19: 323–327, 1987.
- Rauh J, Pluntke S, Müller C: Paravenöse Zytostatikainjektion: Prophylaxe und Sofortmaßnahmen im Notfall. MMW Fortschr Med 146: 682–686, 2004.

- Rudolph R, Suzuki M, Luce JK: Experimental skin necrosis produced by adriamycin. Cancer Treat Rep 63: 529–537, 1979.
- Schulmeister L, Camp-Sorrell D: Chemotherapy extravasation from implanted ports. Oncol Nurs Forum 27: 531–538, 2000.
- Schwartsmann G, Sander EB, Vinholes J, et al: N-acetylcysteine protects skin lesion induced by local extravasation of doxorubicin in a rat model. Am J Pediatr Hematol Oncol 14: 280–281, 1992.
- Seyfer AE, Solimando DA: Toxic lesions of the hand associated with chemotherapy. J Hand Surg 8: 39–42, 1983.
- Svingen BA, Powis G, Appel PL, et al: Protection against adriamycin-induced skin necrosis in the rat by dimethyl sulfoxide and α-tocopherol. Cancer Res 41: 3395–3399, 1981.
- Upton PG, Yamaguchi KT, Myers S, et al: Effects of antioxidants and hyperbaric oxygen in ameliorating experimental doxorubicin skin toxicity in the rat. Cancer Treat Rep 70: 503–507, 1986.
- Vogelzang NJ: "Adriamycin flare": a skin reaction resembling extravasation. Cancer Treat Rep 63: 2067–2069, 1979.
- Wolgemuth RL, Myers CA, Luce JK, et al: Doxorubicin extravasation ulceration: animal model development and testing of potential antidotes. Proc AACR 23: 171, 1982.
- Yilmaz M, Demirdover C, Mola F: Treatment options in extravasation injury: an experimental study in rats. Plast Reconstr Surg 109: 2418–2423, 2002.
- Zweig JI, Kabakow B, Wallach RC, et al: Rational effective medical treatment of skin ulcers due to adriamycin. Cancer Treat Rep 63: 2101–2103, 1979.

Revisions by Elisabeth Nogler-Semenitz

D

Doxorubicin liposomal, Doxorubicin pegylated liposomal

CONSENSUS

Type of damage: irritant

Recommended treatment:

General measures:

1. Stop injection/infusion immediately
2. Get extravasation kit
3. Put on (sterile) gloves
4. Replace infusion lead or syringe with 5 ml disposable syringe and aspirate slowly as much as possible of the extravasated drug; **Cave!** do not exert pressure on extravasation area
5. Remove i.v. access while aspirating
6. If blisters occur: aspirate with 1 ml syringe and s.c. cannula, use new equipment for every new attempt at aspiration
7. Elevate limb and immobilise
8. Start **substance specific measures**
9. Complete extravasation documentation sheet (mention extent of extravasation)
10. Inform and instruct the patient and relatives
11. Regular control (aftercare)

Substance specific measures:

Topical cooling:

1. Apply cold, dry pack immediately for at least 1 hour (for example, using a cold-hot pack)
2. Continue several times daily for 15 minutes each time

Cave! after extravasation:

1. No flushing of i.v. access
2. No moist compresses
3. No alcohol compresses
4. No occlusive dressings

Type of damage reported in literature:

Irritant [2,8,17]

Exfoliant [11]

Low risk of necrosis [9]

Potentially vesicant [6]

Vesicant [5,10,12], with low risk of necrosis [18]

Symptoms and clinical course reported in literature:

Initial symptoms: Swelling, erythema, (8 patients) [2] persistent for months (1 patient) [4]

Delayed-onset symptoms: No data available

Residual findings: No data available

Single case report: Extravasation of up to 80 mg pegylated liposomal doxorubicin in application via port system. Initially no swelling or erythema, haematoma 1 week later, followed by necrosis with yellow coating, then eschar formation over necrosis [5]

Measures reported in literature:

Successful treatment:
- Cooling with ice for at least 30–60 minutes (8 patients) [2]
- Infiltration of heparin, cooling with ice, venous ointment (1 patient) [4]

Unsuccessful treatment:
- Cooling with ice [5]

Outcome of treatment not reported:
- Immediate treatment: infiltration of 2–5 ml sodium bicarbonate (8.4%), infiltration with 4–8 mg dexamethasone, DMSO every 3–4 hours for 3–14 days [6]

- Immediate topical cooling for 24 hours alternating with 1.5 ml topical DMSO (50%) every 6 hours; DMSO over 14 days [9]

- 100 mg hydrocortisone s.c. and i.v., hydrocortisone applied topically, ice pack. There are indications that doxorubicin is released from the liposome within 2–3 weeks, hence DMSO should be applied 8–12 hours after the extravasation event, every 2 hours over 24 hours, followed by 4 × daily over 10–14 days [11]

- Application of cold 4 × daily for 20 minutes over 3–4 days [14]

- Application of cold [17] for 30 minutes [8,12,15,16]

Particular remarks:

Animal experiments: non-vesicant [1,3]; possible mechanism: liposomal complex remains stable until resorption, thus preventing reaction of free doxorubicin with tissue [1–3,7,8]

Heparin, venous ointment: positive effect not sufficiently proved

Cooling: positive effects have been reported [2,4]

The European Medicines Agency (EMEA) has a report of necrosis after extravasation of pegylated liposomal doxorubicin [11]

In 9 cases of extravasation with liposomal doxorubicin (Myocet®), no serious skin damage, ulceration, or necroses were found [14]

Animal studies [1, 3] were conducted with liposomal doxorubicin that had been produced in the laboratory. It is assumed that pegylated liposomal doxorubicin leads to identical reactions as liposomal doxorubicin in the event of an extravasation.

D

Conclusion:

The liposomal formulation seems to be less damaging than conventional doxorubicin [8]; doxorubicin liposomal is therefore classified as irritant

Owing to little experience with extravasations of (pegylated) doxorubicin liposomal, a final classification of the type of damage is not possible

Exclusively, the application of topical cooling is recommended; the lipid solving attribute of DMSO may cause a release of doxorubicin from the liposomes and may result in greater damage [1,8]

Original articles

[1] Forssen EA, Tökes´ ZA: Attenuation of dermal toxicity of doxorubicin by liposome encapsulation. Cancer Treat Rep 67: 481–484, 1983.
[2] Madhavan S, Northfelt DW: Lack of vesicant injury following extravasation of liposomal doxorubicin. J Natl Cancer Inst 87: 1556–1557, 1995.
[3] Balazsovits JA, Mayer LD, Bally MB, et al: Analysis of the effect of liposome encapsulation on the vesicant properties, acute and cardiac toxicities, and antitumor efficacy of doxorubicin. Cancer Chemother Pharmacol 23: 81–86, 1989.
[4] Schmidmair M: personal communication, May 1999.
[5] Lokich J: Doxil extravasation injury: a case report. Ann Oncol 10: 735–736, 1999.

Secondary literature

[6] van Gemmern R: Gewebstoxizität und Paravasatbehandlung neuer Zytostatika. Krankenhauspharmazie 17: 471–473, 1996.
[7] Dezube BJ: Safety assessment: Doxil® (doxorubicin HCl liposome injection) in refractory AIDS-related Kaposi s sarcoma. Doxil Clinical Series 1: 1–7, 1997.
[8] Mullin S, Beckwith MC, Tyler LS: Prevention and management of antineoplastic extravasation injury. Hosp Pharm 35: 57–76, 2000.
[9] Dorr RT: Antidotes to vesicant chemotherapy extravasations. Blood Rev 4: 41–60, 1990.

[10] Bertelli G: Prevention and management of extravasation of cytotoxic drugs. Drug Safety 12: 245–255, 1995.
[11] Stanley A: Managing complications of chemotherapy administration. In: Allwood M, Stanley A, Wright P (eds) The Cytotoxics Handbook. Radcliffe Medical Press, 4th edition: 119–193, 2002.
[12] Gain M, Melzer S, Meyer-Jürshof A, et al: Pegyliertes liposomales Doxorubicin: Behandlung von Paravasaten. In: Gain M, et al (eds) ADKA-Zytostatika-Handbuch, Pharmazeutisch-wissenschaftliche Monographien. Verlag Heiner Biller, vol 7: 49, 2003.
[13] Gain M, Melzer S, Meyer-Jürshof A, et al: Liposomales Doxorubicin: Behandlung von Paravasaten. In: Gain M, et al (eds) ADKA-Zytostatika-Handbuch, Pharmazeutisch-wissenschaftliche Monographien. Verlag Heiner Biller, vol 7: 38, 2003.
[14] Krämer I, Stützle M: Zytostatika-Paravasation – Wie ist vorzugehen? Krankenhauspharmazie 23: 261–268, 2002.
[15] Summary of product characteristics Myocet® (Germany), Elan Pharma, October 2002.
[16] Summary of product characteristics Caelyx® (Austria), SP Europe, Belgien, January 2003.
[17] Jordan K, Grothe W, Schmoll HJ: Paravasation von Zytostatika: Prävention und Therapie. Dtsch Med Wochenschr 130: 33–37, 2005.
[18] Ener RA, Meglathery SB, Styler M: Extravasation of systemic hemato-oncological therapies. Ann Oncol 15: 858–862, 2004.

Further reading:

- Krämer I: Onkologische Pharmazie. In: Jaehde U, Radziwill R, Mühlebach S, et al (eds) Lehrbuch der Klinischen Pharmazie. Wissenschaftliche Verlagsgesellschaft mbH, 2nd edition: 307–336, 2003.

Revisions by Elisabeth Nogler-Semenitz

D

Epirubicin

CONSENSUS

Type of damage: vesicant

Recommended treatment:

General measures:

1. Stop injection/infusion immediately
2. Get extravasation kit
3. Put on (sterile) gloves
4. Replace infusion lead or syringe with 5 ml disposable syringe and aspirate slowly as much as possible of the extravasated drug; **Cave!** do not exert pressure on extravasation area
5. Remove i.v. access while aspirating
6. If blisters occur: aspirate with 1 ml syringe and s.c. cannula, use new equipment for every new attempt at aspiration
7. Elevate limb and immobilise
8. Start **substance specific measures**
9. Ensure adequate analgesia
10. Complete extravasation documentation sheet (mention extent of extravasation)
11. Inform and instruct the patient and relatives
12. Regular control (aftercare)
13. Always consult a (plastic) surgeon within 24 hours

Substance specific measures:

DMSO:

1. Apply DMSO (99%) every 8 hours (e.g. with a sterile gauze pad) without pressure
2. Allow to air-dry – **Cave!** do not cover
3. Continue for a minimum of 7 days

Immediately afterwards topical cooling:

1. Apply cold, dry pack immediately for at least 1 hour (for example, using a cold-hot pack)
2. Continue several times daily for 15 minutes each time

or as alternative intervention to DMSO/cooling

Dexrazoxane:

1. Administer 1000 mg dexrazoxane /m^2 i.v. within six hours after extravasation
2. Repeat the i.v. treatment on day 2 (1000 mg dexrazoxane /m^2) and on day 3 (500 mg dexrazoxane /m^2)

Cave! after extravasation:

1. No flushing of i.v. access
2. No moist compresses
3. No alcohol compresses
4. No occlusive dressings

Type of damage reported in literature: Vesicant [1,2,12–20,22]

Symptoms and clinical course reported in literature:

Initial symptoms: Pain, erythema (1 patient) [6]

Delayed-onset symptoms: Blistering, swelling, erythema (1 patient) [6], thrombophlebitis [15], necroses [15] (2 patients) [2,6]

Residual findings: Induration [2], hyperpigmentation [2, 5], dry crust (1 patient) [7]

Single case report: Extravasation in patient with Port-a-cath system: pain, fever, pleural effusions, after 12 months symptom-free (1 patient) [9]

Measures reported in literature:

Successful treatment:

- 4 drops DMSO (99%) per 10 cm^2 applied topically to an area twice the size of the affected area, repeat every 8 hours for 1 week or until symptoms have subsided; local cooling (cold-hot pack) for 60 minutes, every 8 hours for 3 days (19 patients [1,12] and 42 patients [2])

E

- 5–90 minutes after extravasation: infiltration of 500 mg hydrocortisone, application of betamethasone-gentamicin ointment every 12 hours for 2 days, then every 24 hours until healing is complete (11 and 12 patients) [4,5]; more than 5 days after extravasation: application of keratolytic ointment containing salicylic acid for 5 hours (8 patients) [4]; additionally infiltration of sodium thiosulfate solution (2%) followed by massage reduced the time of healing from 16 to 9 days (11 patients) [5]

- Ice cooling, DMSO (99%) applied topically, after 20 minutes, application of DMSO stopped because of pain and erythema. Hydrocortisone applied topically, cooling over 12 hours. 1000 mg dexrazoxane i.v. over 15 minutes, followed by daily hydrocortisone applied topically [7]

- Dexrazoxane 1000 mg/m^2 within 5 hours after extravasation event on day 1, 1000 mg/m^2 on day 2, 500 mg/m^2 on day 3. Healing complete after 3 months, only side effect: temporary raise in liver transaminases and leucopenia [8]

- Symptomatic therapy (1 patient with central venous extravasation) [9]

- Administration of dexrazoxane within 6 hours after extravasation, 1000 mg dexrazoxane /m^2 i.v. on day 1 to be repeated on day 2 (1000 mg/m^2) and on day 3 (500 mg/m^2) (40 patients) [10]

Unsuccessful treatment:

- Infiltration of prednisolone s.c., after 7 days: 3 × daily DMSO (99%) and ice packs over 1 hour, additionally, hyaluronic acid-gauze dressing, antibiotics i.m. (1 patient) [6]

Outcome of treatment not reported:

- Bromelin, trypsin, and rutin combination: 1 tablet 3 × daily p.o. over 1 month. At the start of treatment within 24 hours: cold compresses and hydrocortisone (3 patients) [11]

- Topical DMSO every 6–8 hours for several days, topical cooling [12]

- Ice packs over 1–3 days, topical application of DMSO (70–100%) every 3–4 hours for 3–14 days, early consultation of plastic surgeon [13]

- DMSO (99%) every 6 hours over 3–14 days, immediate cold compresses for 20 minutes, then 4 × daily for 20 minutes over 3–4 days[14]

- 4 drops DMSO (99%) per 10 cm^2 skin surface (treatment area: twice the size of the extravasation area), every 8 hours for at least 14 days, optional topical cooling with ice packs sequentially to DMSO treatment; in case of persistent pain or development of skin necrosis or ulceration consider surgical débridement [15,19]

- On the first day DMSO every 2 hours, topical hydrocortisone (1%), and cold compresses for 30 minutes, for 7–10 days alternating DMSO or topical hydrocortisone at 3 hourly intervals [17]

- DMSO (99%) applied topically to an area twice the size of the affected area, every 6 hours over 14 days, optional ice pack for 15 minutes every 6 hours for 2 days [18]

- Immediate cooling over 24 hours alternating 1.5 ml DMSO (50%) applied topically every 6 hours; DMSO for 14 days [20]

E

- Dry cold applied immediately for 1 hour, subsequently several times daily over 15 minutes; DMSO (99%) every 8 hours over 8 days; maintain therapy free interval between cold pack and DMSO [21]
- 1–2 ml DMSO (50–99%) applied topically to an area twice the size of the affected area, every 6–8 hours over 7–14 days, ice packs [22]

E

Particular remarks:

With regard to the risk of necrosis and the treatment after extravasation, epirubicin is often compared with doxorubicin [12–14]

Recall phenomenon: renewed ulceration of a healed extravasate lesion after a second application 1 month later (1 patient) [2]

Corticosteroids: positive effect is questionable, because extravasations are only rarely accompanied by inflammatory processes [12,13,19] (see chapter "Histopathological investigations")

DMSO and cooling: reports about a positive effect in preventing necroses exists [1,2]. Cave! Local cooling alone is not sufficient [19]

Gentamicin: only for prophylaxis of secondary infection, no causal treatment of extravasation

Sodium thiosulfate: positive effect not sufficiently proved—invasive measure! [5]

Conclusion:

In analogy to the chemically related compound doxorubicin, epirubicin is classified as vesicant

The non-invasive measures DMSO and topical cooling are well established after extravasation of doxorubicin; therefore, they are also recommended for epirubicin; as an alternative intervention, the i.v. administration of dexrazoxane has proven to be effective, if started within 6 hours after the extravasation event

Original articles

[1] Bertelli G, Dini D, Forno G, et al: Dimethylsulphoxide and cooling after extravasation of antitumour agents. Lancet 341: 1098–1099, 1993.
[2] Bertelli G, Gozza A, Forno GB, et al: Topical dimethylsulfoxide for the prevention of soft tissue injury after extravasation of vesicant cytotoxic drugs: a prospective clinical study. J Clin Oncol 13: 2851–2855, 1995.
[3] Kappel B, Hindenburg AA, Taub RN: Treatment of anthracycline extravasation – a warning against the use of sodium bicarbonate. J Clin Oncol 5: 825–826, 1987.
[4] Tsavaris NB, Karagiaouris P, Tzannou I, et al: Conservative approach to the treatment of chemotherapy-induced extravasation. J Dermatol Surg Oncol 16: 519–522, 1990.
[5] Tsavaris NB, Komitsopoulou P, Karagiaouris P, et al: Prevention of tissue necrosis due to accidental extravasation of cytostatic drugs by a conser-vative approach. Cancer Chemother Pharmacol 30: 330–333, 1992.
[6] Dini D, Forno G, Gozza A, et al: Combined management in the treatment of epidoxorubicin extravasation: a case report. Support Care Cancer 3: 150–152, 1995.
[7] Bos AME, van der Graaf WTA, Willemse PHB: A new conservative approach to extravasation of anthracyclines with dimethylsulfoxide and dexrazoxane. Act Oncol 40: 541–542, 2001.
[8] Langer SW, Sehested M, Jansen PB, et al: Dexrazoxane in anthracycline extravasation. J Clin Oncol 18: 3064, 2000.
[9] Bozkurt AK, Uzel B, Akman C, et al: Intrathoracic extravasation of antineoplastic agents. Am J Clin Oncol 26: 121–123, 2003.
[10] Mouridsen HT, Langer SW, Buter J, et al: Treatment of anthracycline extravasation with Savene (dexrazoxane): results from two prospective cilinical multicentre studies. Ann Oncol 18: 546-550, 2007.
[11] Parikh PM, Ranjan S, Swami A, et al: Phlogenzym® is safe and effective in reducing morbidity of vesicant chemotherapy extravasation. A prospective study. Int J Immunother 17: 163–170, 2001.

Secondary literature

[12] Bertelli G: Prevention and management of extravasation of cytotoxic drugs. Drug Safety 12: 245–255, 1995.
[13] Schneider G: Paravasate von Zytostatika. Diagnostik und Therapie. Aina S. Schneider Verlag, 6th edition: 1–17, 1999.
[14] Krämer I, Stützle M: Zytostatika-Paravasation – Wie ist vorzugehen? Krankenhauspharmazie 23: 261–268, 2002.

E

[15] Gain M, Melzer S, Meyer-Jürshof A, et al: Epirubicin: Behandlung von Paravasaten. In: Gain M, et al (eds) ADKA-Zytostatika-Handbuch, Pharmazeutisch-wissenschaftliche Monographien. Verlag Heiner Biller, vol 6: 37–38, 2002.
[16] Dorr RT, Von Hoff DD: Drug monographs: epirubicin. In: Dorr RT, Von Hoff DD (eds) Cancer Chemotherapy Handbook. Appleton & Lange, 2nd edition: 434–439, 1994.
[17] Stanley A: Managing complications of chemotherapy administration. In: Allwood M, Stanley A, Wright P (eds) The Cytotoxics Handbook. Radcliffe Medical Press, 4th edition: 119–193, 2002.
[18] Mullin S, Beckwith MC, Tyler LS: Prevention and management of antineoplastic extravasation injury. Hosp Pharm 35: 57–76, 2000.
[19] Kraft A, Weinig S, Edinger M, et al: Anthrazyklin-Extravasate. Der Onkologe 6: 674–686, 2000.
[20] Dorr RT: Antidotes to vesicant chemotherapy extravasations. Blood Rev 4: 41–60, 1990.
[21] Jordan K, Grothe W, Schmoll HJ: Paravasation von Zytostatika: Prävention und Therapie. Dtsch Med Wochenschr 130: 33–37, 2005.
[22] Ener RA, Meglathery SB, Styler M: Extravasation of systemic hemato-oncological therapies. Ann Oncol 15: 858–862, 2004.

Further reading:

- Alley E, Green R, Schuchter L: Cutaneous toxicities of cancer therapy. Curr Opin Oncol 14: 212–216, 2002.
- Fenchel K, Karthaus M: Zytostatika-Paravasate – gibt es neue Empfehlungen zum therapeutischen Vorgehen? Wien Med Wochenschr 151: 44–46, 2001.
- Kahn MS, Holmes JD: Reducing the morbidity from extravasation injuries. Ann Plast Surg 48: 628–632, 2002.
- Krämer I: Zehn Jahre Dokumentation von Zytostatika-Paravasat-Ereignissen: Auswertung von 175 Paravasate-Dokumentationen. Krankenhauspharmazie 23: 269–274, 2002.
- Krämer I: Onkologische Pharmazie. In: Jaehde U, Radziwill R, Mühlebach S, et al (eds) Lehrbuch der Klinischen Pharmazie. Wissenschaftliche Verlagsgesellschaft mbH, 2nd edition: 307–336, 2003.
- Preuss P, Partoft S: Cytostatic extravasations. Ann Plast Surg 19: 323–327, 1987.
- Rauh J, Pluntke S, Müller C: Paravenöse Zytostatikainjektion: Prophylaxe und Sofortmaßnahmen im Notfall. MMW Fortschr Med 146: 682–686, 2004.

E

- Rauthe G, Altmann C: Venous port systems in the field of gynaecological oncology. Eur J Gynaec Oncol 21: 173–178, 1998.
- Schrijvers DL: Extravasation: a dreaded complication of chemotherapy. Ann Oncol 14: iii26–iii30, 2003.
- Webster PJ, D'Souza D: Extravasation of epirubicin/vincristine and ifosfamide/mesna from a central venous catheter. J Oncol Pharm Practice 1: 41–44, 1995.

Revisions by Elisabeth Nogler-Semenitz

Estramustine

CONSENSUS

Type of damage: non-vesicant

Recommended treatment:

General measures:

1. Stop injection/infusion immediately
2. Get extravasation kit
3. Put on (sterile) gloves
4. Replace infusion lead or syringe with 5 ml disposable syringe and aspirate slowly as much as possible of the extravasated drug; **Cave!** do not exert pressure on extravasation area
5. Remove i.v. access while aspirating
6. Elevate limb and immobilise
7. Complete extravasation documentation sheet (mention extent of extravasation)
8. Inform and instruct the patient and relatives
9. Regular control (aftercare)

Substance specific measures: none

Cave! after extravasation:

1. No flushing of i.v. access
2. No moist compresses
3. No alcohol compresses
4. No occlusive dressings

Type of damage reported in literature:

Unknown tissue toxic potential [9]

Non-vesicant [1]

Irritant [8]

Vesicant [3,5]

Symptoms and clinical course reported in literature:

No data available

Measures reported in literature:

Successful treatment:
- No data available

Unsuccessful treatment:
- No data available

Outcome of treatment not reported:
- Glucose 5% (no further details about type of administration), cooling with ice or local anaesthetic, corticosteroids applied topically [2]

- Infiltration with isotonic glucose solution [7] or isotonic saline solution [8], ice cooling or local anaesthetic, corticosteroids applied topically if required [7,8]

- Topical cooling 4 × daily for 20 minutes over 3–4 days [9]

- No specific measures mentioned [1,5]

Particular remarks:

Results of literature search: no animal experiments or clinical studies regarding extravasation have been published

Thrombophlebitis at the injection site [2,4,6] is not associated with extravasation

Conclusion:

Although estramustine is classified as irritant/vesicant in some of the literature, no clinical case of tissue damage after extravasation has been documented; the substance is therefore classified as non-vesicant

Owing to little or no experience with extravasations of estramustine, a final classification of the type of damage is not possible

No substance specific measures can be recommended

Original articles

–

Secondary literature

[1] Pharmacia & Upjohn, personal communication, November 1998.
[2] Summary of product characteristics Estracyt® (Austria), Pfizer, March 2004.
[3] Dorr RT: Extravasation of vesicant antineoplastics: clinical and experimental findings. Ariz Med 38: 271–275, 1981.
[4] Dorr RT, Von Hoff DD: Drug monographs: estramustine phosphate. In: Dorr RT, Von Hoff DD (eds) Cancer Chemotherapy Handbook. Appleton & Lange, 2nd edition: 443–446, 1994.
[5] Schneider SM, Distelhorst CW: Chemotherapy-induced emergencies. Semin Oncol 16: 572–578, 1989.
[6] Information for hospital pharmacists Estracyt® (Germany), Pharmacia & Upjohn, August 1997.
[7] Summary of product characteristics Estracyt® (Switzerland), Pfizer, April 2003.
[8] Gain M, Melzer S, Meyer-Jürshof A, et al: Estramustin: Behandlung von Paravasaten. In: Gain M, et al (eds) ADKA-Zytostatika-Handbuch, Pharmazeutisch-wissenschaftliche Monographien. Verlag Heiner Biller, vol 6: 30–31, 2002.
[9] Krämer I, Stützle M: Zytostatika-Paravasation – Wie ist vorzugehen? Krankenhauspharmazie 23: 261–268, 2002.

Revisions by Patrizia Fürst-Weger

Etoposide

CONSENSUS

Type of damage: irritant

Recommended treatment:

General measures:

1. Stop injection/infusion immediately
2. Get extravasation kit
3. Put on (sterile) gloves
4. Replace infusion lead or syringe with 5 ml disposable syringe and aspirate slowly as much as possible of the extravasated drug; **Cave!** do not exert pressure on extravasation area
5. Remove i.v. access while aspirating
6. If blisters occur: aspirate with 1 ml syringe and s.c. cannula, use new equipment for every new attempt at aspiration
7. Elevate limb and immobilise
8. Complete extravasation documentation sheet (mention extent of extravasation)
9. Inform and instruct the patient and relatives
10. Regular control (aftercare)

Substance specific measures: none

Cave! after extravasation:

1. No flushing of i.v. access
2. No moist compresses
3. No alcohol compresses
4. No occlusive dressings

E

Type of damage reported in literature:

Non-vesicant [3,8]

Weak irritant (not vesicant) [15]

Irritant [6,9,10,13–15,21,23] and/or weak vesicant in case of extravasation of large amounts and high concentrations [7]

Low necrotic potential [4,5,20]

Vesicant [11]

Symptoms and clinical course reported in literature:

Initial symptoms: Erythema, pain, induration (30 patients) [2], inflammatory reactions [18]

Delayed-onset symptoms: No data available

Residual findings: No data available

According to the summary of product characteristics no ulcerations occur [18]

Measures reported in literature:

Successful treatment:
- Animal experiments: NaCl 0.9% or hyaluronidase i.d. [1]

Unsuccessful treatment:
- No data available

Outcome of treatment not reported:
- After extravasation in the context of combination chemotherapy with cisplatin, etoposide, and vindesine (extravasated substance not identified): local treatment with glucocorticoid (1 patient) [2]

- After extravasation in the context of combination chemotherapy with cisplatin and etoposide, carboplatin and etoposide, or ifosfamide and etoposide (extravasated substance not identified): no specific measures mentioned (1 patient each) [2]

- Optional local infiltration of corticosteroids, warm to hot compresses for 1 hour [3]
- 150 IU hyaluronidase in 1–3 ml NaCl 0.9% injected into site [4, 9]
- Mild, dry heat over 1–2 hours, 150–900 IU hyaluronidase s.c., alternatively: DMSO every 3–4 hours for 1–3 days administered locally [5]
- Warm compresses immediately applied for 30–60 minutes, then for 24 hours alternating every 15 minutes (with/without compresses), 150 IU hyaluronidase s.c. [7]
- 100 mg hydrocortisone s.c. and i.v., respectively, ice or cold pack 4 × daily for 15–20 minutes, topical hydrocortisone [8, 13]
- 100 mg hydrocortisone s.c. and i.v., additionally, hydrocortisone applied topically, ice packs [10]
- 150-900 IU hyaluronidase s.c. or i.d. [10], and warm compresses [15]
- 150 IU hyaluronidase s.c. in case of extravasation of ≥50% of the planned total dosis [19]
- Mild heat over 1–2 hours, in severe cases additionally 150 IU hyaluronidase s.c. [23]
- No specific measures mentioned [2 (27 patients),14,16]

Particular remarks: Animal experiments: ulceration after i.d. undiluted administration is due to the excipients; less ulcerogenic effect with diluted solutions [1,11]

E

Phlebitis [4,5,7,10,17,18] and hypersensitivity reactions [10,12,18,21] are not associated with extravasation; these symptoms are most likely to be due to the excipients in the formulation (polysorbate 80, ethanol, and polyethylenglycol 300 [18,21])

Recall phenomena described after radiotherapy [21,22]

In formulations that contain benzyl alcohol, extravasation of etoposide may initially be painless and remain unnoticed (local anaesthetic effect) [23]

Hyaluronidase and NaCl 0.9%: positive effect reported only in animal experiment [1]; disadvantage: invasive measure

There is no clinical evidence for the application of hyaluronidase after extravasation of etoposide, in spite of recent reports in the literature [10,23]

Cooling: avoid cooling since crystallisation of etoposide may occur [6]

Heat: increased absorption [6,15]

Conclusion:

Although etoposide is classified as vesicant in some of the literature, no clinical case of necrosis after extravasation has been documented; the substance is classified as irritant due to the excipients in the formulation

Symptoms mentioned in the secondary literature, such as necroses, could not be verified in clinical case reports

Positive results of substance specific measures have not been described so far; until further data become available no substance specific measures can be recommended

Original articles

[1] Dorr RT, Alberts DS: Skin ulceration potential without therapeutic anticancer activity for epipodophyllotoxin commercial diluents. Invest New Drugs 1: 151–159, 1983.
[2] Krämer I: Zehn Jahre Dokumentation von Zytostatika-Paravasat-Ereignissen: Auswertung von 175 Paravasate-Dokumentationen. Krankenhauspharmazie 23: 269–274, 2002.

E

Secondary literature

[3] Ignoffo RJ, Friedman MA: Therapy of local toxicities caused by extravasation of cancer chemotherapeutic drugs. Cancer Treat Rev 7: 17–27, 1980.
[4] Dorr RT: Antidotes to vesicant chemotherapy extravasations. Blood Rev 4: 41–60, 1990.
[5] Schneider G: Paravasate von Zytostatika. Diagnostik und Therapie. Aina S. Schneider Verlag, 6th edition: 1–17, 1999.
[6] Krämer I: Zytostatika-Paravasate-Set. Krankenhauspharmazie 13: 154–160, 1992.
[7] Dorr RT: Pharmacologic management of vesicant chemotherapy extravasations. In: Dorr RT, Von Hoff DD (eds) Cancer Chemotherapy Handbook. Appleton & Lange, 2nd edition: 109–118, 1994.
[8] Donislawski S, Gain M, Meyer-Jürshof A, et al: Etoposid: Behandlung von Paravasaten. In: Donislawski S, et al (eds) ADKA-Zytostatika-Handbuch, Pharmazeutisch-wissenschaftliche Monographien. Verlag Heiner Biller, vol 2: 33, 1994.
[9] Bristol-Myers Squibb, personal communication, January 1999.
[10] Stanley A: Managing complications of chemotherapy administration. In: Allwood M, Stanley A, Wright P (eds) The Cytotoxics Handbook. Radcliffe Medical Press, 4th edition: 119–193, 2002.
[11] Bertelli G: Prevention and management of extravasation of cytotoxic drugs. Drug Safety 12: 245–255, 1995.
[12] Bokemeyer C: Dermatoxizität antineoplastischer Substanzen. In: Schmoll HJ, Höffken K, Possinger K (eds) Kompendium Internistische Onkologie. Standards in Diagnostik und Therapie. Springer, vol 1, 3rd edition: 1411–1426, 1999.
[13] Gain M, Melzer S, Meyer-Jürshof A, et al: Allgemeiner Teil: Behandlung von Paravasaten. In: Gain M, et al (eds) ADKA-Zytostatika-Handbuch, Pharmazeutisch-wissenschaftliche Monographien. Verlag Heiner Biller, vol 1, 2nd edition: A42–44, 1997.
[14] Mullin S, Beckwith MC, Tyler LS: Prevention and management of antineoplastic extravasation injury. Hosp Pharm 35: 57–76, 2000.
[15] Schneider SM, Distelhorst CW: Chemotherapy-induced emergencies. Semin Oncol 16: 572–578, 1989.

[16] Barth J: Paravasate und deren Behandlung. In: Barth J (ed) Zytostatika-Herstellung in der Apotheke. Deutscher Apotheker Verlag, chapter VI-3: 1–9, 2000.
[17] Dorr RT, Von Hoff DD: Drug monographs: etoposide. In: Dorr RT, Von Hoff DD (eds) Cancer Chemotherapy Handbook. Appleton & Lange, 2nd edition: 459–472, 1994.
[18] Summary of product characteristics Vepesid® (Germany), Bristol-Myers Squibb, February 2005.
[19] Albanell J, Baselga J: Systemic therapy emergencies. Semin Oncol 27: 347–361, 2000.
[20] Ener RA, Meglathery SB, Styler M: Extravasation of systemic hemato-oncological therapies. Ann Oncol 15: 858–862, 2004.
[21] Alley E, Green R, Schuchter L: Cutaneous toxicities of cancer therapy. Curr Opin Oncol 14: 212–216, 2002.
[22] Koppel RA, Boh EE: Cutaneous reactions to chemotherapeutic agents. Am J Med Sci 321: 327–335, 2001.
[23] Krämer I, Stützle M: Zytostatika-Paravasation – Wie ist vorzugehen? Krankenhauspharmazie 23: 261–268, 2002.

Further reading:

- Fenchel K, Karthaus M: Zytostatika-Paravasate – gibt es neue Empfehlungen zum therapeutischen Vorgehen? Wien Med Wochenschr 151: 44–46, 2001.
- Jordan K, Grothe W, Schmoll HJ: Paravasation von Zytostatika: Prävention und Therapie. Dtsch Med Wochenschr 130: 33–37, 2005.
- Kassner E: Evaluation and treatment of chemotherapy extravasation injuries. J Pediatr Oncol Nurs 17: 135–148, 2000.
- Krämer I: Onkologische Pharmazie. In: Jaehde U, Radziwill R, Mühlebach S, et al (eds) Lehrbuch der Klinischen Pharmazie. Wissenschaftliche Verlagsgesellschaft mbH, 2nd edition: 307–336, 2003.
- Langstein HN, Duman H, Seelig D, et al: Retrospective study of the management of chemotherapeutic extravasation injury. Ann Plast Surg 49: 369–374, 2002.
- Otto J, Goebell PJ, Otto T: Urologischer Notfall in der Onkologie. Der Onkologe 10: 351–357, 2004.
- Rauh J, Pluntke S, Müller C: Paravenöse Zytostatikainjektion: Prophylaxe und Sofortmaßnahmen im Notfall. MMW Fortschr Med 146: 682–686, 2004.
- Schrijvers DL: Extravasation: a dreaded complication of chemotherapy. Ann Oncol 14: iii26–iii30, 2003.

E

- Sewell G: Investigational drugs: etoposide. In: Allwood M, Stanley A, Wright P (eds) The Cytotoxics Handbook. Radcliffe Medical Press, 4th edition: 339–342, 2002.
- Whang SW, Lee SH, Elias PM, et al: Intralesional steroids reduce inflammation from extravasated chemotherapeutic agents. Br J Dermatol 145: 680–682, 2001.

Revisions by Ines Mader

Etoposide phosphate

CONSENSUS

Type of damage: non-vesicant

Recommended treatment:

General measures:

1. Stop injection/infusion immediately
2. Get extravasation kit
3. Put on (sterile) gloves
4. Replace infusion lead or syringe with 5 ml disposable syringe and aspirate slowly as much as possible of the extravasated drug; **Cave!** do not exert pressure on extravasation area
5. Remove i.v. access while aspirating
6. Elevate limb and immobilise
7. Complete extravasation documentation sheet (mention extent of extravasation)
8. Inform and instruct the patient and relatives
9. Regular control (aftercare)

Substance specific measures: none

Cave! after extravasation:

1. No flushing of i.v. access
2. No moist compresses
3. No alcohol compresses
4. No occlusive dressings

Type of damage reported in literature:

Minor tissue toxic potential [1]

Inflammatory [4]

Symptoms and clinical course reported in literature:

Initial symptoms: According to the summary of product characteristics rarely irritations and inflammation [2]

Delayed-onset symptoms: No data available

Residual findings: No data available

According to the summary of product characteristics no ulceration occur [2]

Measures reported in literature:

Successful treatment:
- No data available

Unsuccessful treatment:
- No data available

Outcome of treatment not reported:
- 150 IU hyaluronidase in 1–3 ml NaCl 0.9% s.c. [1]

- 100 mg hydrocortisone i.v. and s.c., topical hydrocortisone, intermittent ice packs over 24 hours, after the local reaction has subsided, heat and compression [4]

- Local, mild heat for 1–2 hours, in severe cases 150 IU hyaluronidase s.c. [5]

Particular remarks:

Results of literature search: no animal studies or clinical studies regarding extravasation have been published

Phlebitis at the injection site [2] is not associated with extravasation

Anaphylactoid reactions to etoposide phosphate or more rarely to dextran 40 (excipient) are possible [2]

Etoposide phosphate is an atoxic prodrug [1] and is activated by phosphatases [3]; in cases of extravasation no problems are therefore to be expected

Since the formulation does not contain excipients such as ethanol or polysorbate 80, the risk of tissue damage is lower than in etoposide [1, 5]

E

Conclusion: Since no clinical case of tissue damage after extravasation of etoposide phosphate has been documented in the literature, the substance is classified as non-vesicant

Owing to little experience with extravasations of etoposide phosphate, a final classification of the type of damage is not possible

Original articles

–

Secondary literature

[1] Bristol-Myers Squibb, personal communication, January 1999.
[2] Summary of product characteristics Etopofos® (Germany), Bristol-Myers Squibb, February 2005.
[3] Hande KR: Etoposide: four decades of development of a topoisomerase II inhibitor. Eur J Cancer 43: 1514–1521, 1998.
[4] Stanley A: Managing complications of chemotherapy administration. In: Allwood M, Stanley A, Wright P (eds) The Cytotoxics Handbook. Radcliffe Medical Press, 4th edition: 119–193, 2002.
[5] Krämer I, Stützle M: Zytostatika-Paravasation – Wie ist vorzugehen? Krankenhauspharmazie 23: 261–268, 2002.

Further reading:

– Stanley A: Investigational drugs: etoposide phosphate. In: Allwood M, Stanley A, Wright P (eds) The Cytotoxics Handbook. Radcliffe Medical Press, 4th edition: 343–345, 2002.

Revisions by Ines Mader

Fludarabine

CONSENSUS

Type of damage: non-vesicant

Recommended treatment:

General measures:

1. Stop injection/infusion immediately
2. Get extravasation kit
3. Put on (sterile) gloves
4. Replace infusion lead or syringe with 5 ml disposable syringe and aspirate slowly as much as possible of the extravasated drug; **Cave!** do not exert pressure on extravasation area
5. Remove i.v. access while aspirating
6. Elevate limb and immobilise
7. Complete extravasation documentation sheet (mention extent of extravasation)
8. Inform and instruct the patient and relatives
9. Regular control (aftercare)

Substance specific measures: none

Cave! after extravasation:

1. No flushing of i.v. access
2. No moist compresses
3. No alcohol compresses
4. No occlusive dressings

Type of damage reported in literature:	Non-vesicant [1–4,7–9] Weak irritant (not vesicant) [6] Vesicant [5]
Symptoms and clinical course reported in literature:	No data available
Measures reported in literature:	**Successful treatment:** – No data available **Unsuccessful treatment:** – No data available **Outcome of treatment not reported:** – 1500 IU hyaluronidase s.c., application of heat and compression [1] – Cooling [5] 4 × daily for 20 minutes over 3–4 days [8] – No specific measures mentioned [2,4,6,7,9]
Particular remarks:	Results of literature search: no clinical studies regarding extravasation have been published Animal experiments: no relevant local reactions after extravascular, i.a., or i.m. administration of an aqueous solution of 7.5 mg/ml [3]
Conclusion:	Although fludarabine is classified as irritant/ vesicant in some of the literature, no clinical case of tissue damage after extravasation has been documented; the substance is therefore classified as non-vesicant No substance specific measures are required

F

Original articles

–

Secondary literature

[1] Stanley A: Managing complications of chemotherapy administration. In: Allwood M, Stanley A, Wright P (eds) The Cytotoxics Handbook. Radcliffe Medical Press, 4th edition: 119–193, 2002.
[2] van Gemmern R: Gewebstoxizität und Paravasatbehandlung neuer Zytostatika. Krankenhauspharmazie 17: 471–473, 1996.
[3] Summary of product characteristics Fludara® (Austria), Schering, February 2003.
[4] Gain M, Melzer S, Meyer-Jürshof A, et al: Allgemeiner Teil: Behandlung von Paravasaten. In: Gain M, et al (eds) ADKA-Zytostatika-Handbuch, Pharmazeutisch-wissenschaftliche Monographien. Verlag Heiner Biller, vol 1, 2nd edition: A42–44, 1997.
[5] Berdel WE, Schmoll HJ, Büchele T, et al: Prävention und Therapie von Paravasaten/Extravasaten. In: Schmoll HJ, Höffken K, Possinger K (eds) Kompendium Internistische Onkologie. Standards in Diagnostik und Therapie. Springer, vol 1, 3rd edition: 1689–1701, 1999.
[6] Barth J: Paravasate und deren Behandlung. In: Barth J (ed) Zytostatika-Herstellung in der Apotheke. Deutscher Apotheker Verlag, chapter VI-3: 1–9, 2000.
[7] Jordan K, Grothe W, Schmoll HJ: Paravasation von Zytostatika: Prävention und Therapie. Dtsch Med Wochenschr 130: 33–37, 2005.
[8] Krämer I, Stützle M: Zytostatika-Paravasation – Wie ist vorzugehen? Krankenhauspharmazie 23: 261–268, 2002.
[9] Fenchel K, Karthaus M: Zytostatika-Paravasate – gibt es neue Empfehlungen zum therapeutischen Vorgehen? Wien Med Wochenschr 151: 44–46, 2001.

Further reading:

- Rauh J, Pluntke S, Müller C: Paravenöse Zytostatikainjektion: Prophylaxe und Sofortmaßnahmen im Notfall. MMW Fortschr Med 146: 682–686, 2004.
- Schrijvers DL: Extravasation: a dreaded complication of chemotherapy. Ann Oncol 14: iii26–iii30, 2003.

Revisions by Sabine Wassertheurer

F

5-Fluorouracil

CONSENSUS

Type of damage: non-vesicant
irritant if used in undiluted form (pH)

Recommended treatment:

General measures:

1. Stop injection/infusion immediately
2. Get extravasation kit
3. Put on (sterile) gloves
4. Replace infusion lead or syringe with 5 ml disposable syringe and aspirate slowly as much as possible of the extravasated drug; **Cave!** do not exert pressure on extravasation area
5. Remove i.v. access while aspirating
6. If blisters occur: aspirate with 1 ml syringe and s.c. cannula, use new equipment for every new attempt at aspiration
7. Elevate limb and immobilise
8. Complete extravasation documentation sheet (mention extent of extravasation)
9. Inform and instruct the patient and relatives
10. Regular control (aftercare)

Substance specific measures: none

Cave! after extravasation:

1. No flushing of i.v. access
2. No moist compresses
3. No alcohol compresses
4. No occlusive dressings

Type of damage reported in literature:

Non-vesicant [15,20,23,26,29]

Weak irritant (not vesicant) [27]

Inflammatory [18]

Irritant [25,31] and/or weak vesicant in large amounts and at high concentrations [21]

Low risk of necroses [19,28,30]

Vesicant [3,5,7,16,22,24]

F

Symptoms and clinical course reported in literature:

Continuous central venous application (Hickman catheter, port-a-cath):

Initial symptoms: Slight fever, pleural pain (1 patient) [1]; presternal pain (1 patient receiving combination chemotherapy with epirubicin) [2]; swelling above access port (1 patient) [7]; hyperthermia, erythema, oedema (1 patient) [11]

Delayed-onset symptoms: Pericardial effusion and tachycardias over weeks and months (1 patient) [1]; increased presternal pain, pleural and pericardial effusions (1 patient receiving combination chemotherapy with epirubicin) [2]; chest pain, lung infiltrate (1 patient) [5]; skin necrosis (1 patient) [7]

Residual findings: Fibrotically reduced pulmonary lobe (1 patient) [5]

Single case report in peripheral venous application: Within a week erythema, pain; after another week hyperpigmentation and 2 small ulcers, healing with scarring, regaining of joint mobility (1 patient) [3]

Measures reported in literature:

Successful treatment:

- 4 drops of DMSO (99%) per 10 cm^2 applied topically on an area twice the size of the affected area, repeat every 8 hours over 1 week or until symptoms have subsided; local cooling for 60 minutes, every 8 hours for 3 days (cold-hot pack) (5 patients) [6]

- Cold compresses over 24 hours (1 patient) [13]
- Cold pack, oral antibiotics (1 patient) [11]
- Intralesional steroid injections (3 patients) [12]

Unsuccessful treatment:
- No substance specific measure mentioned (1 patient each) [3, 5, 7]

F

Outcome of treatment not reported:
- Optional local infiltration of corticosteroids, warm to hot compresses for 1 hour [15]
- If local symptoms develop, hydrocortisone (1%) or heparin to be applied topically combined with cold compresses (either once for 45 minutes or 20 minutes per day for 3 days) or warm compresses [16]
- 100 mg hydrocortisone s.c. and i.v., respectively, additionally topical hydrocortisone, intermittent ice pack over 24 hours; after local reaction has subsided application of heat and compression [18]
- 100 mg hydrocortisone s.c. and i.v., respectively, ice or cold pack 4 × daily over 15–20 minutes, topical hydrocortisone [20,26]
- Topical cooling [24] 4 × daily for 20 minutes over 3–4 days [31]
- No specific measures mentioned [14 (32 patients),19,21–23,27–30]

Particular remarks: Results of literature search: no animal experiments regarding extravasation have been published

After continuous central venous application subsequent pericarditis [1], pneumonitis [2,5], and after hepatic arterial chemoperfusion subsequent gastrointestinal haemorrhage [4] have been reported; in these cases substance specific as well as mechanical causes are discussed as underlying the perforation of the vessel; in one case, the base plate of a dual port perforated after only 3 venipunctures [11]

Because of the high pH, an irritant effect cannot be ruled out [31]; especially in continuous central venous application of undiluted solutions

Ulceration during peripheral venous application represents some idiosyncratic reaction [3]

Hypersensitivity reactions and recall phenomena after irradiation have been described [32]

Delayed phlebitis at the injection site [15], erythematous lesion over the veins after i.v. administration of 5-fluorouracil (1 patient) [10] as well as partly reversible hyperpigmentation of the skin in the area of the veins used for infusion [8–10,15,17,32,33] are not associated with extravasation

Corticosteroids: positive effect is questionable, because extravasations are only rarely accompanied by inflammatory processes (see chapter "Histopathological investigations")

DMSO and topical cooling: positive effects in preventing tissue damage have been reported [6]

Cooling alone: positive effect not sufficiently proved (2 patients) [11,13]

Conclusion:

5-Fluorouracil is controversially classified in the literature; considering the frequency of its use only 3 case reports of tissue damage after extravasation have been documented, which were not conclusively due to 5-fluorouracil; the substance is therefore classified as non-vesicant

In case of undiluted, continuous central venous application of 5-fluorouracil, several cases of tissue damage have been reported [1,2,5,7]; the classification is therefore irritant in the context of central venous application

No substance specific measures – such as DMSO and topical cooling – are required

F

Original articles

[1] Cathcart-Rake WF, Mowery WE: Intrapericardial infusion of 5-fluorouracil. An unusual complication of a Hickman catheter. Cancer 67: 735–737, 1991.
[2] Rodier JM, Malbec L, Lauraine EP, et al: Mediastinal infusion of epirubicin and 5-fluorouracil. A complication of totally implantable central venous systems. Report of a case. J Cancer Res Clin Oncol 122: 566–567, 1996.
[3] Teta JB, O'Connor L: Local tissue damage from 5-fluorouracil extravasation. Oncol Nurs Forum 11: 77, 1984.
[4] Ross WB, Morris DL, Clingan PR: Major upper gastrointestinal haemorrhage associated with hepatic arterial chemoperfusion. Aust N Z J Surg 66: 816–819, 1996.
[5] Manheimer F, Aranda CP, Smith RL: Necrotizing pneumonitis caused by 5-fluorouracil infusion. A complication of a Hickman catheter. Cancer 70: 554–556, 1992.
[6] Bertelli G, Gozza A, Forno GB, et al: Topical dimethylsulfoxide for the prevention of soft tissue injury after extravasation of vesicant cytotoxic drugs: a prospective clinical study. J Clin Oncol 13: 2851–2855, 1995.
[7] Reed WP, Newman KA, Applefeld MM, et al: Drug extravasation as a complication of venous access ports. Ann Intern Med 102: 788–790, 1985.
[8] Seyfer AE, Solimando DA: Toxic lesions of the hand associated with chemotherapy. J Hand Surg 8: 39–42, 1983.

[9] Hrushesky WJ: Serpentine supravenous 5-fluorouracil (NSC-19893) hyperpigmentation. Cancer Treat Rep 60: 639, 1976.
[10] Pujol RM, Rocamora V, Lopez-Pousa A, et al: Persistent supravenous erythematous eruption: a rare local complication of intravenous 5-fluorouracil therapy. J Am Acad Dermatol 39: 839–842, 1998.
[11] Nesti SP, Kavac R: 5-Fluorouracil extravasation following port failure. J Intrav Nurs 23: 176–180, 2000.
[12] Whang SW, Lee SH, Elias PM, et al: Intralesional steroids reduce inflammation from extravasated chemotherapeutic agents. Br J Dermatol 145: 680–682, 2001.
[13] Langstein HN, Duman H, Seelig D, et al: Retrospective study of the management of chemotherapeutic extravasation injury. Ann Plast Surg 49: 369–374, 2002.
[14] Krämer I: Zehn Jahre Dokumentation von Zytostatika-Paravasat-Ereignissen: Auswertung von 175 Paravasate-Dokumentationen. Krankenhauspharmazie 23: 269–274, 2002.

F

Secondary literature

[15] Ignoffo RJ, Friedman MA: Therapy of local toxicities caused by extravasation of cancer chemotherapeutic drugs. Cancer Treat Rev 7: 17–27, 1980.
[16] Cox K, Stuart-Harris R, Abdini G, et al: The management of cytotoxic-drug extravasation: guide-lines drawn up by a working party for the Clinical Oncological Society of Australia. Med J Aust 148: 185–189, 1988.
[17] Krämer I: Zytostatika-Paravasate-Set. Krankenhauspharmazie 13: 154–160, 1992.
[18] Stanley A: Managing complications of chemotherapy administration. In: Allwood M, Stanley A, Wright P (eds) The Cytotoxics Handbook. Radcliffe Medical Press, 4th edition: 119–193, 2002.
[19] Schneider G: Paravasate von Zytostatika. Diagnostik und Therapie. Aina S. Schneider Verlag, 6th edition: 1–17, 1999.
[20] Gain M, Melzer S, Meyer-Jürshof A, et al: Allgemeiner Teil: Behandlung von Paravasaten. In: Gain M, et al (eds) ADKA-Zytostatika-Handbuch, Pharmazeutisch-wissenschaftliche Monographien. Verlag Heiner Biller, vol 1, 2nd edition: A42–44, 1997.
[21] Dorr RT: Pharmacologic management of vesicant chemotherapy extravasations. In: Dorr RT, Von Hoff DD (eds) Cancer Chemotherapy Handbook. Appleton & Lange, 2nd edition: 109–118, 1994.
[22] Bertelli G: Prevention and management of extravasation of cytotoxic drugs. Drug Safety 12: 245–255, 1995.

[23] Schneider SM, Distelhorst CW: Chemotherapy-induced emergencies. Semin Oncol 16: 572–578, 1989.
[24] Berdel WE, Schmoll HJ, Büchele T, et al: Prävention und Therapie von Paravasaten/Extravasaten. In: Schmoll HJ, Höffken K, Possinger K (eds) Kompendium Internistische Onkologie. Standards in Diagnostik und Therapie. Springer, vol 1, 3rd edition: 1689–1701, 1999.
[25] Mullin S, Beckwith MC, Tyler LS: Prevention and management of antineoplastic extravasation injury. Hosp Pharm 35: 57–76, 2000.
[26] Gain M, Melzer S, Meyer-Jürshof A, et al: Fluorouracil: Behandlung von Paravasaten. In: Gain M, et al (eds) ADKA-Zytostatika-Handbuch, Pharmazeutisch-wissenschaftliche Monographien. Verlag Heiner Biller, vol 1, 2nd edition: 57, 1997.
[27] Barth J: Paravasate und deren Behandlung. In: Barth J (ed) Zytostatika-Herstellung in der Apotheke. Deutscher Apotheker Verlag, chapter VI-3: 1–9, 2000.
[28] Dorr RT: Antidotes to vesicant chemotherapy extravasations. Blood Rev 4: 41–60, 1990.
[29] Jordan K, Grothe W, Schmoll HJ: Paravasation von Zytostatika: Prävention und Therapie. Dtsch Med Wochenschr 130: 33–37, 2005.
[30] Ener RA, Meglathery SB, Styler M: Extravasation of systemic hemato-oncological therapies. Ann Oncol 15: 858–862, 2004.
[31] Krämer I, Stützle M: Zytostatika-Paravasation – Wie ist vorzugehen? Krankenhauspharmazie 23: 261–268, 2002.
[32] Koppel RA, Boh EE: Cutaneous reactions to chemotherapeutic agents. Am J Med Sci 321: 327–335, 2001.
[33] Alley E, Green R, Schuchter L: Cutaneous toxicities of cancer therapy. Curr Opin Oncol 14: 212–216, 2002.

Further reading:

- Fenchel K, Karthaus M: Zytostatika-Paravasate – gibt es neue Empfehlungen zum therapeutischen Vorgehen? Wien Med Wochenschr 151: 44–46, 2001.
- Rauh J, Pluntke S, Müller C: Paravenöse Zytostatikainjektion: Prophylaxe und Sofortmaßnahmen im Notfall. MMW Fortschr Med 146: 682–686, 2004.
- Schrijvers DL: Extravasation: a dreaded complication of chemotherapy. Ann Oncol 14: iii26–iii30, 2003.
- Schulmeister L, Camp-Sorrell D: Chemotherapy extravasation from implanted ports. Oncol Nurs Forum 27: 531–538, 2000.

Revisions by Sabine Wassertheurer

F

Fotemustine

CONSENSUS

Type of damage: irritant

Recommended treatment:

General measures:

1. Stop injection/infusion immediately
2. Get extravasation kit
3. Put on (sterile) gloves
4. Replace infusion lead or syringe with 5 ml disposable syringe and aspirate slowly as much as possible of the extravasated drug; **Cave!** do not exert pressure on extravasation area
5. Remove i.v. access while aspirating
6. If blisters occur: aspirate with 1 ml syringe and s.c. cannula, use new equipment for every new attempt at aspiration
7. Elevate limb and immobilise
8. Complete extravasation documentation sheet (mention extent of extravasation)
9. Inform and instruct the patient and relatives
10. Regular control (aftercare)

Substance specific measures: none

Cave! after extravasation:

1. No flushing of i.v. access
2. No moist compresses
3. No alcohol compresses
4. No occlusive dressings

Type of damage mentioned in literature:

Unknown tissue toxic potential [6]

Irritant [4,5,7]

Symptoms and clinical course reported in literature:

No data available

F

Measures reported in literature:

Successful treatment:
- No data available

Unsuccessful treatment:
- No data available

Outcome of treatment not reported:
- Flushing of the vein with glucose 5%, cooling with ice, corticosteroids s.c. and i.d. in allergic reactions [1,3,5]
- Topical cooling 4 × daily for 20 minutes over 3–4 days [6]
- No specific measures mentioned [4,7]

Particular remarks:

Results of literature search: no animal experiments or clinical studies regarding extravasation have been published

Phlebitis at the injection site [1,2] is not associated with extravasation; the symptoms are likely to be due to the excipient ethanol [2] in the reconstituted drug

A duration of infusion of less than 1 hour results in reduced tolerance of the substance, especially in an irritation of the intima at the injection site [2]

Conclusion: Although fotemustine is classified as irritant in the literature, no clinical case of irritation of tissue after extravasation has been documented; the classification as irritant is therefore due to the ethanol content in the reconstituted formulation

Positive results of substance specific measures have not been described so far; until further data become available no substance specific measures can be recommended

F

Original articles

–

Secondary literature

[1] van Gemmern R: Gewebstoxizität und Paravasatbehandlung neuer Zytostatika. Krankenhauspharmazie 17: 471–473, 1996.
[2] Summary of product characteristics Muphoran® (Austria), Servier, February 1999.
[3] Servier Pharma, personal communication, September 1998.
[4] Gain M, Melzer S, Meyer-Jürshof A, et al: Allgemeiner Teil: Behandlung von Paravasaten. In: Gain M, et al (eds) ADKA-Zytostatika-Handbuch, Pharmazeutisch-wissenschaftliche Monographien. Verlag Heiner Biller, vol 1, 2nd edition: A42–44, 1997.
[5] Berdel WE, Schmoll HJ, Büchele T, et al: Prävention und Therapie von Paravasaten/Extravasaten. In: Schmoll HJ, Höffken K, Possinger K (eds) Kompendium Internistische Onkologie. Standards in Diagnostik und Therapie. Springer, vol 1, 3rd edition: 1689–1701, 1999.
[6] Krämer I, Stützle M: Zytostatika-Paravasation – Wie ist vorzugehen? Krankenhauspharmazie 23: 261–268, 2002.
[7] Jordan K, Grothe W, Schmoll HJ: Paravasation von Zytostatika: Prävention und Therapie. Dtsch Med Wochenschr 130: 33–37, 2005.

Further reading:

- Rauh J, Pluntke S, Müller C: Paravenöse Zytostatikainjektion: Prophylaxe und Sofortmaßnahmen im Notfall. MMW Fortschr Med 146: 682–686, 2004.

Revisions by Patrizia Fürst-Weger

Gemcitabine

CONSENSUS

Type of damage: irritant

Recommended treatment:

General measures:

1. Stop injection/infusion immediately
2. Get extravasation kit
3. Put on (sterile) gloves
4. Replace infusion lead or syringe with 5 ml disposable syringe and aspirate slowly as much as possible of the extravasated drug; **Cave!** do not exert pressure on extravasation area
5. Remove i.v. access while aspirating
6. If blisters occur: aspirate with 1 ml syringe and s.c. cannula, use new equipment for every new attempt at aspiration
7. Elevate limb and immobilise
8. Complete extravasation documentation sheet (mention extent of extravasation)
9. Inform and instruct the patient and relatives
10. Regular control (aftercare)

Substance specific measures: none

Cave! after extravasation:

1. No flushing of i.v. access
2. No moist compresses
3. No alcohol compresses
4. No occlusive dressings

Type of damage reported in literature:

Non-vesicant [4]

No tissue toxic potential [14]

Weak irritant (not vesicant) [10]

Irritant [7–9,12,13]

Vesicant [7]

Symptoms and clinical course reported in literature:

Initial symptoms: Pain, erythema, inflammation, oedema [1]

Delayed-onset symptoms: No data available

Residual findings: No data available

Measures reported in literature:

Successful treatment:
- Cold compresses over 24 hours (1 patient) [2]

Unsuccessful treatment:
- No data available

Outcome of treatment not reported:
- 1500 IU hyaluronidase s.c, application of heat and compression [4]
- Topical cooling [7] 4 × daily for 20 minutes over 3–4 days [14]
- No specific measures mentioned [3,5,6, 8–13]

Particular remarks:

Results of literature search: no animal experiments regarding extravasation have been published

No necroses after extravasation had been documented worldwide until May 2003 [6]

Cooling: a positive effect has been reported [2]

G

Conclusion: Although gemcitabine is classified as non-vesicant in some of the literature, the occurrence of phlebitis [1, 5] implies irritant potential of the substance; gemcitabine is therefore classified as irritant

Positive results of substance specific measures, e.g. cooling, have not been proved sufficiently; until further data become available no substance specific measures can be recommended

G

Original articles

[1] Aapro MS, Martin C, Hatty S: Gemcitabine – a safety review. Anti-Cancer Drugs 9: 191–201, 1998.
[2] Langstein HN, Duman H, Seelig D, et al: Retrospective study of the management of chemotherapeutic extravasation injury. Ann Plast Surg 49: 369–374, 2002.
[3] Krämer I: Zehn Jahre Dokumentation von Zytostatika-Paravasat-Ereignissen: Auswertung von 175 Paravasate-Dokumentationen. Krankenhauspharmazie 23: 269–274, 2002.

Secondary literature

[4] Stanley A: Managing complications of chemotherapy administration. In: Allwood M, Stanley A, Wright P (eds) The Cytotoxics Handbook. Radcliffe Medical Press, 4th edition: 119–193, 2002.
[5] van Gemmern R: Gewebstoxizität und Paravasatbehandlung neuer Zytostatika. Krankenhauspharmazie 17: 471–473, 1996.
[6] Eli Lilly, peronal communication, April 2005.
[7] Berdel WE, Schmoll HJ, Büchele T, et al: Prävention und Therapie von Paravasaten/Extravasaten. In: Schmoll HJ, Höffken K, Possinger K (eds) Kompendium Internistische Onkologie. Standards in Diagnostik und Therapie. Springer, vol 1, 3rd edition: 1689–1701, 1999.
[8] Gain M, Melzer S, Meyer-Jürshof A, et al: Allgemeiner Teil: Behandlung von Paravasaten. In: Gain M, et al (eds) ADKA-Zytostatika-Handbuch, Pharmazeutisch-wissenschaftliche Monographien. Verlag Heiner Biller, vol 1, 2nd edition: A42–44, 1997.
[9] Mullin S, Beckwith MC, Tyler LS: Prevention and management of antineoplastic extravasation injury. Hosp Pharm 35: 57–76, 2000.

[10] Barth J: Paravasate und deren Behandlung. In: Barth J (ed) Zytostatika-Herstellung in der Apotheke. Deutscher Apotheker Verlag, chapter VI-3: 1–9, 2000.

[11] Gain M, Melzer S, Meyer-Jürshof A, et al: Gemcitabin: Behandlung von Paravasaten. In: Gain M, et al (eds) ADKA-Zytostatika-Handbuch, Pharmazeutisch-wissenschaftliche Monographien. Verlag Heiner Biller, vol 5: 37–38, 2001.

[12] Jordan K, Grothe W, Schmoll HJ: Paravasation von Zytostatika: Prävention und Therapie. Dtsch Med Wochenschr 130: 33–37, 2005.

[13] Ener RA, Meglathery SB, Styler M: Extravasation of systemic hemato-oncological therapies. Ann Oncol 15: 858–862, 2004.

[14] Krämer I, Stützle M: Zytostatika-Paravasation – Wie ist vorzugehen? Krankenhauspharmazie 23: 261–268, 2002.

G

Further reading:

- Fenchel K, Karthaus M: Zytostatika-Paravasate – gibt es neue Empfehlungen zum therapeutischen Vorgehen? Wien Med Wochenschr 151: 44–46, 2001.
- Rauh J, Pluntke S, Müller C: Paravenöse Zytostatikainjektion: Prophylaxe und Sofortmaßnahmen im Notfall. MMW Fortschr Med 146: 682–686, 2004.
- Schrijvers DL: Extravasation: a dreaded complication of chemotherapy. Ann Oncol 14: iii26–iii30, 2003.

Revisions by Sabine Wassertheurer

Idarubicin

CONSENSUS

Type of damage: vesicant

Recommended treatment:

General measures:

1. Stop injection/infusion immediately
2. Get extravasation kit
3. Put on (sterile) gloves
4. Replace infusion lead or syringe with 5 ml disposable syringe and aspirate slowly as much as possible of the extravasated drug; **Cave!** do not exert pressure on extravasation area
5. Remove i.v. access while aspirating
6. If blisters occur: aspirate with 1 ml syringe and s.c. cannula, use new equipment for every new attempt at aspiration
7. Elevate limb and immobilise
8. Start **substance specific measures**
9. Ensure adequate analgesia
10. Complete extravasation documentation sheet (mention extent of extravasation)
11. Inform and instruct the patient and relatives
12. Regular control (aftercare)
13. Always consult a (plastic) surgeon within 24 hours

Substance specific measures:

DMSO:

1. Apply DMSO (99%) every 8 hours (e.g. with a sterile gauze pad) without pressure
2. Allow to air-dry – **Cave!** do not cover
3. Continue for a minimum of 7 days

Immediately afterwards topical cooling:

1. Apply cold, dry pack immediately for at least 1 hour (for example, using a cold-hot pack)
2. Continue several times daily for 15 minutes each time

or as alternative intervention to DMSO/cooling

Dexrazoxane:

1. Administer 1000 mg dexrazoxane /m^2 i.v. within six hours after extravasation
2. Repeat the i.v. treatment on day 2 (1000 mg dexrazoxane /m^2) and on day 3 (500 mg dexrazoxane /m^2)

Cave! after extravasation:

1. No flushing of i.v. access
2. No moist compresses
3. No alcohol compresses
4. No occlusive dressings

Type of damage reported in literature: Vesicant [5–12]

Symptoms and clinical course reported in literature: No data available

Measures reported in literature:

Successful treatment:
- No data available

Unsuccessful treatment:
- No data available

Outcome of treatment not reported:
- Topical DMSO every 6–8 hours for several days, topical cooling [5]

- DMSO (99%) every 6 hours over 3–14 days, immediate cold compresses for 20 minutes, then 4 × daily for 20 minutes over 3–4 days[6]

- Ice packs over 1–3 days, topical application of DMSO (70–100%) every 3–4 hours for 3–14 days, early consultation of plastic surgeon [7]

- On the first day DMSO every 2 hours, topical hydrocortisone (1%) and cold compresses for 30 minutes, over 14 days every 3 hours alternating DMSO and topical hydrocortisone [7]
- 4 drops DMSO (99%) per 10 cm^2 skin surface (treatment area: twice the size of the extravasation area), every 8 hours for at least 14 days, optional topical cooling with ice packs sequentially to DMSO treatment; in case of persistent pain or development of skin necrosis or ulceration consider surgical débridement [10,11]
- Apply dry cold immediately for 1 hour, followed by several times daily over 15 minutes; DMSO (99%) every 8 hours over 8 days; maintain therapy free interval between cooling and DMSO [12]
- 1–2 ml DMSO (50–99%) to be applied immediately to an area twice the size of the extravasation area, every 6–8 hours over 7–14 days, ice packs [13]
- No specific measures mentioned [9]

Particular remarks:

After slight extravasation in 2 patients surgical intervention was not necessary – no further details about course and treatment [1]

Concerning the risk of necrosis and treatment after extravasation, idarubicin is often compared with doxorubicin, daunorubicin, and epirubicin [6–7]

Dexrazoxane: after experimental extravasation, systemic administration of dexrazoxane reduced the size of the skin lesion and shortened the healing period [4].

Conclusion:

In analogy to the chemically related substance doxorubicin, idarubicin is classified as vesicant

The non-invasive measures DMSO and topical cooling [2,3] are well-established after extravasation of doxorubicin; therefore they are also recommended for idarubicin

Although the efficacy of dexrazoxane has not been proven after extravasation of daunorubicin in terms of clinical evidence, the administration schedule of dexrazoxane established after extravasation of doxorubicin and epirubicin is applied to all anthracyclines

Original articles

[1] Lu K, Savaraj N, Kavanagh J, et al: Clinical pharmacology of 4-demethoxydaunorubicin (DMDR). Cancer Chemother Pharmacol 17: 143–148, 1986.
[2] Bertelli G, Gozza A, Forno GB, et al: Topical dimethylsulfoxide for the prevention of soft tissue injury after extravasation of vesicant cytotoxic drugs: a prospective clinical study. J Clin Oncol 13: 2851–2855, 1995.
[3] Bertelli G, Dini D, Forno G, et al: Dimethylsulphoxide and cooling after extravasation of antitumour agents. Lancet 341: 1098–1099, 1993.
[4] Langer SW, Sehested M, Jensen PB: Treatment of anthracycline extravasation with dexrazoxane. Clin Cancer Res 6: 3680–3686, 2000.

Secondary literature

[5] Bertelli G: Prevention and management of extravasation of cytotoxic drugs. Drug Safety 12: 245–255, 1995.
[6] Krämer I, Stützle M: Zytostatika-Paravasation – Wie ist vorzugehen? Krankenhauspharmazie 23: 261–268, 2002.
[7] Schneider G: Paravasate von Zytostatika. Diagnostik und Therapie. Aina S. Schneider Verlag, 6th edition: 1–17, 1999.
[8] Stanley A: Managing complications of chemotherapy administration. In: Allwood M, Stanley A, Wright P (eds) The Cytotoxics Handbook. Radcliffe Medical Press, 4th edition: 119–193, 2002.
[9] Mullin S, Beckwith MC, Tyler LS: Prevention and management of antineoplastic extravasation injury. Hosp Pharm 35: 57–76, 2000.
[10] Gain M, Melzer S, Meyer-Jürshof A, et al: Idarubicin: Behandlung von Paravasaten In: Gain M, et al (eds) ADKA-Zytostatika-Handbuch, Pharmazeutisch-wissenschaftliche Monographien. Verlag Heiner Biller, vol 7, 34–35, 2003.

[11] Kraft A, Weinig S, Edinger M, et al: Anthrazyklin-Extravasate. Der Onkologe 6: 674–686, 2000.
[12] Jordan K, Grothe W, Schmoll HJ: Paravasation von Zytostatika: Prävention und Therapie. Dtsch Med Wochenschr 130: 33–37, 2005.
[13] Ener RA, Meglathery SB, Styler M: Extravasation of systemic hemato-oncological therapies. Ann Oncol 15: 858–862, 2004.

Further reading:

- Alley E, Green R, Schuchter L: Cutaneous toxicities of cancer therapy. Curr Opin Oncol 14: 212–216, 2002.
- Fenchel K, Karthaus M: Zytostatika-Paravasate – gibt es neue Empfehlungen zum therapeutischen Vorgehen? Wien Med Wochenschr 151: 44–46, 2001.
- Krämer I: Onkologische Pharmazie. In: Jaehde U, Radziwill R, Mühlebach S, et al (eds) Lehrbuch der Klinischen Pharmazie. Wissenschaftliche Verlagsgesellschaft mbH, 2nd edition: 307–336, 2003.
- Kurul S, Saip P, Aydin T: Totally implantable venous-access ports: local problems and extravasation injury. Lancet Oncol 3: 684–692, 2002.
- Rauh J, Pluntke S, Müller C: Paravenöse Zytostatikainjektion: Prophylaxe und Sofortmaßnahmen im Notfall. MMW Fortschr Med 146: 682–686, 2004.
- Schrijvers DL: Extravasation: a dreaded complication of chemotherapy. Ann Oncol 14: iii26–iii30, 2003.

Revisions by Elisabeth Nogler-Semenitz

Ifosfamide

CONSENSUS

Type of damage: non-vesicant

Recommended treatment:

General measures:

1. Stop injection/infusion immediately
2. Get extravasation kit
3. Put on (sterile) gloves
4. Replace infusion lead or syringe with 5 ml disposable syringe and aspirate slowly as much as possible of the extravasated drug; **Cave!** do not exert pressure on extravasation area
5. Remove i.v. access while aspirating
6. Elevate limb and immobilise
7. Complete extravasation documentation sheet (mention extent of extravasation)
8. Inform and instruct the patient and relatives
9. Regular control (aftercare)

Substance specific measures: none

Cave! after extravasation:

1. No flushing of i.v. access
2. No moist compresses
3. No alcohol compresses
4. No occlusive dressings

Type of damage reported in literature:

Non-vesicant [8–12]

Weak irritant (not vesicant) [16]

Irritant [5,14,18,19]

Symptoms and clinical course reported in literature:

Initial symptoms: No data available

Delayed-onset symptoms: One day after infusion of ifosfamide: inflammation, pain (1 patient) [5]

Residual findings: No data available

Measures reported in literature:

Successful treatment:

- 4 drops DMSO (99%) per 10 cm^2 applied topically to an area twice the size of the affected area, repeat every 8 hours for 1 week or until symptoms have subsided; local cooling for 60 minutes, every 8 hours for 3 days (cold-hot pack) (10 patients) [1] and (8 patients) [3,13]

- 150 TRU chondroitin sulfatase in 3 ml NaCl 0.9%: s.c. injections of 0.5 ml each, 2 × at 12 hour intervals (1 patient) [5]

- After extravasation in the context of combination chemotherapy with ifosfamide, cisplatin, and vinorelbine (extravasated substance not identified): intralesional steroid injections (5 patients) [6]

Unsuccessful treatment:

- Diflucortolonvalerate (0.1%) applied topically every 6 hours: pain increased the next day (1 patient) [5]

Outcome of treatment not reported:

- After extravasation in the context of combination chemotherapy with ifosfamide and etoposide (extravasated substance not identified): no specific measure mentioned (1 patient) [7]

I

- 1500 IU hyaluronidase s.c., application of heat and compression [9]
- Topical cooling 4 × daily for 20 minutes over 3–4 days [10]
- Optional local infiltration of corticosteroids, warm to hot compresses for 1 hour [11]
- No specific measures mentioned [7 (3 patients),12,14,16,18,19]

Particular remarks: Animal experiments: blistering in i.d. administration of >50 mg/ml, complete healing after 21 days [2]; this reference is controversial regarding the concentration dependence of ulceration

Ifosfamide is an atoxic prodrug and is activated in the liver; no problems after extravasation are therefore to be expected [4,8,15,17]

Phlebitis at the injection site [15] is not associated with extravasation

Chondroitin sulfatase: positive effect has not been sufficiently proved; disadvantage: invasive measure

Corticosteroids: positive effect is questionable, because extravasations are only rarely accompanied by inflammatory processes (see chapter "Histopathological investigations")

DMSO and topical cooling: positive effects in preventing tissue damage have been reported [1,3]

Conclusion: Considering the very low number (only 1 case report) of documented tissue damage after extravasation and the frequency of its use, ifosfamide is classified as non-vesicant

No substance specific measures – such as DMSO and topical cooling – are required

Original articles

[1] Bertelli G, Gozza A, Forno GB, et al: Topical dimethylsulfoxide for the prevention of soft tissue injury after extravasation of vesicant cytotoxic drugs: a prospective clinical study. J Clin Oncol 13: 2851–2855, 1995.

[2] Marnocha RS, Hutson PR: Intradermal carboplatin and ifosfamide extravasation in the mouse. Cancer 70: 850–853, 1992.

[3] Bertelli G, Dini D, Forno G, et al: Dimethylsulphoxide and cooling after extravasation of antitumour agents. Lancet 341: 1098–1099, 1993.

[4] Brock N, Hilgard P, Peukert M, et al: Basis and new developments in the field of oxazaphosphorines. Cancer Invest 6: 513–532, 1988.

[5] Mateu J, Alzamora M, Franco M, et al: Ifosfamide extravasation. Ann Pharmacother 28: 1243–1244, 1994.

[6] Whang SW, Lee SH, Elias PM, et al: Intralesional steroids reduce inflammation from extravasated chemotherapeutic agents. Br J Dermatol 145: 680–682, 2001.

[7] Krämer I: Zehn Jahre Dokumentation von Zytostatika-Paravasat-Ereignissen: Auswertung von 175 Paravasate-Dokumentationen. Krankenhauspharmazie 23: 269–274, 2002.

I

Secondary literature

[8] Summary of product characteristics Holoxan® (Germany), Baxter, January 2002.

[9] Stanley A: Managing complications of chemotherapy administration. In: Allwood M, Stanley A, Wright P (eds) The Cytotoxics Handbook. Radcliffe Medical Press, 4th edition: 119–193, 2002.

[10] Krämer I, Stützle M: Zytostatika-Paravasation – Wie ist vorzugehen? Krankenhauspharmazie 23: 261–268, 2002.

[11] Ignoffo RJ, Friedman MA: Therapy of local toxicities caused by extravasation of cancer chemotherapeutic drugs. Cancer Treat Rev 7: 17–27, 1980.

[12] Gain M, Melzer S, Meyer-Jürshof A, et al: Allgemeiner Teil: Behandlung von Paravasaten. In: Gain M, et al (eds) ADKA-Zytostatika-Handbuch, Pharmazeutisch-wissenschaftliche Monographien. Verlag Heiner Biller, Vol 1, 2nd edition: A42–44, 1997.

[13] Bertelli G: Prevention and management of extravasation of cytotoxic drugs. Drug Safety 12: 245–255, 1995.

[14] Mullin S, Beckwith MC, Tyler LS: Prevention and management of antineoplastic extravasation injury. Hosp Pharm 35: 57–76, 2000.

[15] Dorr RT, Von Hoff DD: Drug monographs: ifosfamide. In: Dorr RT, Von Hoff DD (eds) Cancer Chemotherapy Handbook. Appleton & Lange, 2nd edition: 558–563, 1994.

[16] Barth J: Paravasate und deren Behandlung. In: Barth J (ed) Zytostatika-Herstellung in der Apotheke. Deutscher Apotheker Verlag, chapter VI-3: 1–9, 2000.
[17] Gain M, Melzer S, Meyer-Jürshof A, et al: Ifosfamid: Behandlung von Paravasaten. In: Gain M, et al (eds) ADKA-Zytostatika-Handbuch, Pharmazeutisch-wissenschaftliche Monographien. Verlag Heiner Biller, vol 5: 26, 2001.
[18] Ener RA, Meglathery SB, Styler M: Extravasation of systemic hemato-oncological therapies. Ann Oncol 15: 858–862, 2004.
[19] Jordan K, Grothe W, Schmoll HJ: Paravasation von Zytostatika: Prävention und Therapie. Dtsch Med Wochenschr 130: 33–37, 2005.

Further reading:

- Fenchel K, Karthaus M: Zytostatika-Paravasate – gibt es neue Empfehlungen zum therapeutischen Vorgehen? Wien Med Wochenschr 151: 44–46, 2001.
- Kassner E: Evaluation and treatment of chemotherapy extravasation injuries. J Pediatr Oncol Nurs 17: 135–148, 2000.
- Rauh J, Pluntke S, Müller C: Paravenöse Zytostatikainjektion: Prophylaxe und Sofortmaßnahmen im Notfall. MMW Fortschr Med 146: 682–686, 2004.
- Schrijvers DL: Extravasation: a dreaded complication of chemotherapy. Ann Oncol 14: iii26–iii30, 2003.

Revisions by Patrizia Fürst-Weger

Irinotecan

CONSENSUS

Type of damage: non-vesicant

Recommended treatment:

General measures:

1. Stop injection/infusion immediately
2. Get extravasation kit
3. Put on (sterile) gloves
4. Replace infusion lead or syringe with 5 ml disposable syringe and aspirate slowly as much as possible of the extravasated drug; **Cave!** do not exert pressure on extravasation area
5. Remove i.v. access while aspirating
6. Elevate limb and immobilise
7. Complete extravasation documentation sheet (mention extent of extravasation)
8. Inform and instruct the patient and relatives
9. Regular control (aftercare)

Substance specific measures: none

Cave! after extravasation:

1. No flushing of i.v. access
2. No moist compresses
3. No alcohol compresses
4. No occlusive dressings

Type of damage reported in literature:	Non-vesicant [7,8] Irritant [3,4,9] Vesicant [5]
Symptoms and clinical course reported in literature:	No data available
Measures reported in literature:	**Successful treatment:** – No data available **Unsuccessful treatment:** – No data available **Outcome of treatment not reported:** – Topical cooling [1,5,6,8] – Ice packs for 15–20 minutes every 4–6 hours over 72 hours and treatment with DMSO or hyaluronidase [2] – Topical cooling 4 × daily for 20 minutes over 3–4 days [8] – 100 mg Hydrocortison i.v. and s.c., respectively, additionally hydrocortisone applied topically, ice pack [9] – No specific measures mentioned [3,4,7]
Particular remarks:	Results of literature search: no animal experiments or clinical studies regarding extravasation have been published
Conclusion:	Although irinotecan has been classified as irritant/vesicant in the literature, no clinical case of tissue damage after extravasation has been documented; the substance is therefore classified as non-vesicant Owing to little experience with extravasations of irinotecan, a final classification of the type of damage is not possible [7]

No substance specific measures can be recommended

Original articles

-

Secondary literature

[1] van Gemmern R: Gewebstoxizität und Paravasatbehandlung neuer Zytostatika. Krankenhauspharmazie 17: 471–473, 1996.
[2] Rhone-Poulenc Rorer, personal communication, August 1998.
[3] Mullin S, Beckwith MC, Tyler LS: Prevention and management of antineoplastic extravasation injury. Hosp Pharm 35: 57–76, 2000.
[4] Gain M, Melzer S, Meyer-Jürshof A, et al: Allgemeiner Teil: Behandlung von Paravasaten. In: Gain M, et al (eds) ADKA-Zytostatika-Handbuch, Pharmazeutisch-wissenschaftliche Monographien. Verlag Heiner Biller, vol 1, 2nd edition: A42–44, 1997.
[5] Berdel WE, Schmoll HJ, Büchele T, et al: Prävention und Therapie von Paravasaten/Extravasaten. In: Schmoll HJ, Höffken K, Possinger K (eds) Kompendium Internistische Onkologie. Standards in Diagnostik und Therapie. Springer, vol 1, 3rd edition: 1689–1701, 1999.
[6] Gain M, Melzer S, Meyer-Jürshof A, et al: Irinotecan: Behandlung von Paravasaten. In: Gain M, et al (eds) ADKA-Zytostatika-Handbuch, Pharmazeutisch-wissenschaftliche Monographien. Verlag Heiner Biller, vol 6: 1–46, 2002.
[7] Jordan K, Grothe W, Schmoll HJ: Paravasation von Zytostatika: Prävention und Therapie. Dtsch Med Wochenschr 130: 33–37, 2005.
[8] Krämer I, Stützle M: Zytostatika-Paravasation – Wie ist vorzugehen? Krankenhauspharmazie 23: 261–268, 2002.
[9] Stanley A: Managing complications of chemotherapy administration. In: Allwood M, Stanley A, Wright P (eds) The Cytotoxics Handbook. Radcliffe Medical Press, 4th edition: 119–193, 2002.

Further reading:

- Ener RA, Meglathery SB, Styler M: Extravasation of systemic hemato-oncological therapies. Ann Oncol 15: 858–862, 2004.
- Summary of product characteristics Campto® (Germany), Pfizer, December 2004.
- Fenchel K, Karthaus M: Zytostatika-Paravasate – gibt es neue Empfehlungen zum therapeutischen Vorgehen? Wien Med Wochenschr 151: 44–46, 2001.

I

- Rauh J, Pluntke S, Müller C: Paravenöse Zytostatikainjektion: Prophylaxe und Sofortmaßnahmen im Notfall. MMW Fortschr Med 146: 682–686, 2004.
- Schrijvers DL: Extravasation: a dreaded complication of chemotherapy. Ann Oncol 14: iii26–iii30, 2003.

Revisions by Ines Mader

Melphalan

CONSENSUS

Type of damage: irritant

Recommended treatment:

General measures:

1. Stop injection/infusion immediately
2. Get extravasation kit
3. Put on (sterile) gloves
4. Replace infusion lead or syringe with 5 ml disposable syringe and aspirate slowly as much as possible of the extravasated drug; **Cave**! do not exert pressure on extravasation area
5. Remove i.v. access while aspirating
6. If blisters occur: aspirate with 1 ml syringe and s.c. cannula, use new equipment for every new attempt at aspiration
7. Elevate limb and immobilise
8. Complete extravasation documentation sheet (mention extent of extravasation)
9. Inform and instruct the patient and relatives
10. Regular control (aftercare)

Substance specific measures: none

Cave! after extravasation:

1. No flushing of i.v. access
2. No moist compresses
3. No alcohol compresses
4. No occlusive dressings

Type of damage reported in literature:

Non-vesicant [2,3,7,14]

Irritant [15,16]

No risk of necroses [4,5]

Vesicant [8]

Symptoms and clinical course reported in literature:

Initial symptoms: No data available

Delayed-onset symptoms: According to the summary of product characteristics local tissue damage [9]—no further information

Residual findings: No data available

Measures reported in literature:

Successful treatment:
- No data available

Unsuccessful treatment:
- No data available

Outcome of treatment not reported:
- 1500 IU hyaluronidase s.c., application of heat and compression [3]
- Topical cooling, anti-inflammatory compresses, NaCl 0.9% (type of application not mentioned); steroids in case of inflammations [6]
- Topical cooling 4 × daily for 20 minutes over 3–4 days [14]
- No specific measures mentioned [2,4,5,7,8,15,16]

Particular remarks:

Results of literature search: no clinical studies regarding extravasation have been published

Animal experiments: ulcerations have been observed in case of undiluted i.d. administration [1]

Pain, phlebitis, and erythema at the injection site after bolus administration of undiluted melphalan solutions (35 patients) [10] are not associated with extravasation; these symptoms are likely to be caused by the excipients in the reconstituted drug (e.g. ethanol [9])

Hypersensitivity reactions with incidence of 2–3% [4,11], radio sensitization [13] and radiation recall [12,13] have been described

Conclusion: Although melphalan is classified as vesicant in some of the literature, no clinical case of necroses after extravasation has been documented; the classification as irritant is due to the excipients in the reconstituted formulation

Positive results of substance specific measures have not been described so far; until further data become available no substance specific measures can be recommended

Original articles

[1] Dorr RT, Alberts DS, Soble M: Lack of experimental vesicant activity for the anticancer agents cisplatin, melphalan, and mitoxantrone. Cancer Chemother Pharmacol 16: 91–94, 1986.

Secondary literature

[2] Dorr RT: Pharmacologic management of vesicant chemotherapy extravasations. In: Dorr RT, Von Hoff DD (eds) Cancer Chemotherapy Handbook. Appleton & Lange, 2nd edition: 109–118, 1994.
[3] Stanley A: Managing complications of chemotherapy administration. In: Allwood M, Stanley A, Wright P (eds) The Cytotoxics Handbook. Radcliffe Medical Press, 4th edition: 119–193, 2002.
[4] Schneider G: Paravasate von Zytostatika. Diagnostik und Therapie. Aina S. Schneider Verlag, 6th edition: 1–17, 1999.
[5] Dorr RT: Antidotes to vesicant chemotherapy extravasations. Blood Rev 4: 41–60, 1990.
[6] Glaxo-Wellcome, personal communication, October 1998.
[7] Gain M, Melzer S, Meyer-Jürshof A, et al: Allgemeiner Teil: Behandlung von Paravasaten. In: Gain M, et al (eds) ADKA-Zytostatika-Handbuch, Pharmazeutisch-wissenschaftliche Monographien. Verlag Heiner Biller, vol 1, 2nd edition: A42–44, 1997.

[8] Mullin S, Beckwith MC, Tyler LS: Prevention and management of antineoplastic extravasation injury. Hosp Pharm 35: 57–76, 2000.
[9] Summary of product characteristics Alkeran® (Germany), GlaxoSmithKline, April 2004.
[10] Glaxo Wellcome, personal communication, October 1999.
[11] Schneider SM, Distelhorst CW: Chemotherapy-induced emergencies. Semin Oncol 16: 572–578, 1989.
[12] Koppel RA, Boh EE: Cutaneous reactions to chemotherapeutic agents. Am J Med Sci 321: 327–335, 2001.
[13] Alley E, Green R, Schuchter L: Cutaneous toxicities of cancer therapy. Curr Opin Oncol 14: 212–216, 2002.
[14] Krämer I, Stützle M: Zytostatika-Paravasation – Wie ist vorzugehen? Krankenhauspharmazie 23: 261–268, 2002.
[15] Ener RA, Meglathery SB, Styler M: Extravasation of systemic hemato-oncological therapies. Ann Oncol 15: 858–862, 2004.
[16] Jordan K, Grothe W, Schmoll HJ: Paravasation von Zytostatika: Prävention und Therapie. Dtsch Med Wochenschr 130: 33–37, 2005.

Further reading:

- Fenchel K, Karthaus M: Zytostatika-Paravasate – gibt es neue Empfehlungen zum therapeutischen Vorgehen? Wien Med Wochenschr 151: 44–46, 2001.
- Rauh J, Pluntke S, Müller C: Paravenöse Zytostatikainjektion: Prophylaxe und Sofortmaßnahmen im Notfall. MMW Fortschr Med 146: 682–686, 2004.
- Schrijvers DL: Extravasation: a dreaded complication of chemotherapy. Ann Oncol 14: iii26–iii30, 2003.

Revisions by Patrizia Fürst-Weger

Methotrexate

CONSENSUS

Type of damage: non-vesicant

Recommended treatment:

General measures:

1. Stop injection/infusion immediately
2. Get extravasation kit
3. Put on (sterile) gloves
4. Replace infusion lead or syringe with 5 ml disposable syringe and aspirate slowly as much as possible of the extravasated drug; **Cave!** do not exert pressure on extravasation area
5. Remove i.v. access while aspirating
6. Elevate limb and immobilise
7. Complete extravasation documentation sheet (mention extent of extravasation)
8. Inform and instruct the patient and relatives
9. Regular control (aftercare)

Substance specific measures: none

Cave! after extravasation:

1. No flushing of i.v. access
2. No moist compresses
3. No alcohol compresses
4. No occlusive dressings

M

Type of damage reported in literature:

Non-vesicant [7,11,12,14,20]

No tissue toxic potential [21]

Weak irritant (not vesicant) [19]

Inflammatory [8]

Irritant [10]

No risk of necrosis [9,18]

Vesicant [15,16]

Symptoms and clinical course reported in literature:

Initial symptoms: No data available

Delayed-onset symptoms: No data available

Residual findings: Stiffness, loss of extensor muscle on fingers (1 patient, MOP protocol [1]; no lasting tissue damage (2 patients) [6]

Measures reported in literature:

Successful treatment:
- Ice packs over 15 minutes 4 × daily over 1–2 days (2 patients) [6]

Unsuccessful treatment:
- 40 days after extravasation a surgical intervention was required (1 patient) [1]

Outcome of treatment not reported:
- After extravasation in the context of combination chemotherapy with methotrexate and vinblastine (extravasated substance not identified): hyaluronidase and dexamethasone i.d., topical cooling (1 patient) [5]

- 100 mg hydrocortisone s.c. and i.v., respectively, additionally topical hydrocortisone, ice packs or cold packs 4 × daily over 15–20 minutes [10,16] or intermittent ice packs over 24 hours and after the local reaction has subsided, application of heat and compression [8]
- If local symptoms develop, hydrocortisone (1%) or heparin to be applied topically [11]
- Optional local infiltration of corticosteroids, warm to hot compresses for 1 hour [12]
- Topical cooling [15] 4 × daily for 20 minutes over 3–4 days [21]
- Folic acid (3 mg/5 ml) [24] (no further data on method of application)
- No specific measures mentioned [7,9,14, 18–20]

M

Particular remarks:

1 case of "necrosis" on the dorsum of hand [1] within the application of a MOP regimen – it is questionable whether the developing necroses was associated with methotrexate

Extravasation of larger volumes of concentrated solutions (6.65 mg/ml and 13 mg/ml) did not result in lasting tissue damage (2 patients) [6]

Animal experiments: no local reactions after s.c. and i.d. administration of methotrexate [4]

Hypersensitivity reactions [22]: especially described after administration of high-dose methotrexate [2,3] and recall phenomenon after irradiation [22,23] are not associated with extravasation

Topical cooling: positive effect described in 2 patients [6]

Conclusion: Since methotrexate is also administered i.m. [13], a tissue-damaging effect is unlikely; the substance is therefore classified as non-vesicant, although it has been described as irritant/vesicant in some of the literature

No substance specific measures are required

Original articles

[1] Upton J, Mulliken JB, Murray JE: Major intravenous extravasation injuries. Am J Surg 137: 497–506, 1979.
[2] Gluck-Kuyt I, Irwin LE: Anaphylactic reaction to high-dose methotrexate. Cancer Treat Rep 63: 797–798, 1979.
[3] Goldberg NH, Romolo JL, Austin EH, et al: Anaphylactoid type reactions in two patients receiving high dose intravenous methotrexate. Cancer 41: 52–55, 1978.
[4] Barr RD, Benton SG, Belbeck LW: Soft-tissue necrosis induced by extravasated cancer chemotherapeutic agents. J Natl Cancer Inst 66: 1129–1136, 1981.
[5] Krämer I: Zehn Jahre Dokumentation von Zytostatika-Paravasat-Ereignissen: Auswertung von 175 Paravasate-Dokumentationen. Krankenhauspharmazie 23: 269–274, 2002.
[6] Ang TS, Siderov J: Extravasation of high-dose methotrexate: a case of nothing. Aust J Hosp Pharm 28: 430–431, 1998.

Secondary literature

[7] Dorr RT: Pharmacologic management of vesicant chemotherapy extravasations. In: Dorr RT, Von Hoff DD (eds) Cancer Chemotherapy Handbook. Appleton & Lange, 2nd edition: 109–118, 1994.
[8] Stanley A: Managing complications of chemotherapy administration. In: Allwood M, Stanley A, Wright P (eds) The Cytotoxics Handbook. Radcliffe Medical Press, 4th edition: 119–193, 2002.
[9] Schneider G: Paravasate von Zytostatika. Diagnostik und Therapie. Aina S. Schneider Verlag, 6th edition: 1–17, 1999.
[10] Gain M, Melzer S, Meyer-Jürshof A, et al: Allgemeiner Teil: Behandlung von Paravasaten. In: Gain M, et al (eds) ADKA-Zytostatika-Handbuch, Pharmazeutisch-wissenschaftliche Monographien. Verlag Heiner Biller, vol 1, 2nd edition: A42–44, 1997.
[11] Cox K, Stuart-Harris R, Abdini G, et al: The management of cytotoxic-drug extravasation: guide-lines drawn up by a working party for the Clinical Oncological Society of Australia. Med J Aust 148: 185–189, 1988.

M

[12] Ignoffo RJ, Friedman MA: Therapy of local toxicities caused by extravasation of cancer chemotherapeutic drugs. Cancer Treat Rev 7: 17–27, 1980.
[13] Summary of product characteristics. Methotrexat "Ebewe" 10mg/ml (Austria), Ebewe, July 2004.
[14] Schneider SM, Distelhorst CW: Chemotherapy-induced emergencies. Semin Oncol 16: 572–578, 1989.
[15] Berdel WE, Schmoll HJ, Büchele T, et al: Prävention und Therapie von Paravasaten/Extravasaten. In: Schmoll HJ, Höffken K, Possinger K (eds) Kompendium Internistische Onkologie. Standards in Diagnostik und Therapie. Springer, vol 1, 3rd edition: 1689–1701, 1999.
[16] Donislawski S, Gain M, Meyer-Jürshof A, et al: Methotrexat: Behandlung von Paravasaten. In: Donislawski S, et al (eds) ADKA-Zytostatika-Handbuch, Pharmazeutisch-wissenschaftliche Monographien. Verlag Heiner Biller, vol 2: 43, 1994.
[17] Dorr RT, Von Hoff DD: Drug monographs: methotrexate. In: Dorr RT, Von Hoff DD (eds) Cancer Chemotherapy Handbook. Appleton & Lange, 2nd edition: 692–705, 1994.
[18] Dorr RT: Antidotes to vesicant chemotherapy extravasations. Blood Rev 4: 41–60, 1990.
[19] Barth J: Paravasate und deren Behandlung. In: Barth J (ed) Zytostatika-Herstellung in der Apotheke. Deutscher Apotheker Verlag, chapter VI-3: 1–9, 2000.
[20] Jordan K, Grothe W, Schmoll HJ: Paravasation von Zytostatika: Prävention und Therapie. Dtsch Med Wochenschr 130: 33–37, 2005.
[21] Krämer I, Stützle M: Zytostatika-Paravasation – Wie ist vorzugehen? Krankenhauspharmazie 23: 261–268, 2002.
[22] Koppel RA, Boh EE: Cutaneous reactions to chemotherapeutic agents. Am J Med Sci 321: 327–335, 2001.
[23] Alley E, Green R, Schuchter L: Cutaneous toxicities of cancer therapy. Curr Opin Oncol 14: 212–216, 2002.
[24] Otto J, Goebell PJ, Otto T: Urologischer Notfall in der Onkologie. Der Onkologe 10: 351–357, 2004.

Further reading:

- Fenchel K, Karthaus M: Zytostatika-Paravasate – gibt es neue Empfehlungen zum therapeutischen Vorgehen? Wien Med Wochenschr 151: 44–46, 2001.
- Khan MS, Holmes JD: Reducing the morbidity from extravasation injuries. Ann Plast Surg 48: 628–632, 2002.

M

- Rauh J, Pluntke S, Müller C: Paravenöse Zytostatikainjektion: Prophylaxe und Sofortmaßnahmen im Notfall. MMW Fortschr Med 146: 682–686, 2004.
- Schrijvers DL: Extravasation: a dreaded complication of chemotherapy. Ann Oncol 14: iii26–iii30, 2003.

Revisions by Sabine Wassertheurer

M

Mitomycin C

CONSENSUS

Type of damage: vesicant

Recommended treatment:

General measures:

1. Stop injection/infusion immediately
2. Get extravasation kit
3. Put on (sterile) gloves
4. Replace infusion lead or syringe with 5 ml disposable syringe and aspirate slowly as much as possible of the extravasated drug; **Cave!** do not exert pressure on extravasation area
5. Remove i.v. access while aspirating
6. If blisters occur: aspirate with 1 ml syringe and s.c. cannula, use new equipment for every new attempt at aspiration
7. Elevate limb and immobilise
8. Start **substance specific measures**
9. Ensure adequate analgesia
10. Complete extravasation documentation sheet (mention extent of extravasation)
11. Inform and instruct the patient and relatives
12. Regular controls (aftercare)
13. Always consult a (plastic) surgeon within 24 hours

Substance specific measures:

DMSO:

1. Apply DMSO (99%) every 8 hours (e.g. with a sterile gauze pad) without pressure
2. Allow to air-dry – **Cave!** do not cover
3. Continue for a minimum of 7 days

Immediately afterwards topical cooling:

1. Apply cold, dry pack immediately for at least 1 hour (for example, using a cold-hot pack)
2. Continue several times daily for 15 minutes each time

Cave! after extravasation:

1. No flushing of i.v. access
2. No moist compresses
3. No alcohol compresses
4. No occlusive dressings

Type of damage reported in literature: Vesicant [1,2,8–12,17–28,30,31]

Symptoms and clinical course reported in literature:

Initial symptoms: No pain, erythema (1 patient)[14]

Delayed-onset symptoms: Pain, cellulitis (1 patient) [3], blister formation after 7 days, erythema, ulceration (1 patient) [14], necroses (14 patients) [1, 2, 8, 10], symptoms sometimes occur only months later, rarely lesions distal to the injection site, which spread over weeks [31]

Residual findings: Induration (1 patient) [4]

Measures reported in literature:

Successful treatment:

- Infiltration of pyridoxine hydrochloride (10%) (approx. 6 patients), in delay of treatment necroses developed (2 patients) [1]
- 4 drops DMSO (99%) per 10 cm^2 applied topically to an area twice the size of the affected area, repeat every 8 hours for 1 week or until symptoms have subsided; local cooling for 60 minutes, every 8 hours for 3 days (cold-hot pack) (4 patients [3,17] and 5 patients [4])

- 5–90 minutes after extravasation: infiltration of 500 mg hydrocortisone, application of betamethasone-gentamicin ointment every 12 hours over 2 days, then every 24 hours until healing is complete (3 and 4 patients) [5,6]; more than 5 days after extravasation: application of keratolytic ointment containing salicylic acid for 5 hours (2 patients) [5]; additionally infiltration of sodium thiosulfate solution (2%) followed by massage reduced the time of healing from 11 to 4 days (3 patients) [6]

- DMSO (90%) and a-tocopherol (10%) applied topically every 12 hours for 48 hours (1 patient) [7]

- 100 mg hydrocortisone s.c. [10]

- DMSO (99%) 2 × daily over 7–14 days (2 patients) [12]

- Hydrocortisone, ice pack [14]

Unsuccessful treatment:

- Injection of 300 mg hydrocortisone, application of Kenalog® (0.1%) 3 × daily, polyethylene dressing; surgical intervention was necessary (1 patient) [2]

- Conservative measures (antibiotics, local corticosteroids) not sufficient, surgical intervention required, in some cases permanently impaired function (8 patients) [8]

- 2 ml DMSO applied once; surgical intervention was required (1 patient) [14]

Outcome of treatment not reported:

- Topical DMSO every 6–8 hours for several days [17]

- Ice packs over 1–3 days, topical application of DMSO (70–100%) every 3–4 hours for 3–14 days, early consultation of plastic surgeon [18]

- DMSO every 6 hours over 1–2 weeks applied locally [19]
- Infiltration of 4 ml sodium thiosulfate (4%) or 1 ml ascorbic acid solution (5%), optional local infiltration of corticosteroids, warm to hot compresses for 1 hour [20]
- Infiltration of 5000 IU heparin in 5 ml NaCl 0.9%; topical DMSO every 6 hours over several days [21]
- 1.5 ml DMSO (50–99%) every 6 hours over 14 days applied locally [22,26]
- On the first day DMSO every 2 hours, topical hydrocortisone (1%) and cold compresses for 30 minutes, over 14 days every 3 hours alternating DMSO and topical hydrocortisone [23]
- DMSO (99%) applied topically to an area twice the size of the affected area, every 6 hours over 14 days, optional ice pack for 15 minutes every 6 hours over 2 days [24]
- 1–2 ml DMSO (50–100%) applied once topically [25]
- 100 mg hydrocortisone s.c. and i.v., respectively, DMSO (70–100%) every 3–4 hours for 14 days (minimum 3 days) applied locally, ice or cold pack 4 × daily for 15–20 minutes, topical hydrocortisone [27]
- Topical cooling immediately for 1 hour, then several times daily over 15 minutes; DMSO (99%) every 8 hours over 8 days, maintain treatment free interval between cooling and DMSO [30]
- 1–2 ml DMSO (50–99%) applied to an area twice the size of the extravasation, every 6-8 hours over 7–14 days [31]

- 5–6 ml sodium thiosulfate (4%) through the access, 0.4–0.8 ml per injection site perilesionally s.c., repeat s.c. administration after several hours, afterwards treatment with DMSO (70–90%) every 6 hours over 3–14 days [28]
- 1.6 ml sodium thiosulfate (25%) in 3 ml aqua ad inj., cold compresses [29]
- Cold compresses over 24 hours (1 patient) [34]

Particular remarks: Delayed development of ulcerations:

- 3 months after extravasation, possibly triggered by strong sunlight [10] or consumption of alcohol [13]
- Weeks after extravasation a new ulceration formed at a different injection site after another infusion of mitomycin C (recall phenomenon)[2,12]
- Ulceration and necroses days to weeks after administration without complications without signs of extravasation (8 and 2 patients) [15,16]

Photosensitivity [32,33], enhanced radiosensitivity and recall phenomenon after radiotherapy, recall of skin toxicity [32]

Hyperpigmentation [16] and hypersensitivity reactions [33] are not associated with extravasation

Corticosteroids: positive effect is questionable, because extravasations are only rarely accompanied by inflammatory processes [17, 18], after exclusive use treatment sometimes unsuccessful [2] (see chapter "Histopathological investigations")

DMSO and topical cooling: positive effects in preventing necroses have been reported [3,4]

Gentamicin: only for prophylaxis of secondary infection, no causal treatment of extravasation

Sodium thiosulfate: positive effect not sufficiently proved; disadvantage: invasive measure [5]

Pyridoxine hydrochloride: injections are particularly painful; positive effects of DMSO (and topical cooling) are better documented [3,4,12]

α-tocopherol: positive effects not sufficiently proved [7]

Conclusion: Because of many reports of necroses in the literature, mitomycin C is classified as vesicant

The well-established and non-invasive measures DMSO and topical cooling are therefore recommended

Original articles

[1] Rentschler R, Wilbur D: Pyridoxine: a potential local antidote for mitomycin-C extravasation. J Surg Oncol 37: 269–271, 1988.

[2] Argenta LC, Manders EK: Mitomycin C extravasation injuries. Cancer 51: 1080–1082, 1983.

[3] Bertelli G, Dini D, Forno G, et al: Dimethylsulphoxide and cooling after extravasation of antitumour agents. Lancet 341: 1098–1099, 1993.

[4] Bertelli G, Gozza A, Forno GB, et al: Topical dimethylsulfoxide for the prevention of soft tissue injury after extravasation of vesicant cytotoxic drugs: a prospective clinical study. J Clin Oncol 13: 2851–2855, 1995.

[5] Tsavaris NB, Komitsopoulou P, Karagiaouris P, et al: Prevention of tissue necrosis due to accidental extravasation of cytostatic drugs by a conservative approach. Cancer Chemother Pharmacol 30: 330–333, 1992.

[6] Tsavaris NB, Karagiaouris P, Tzannou I, et al: Conservative approach to the treatment of chemotherapy-induced extravasation. J Dermatol Surg Oncol 16: 519–522, 1990.

[7] Ludwig CU, Stoll HR, Obrist R, et al: Prevention of cytotoxic drug induced skin ulcers with dimethyl sulfoxide (DMSO) and α-tocopherole. Eur J Cancer Clin Oncol 23: 327–329, 1987.

[8] Khanna AK, Khanna A, Asthana AK, et al: Mitomycin C extravasation ulcers. J Surg Oncol 28: 108–110, 1985.
[9] Bowers DG, Lynch JB: Adriamycin extravasation. Plast Reconstr Surg 61: 86–92, 1978.
[10] Fuller B, Lind M, Bonomi P: Mitomycin C extravasation exacerbated by sunlight. Ann Intern Med 94: 542, 1981.
[11] Moertel CG, Reitemeier RJ, Hahn RG: Mitomycin C therapy in advanced gastrointestinal cancer. JAMA 204: 111–114, 1968.
[12] Alberts DS, Dorr RT: Case report: topical DMSO for mitomycin-C-induced skin ulceration. Oncol Nurs Forum 18: 693–695, 1991.
[13] Aizawa H, Tagami H: Delayed tissue necrosis due to mitomycin C. Acta Derm Venereol 67: 364–366, 1987.
[14] Herrera D, Burnham N: DMSO and extravasation of mitomycin. Oncol Nurs Forum 16: 155, 1989.
[15] Wood HA, Ellerhorst-Ryan JM: Delayed adverse skin reactions associated with mitomycin-C administration. Oncol Nurs Forum 11: 14–18, 1984.
[16] Bartkowski-Dodds L, Reville B: Extensive tissue ulceration due to apparent sensitivity reactions to mitomycin. Cancer Treat Rep 69: 925–927, 1985.

Secondary literature

[17] Bertelli G: Prevention and management of extravasation of cytotoxic drugs. Drug Safety 12: 245–255, 1995.
[18] Schneider G: Paravasate von Zytostatika. Diagnostik und Therapie. Aina S. Schneider Verlag, 6th edition: 1–17, 1999.
[19] Krämer I, Stützle M: Zytostatika-Paravasation – Wie ist vorzugehen? Krankenhauspharmazie 23: 261–268, 2002.
[20] Ignoffo RJ, Friedman MA: Therapy of local toxicities caused by extravasation of cancer chemotherapeutic drugs. Cancer Treat Rev 7: 17–27, 1980.
[21] Gain M, Melzer S, Meyer-Jürshof A, et al: Mitomycin: Behandlung von Paravasaten. In: Gain M, et al (eds) ADKA-Zytostatika-Handbuch, Pharmazeutisch-wissenschaftliche Monographien. Verlag Heiner Biller, vol 1, 2nd edition: 35, 1997.
[22] Dorr RT: Pharmacologic management of vesicant chemotherapy extravasations. In: Dorr RT, Von Hoff DD (eds) Cancer Chemotherapy Handbook. Appleton & Lange, 2nd edition: 109–118, 1994.
[23] Stanley A: Managing complications of chemotherapy administration. In: Allwood M, Stanley A, Wright P (eds) The Cytotoxics Handbook. Radcliffe Medical Press, 4th edition: 119–193, 2002.
[24] Mullin S, Beckwith MC, Tyler LS: Prevention and management of antineoplastic extravasation injury. Hosp Pharm 35: 57–76, 2000.

[25] Schneider SM, Distelhorst CW: Chemotherapy-induced emergencies. Semin Oncol 16: 572–578, 1989.
[26] Dorr RT: Antidotes to vesicant chemotherapy extravasations. Blood Rev 4: 41–60, 1990.
[27] Gain M, Melzer S, Meyer-Jürshof A, et al: Allgemeiner Teil: Behandlung von Paravasaten. In: Gain M, et al (eds) ADKA-Zytostatika-Handbuch, Pharmazeutisch-wissenschaftliche Monographien. Verlag Heiner Biller, vol 1, 2nd edition: A42–44, 1997.
[28] Barth J: Paravasate und deren Behandlung. In: Barth J (ed) Zytostatika-Herstellung in der Apotheke. Deutscher Apotheker Verlag, chapter VI-3: 1–9, 2000.
[29] Cox K, Stuart-Harris R, Abdini G, et al: The management of cytotoxic-drug extravasation: guidelines drawn up by a working party for the Clinical Oncological Society of Australia. Med J Aust 148: 185–189, 1988.
[30] Jordan K, Grothe W, Schmoll HJ: Paravasation von Zytostatika: Prävention und Therapie. Dtsch Med Wochenschr 130: 33–37, 2005.
[31] Ener RA, Meglathery SB, Styler M: Extravasation of systemic hemato-oncological therapies. Ann Oncol 15: 858–862, 2004.
[32] Koppel RA, Boh EE: Cutaneous reactions to chemotherapeutic agents. Am J Med Sci 321: 327–335, 2001.
[33] Alley E, Green R, Schuchter L: Cutaneous toxicities of cancer therapy. Curr Opin Oncol 14: 212–216, 2002.
[34] Langstein HN, Duman H, Seelig D, et al: Retrospective study of the management of chemotherapeutic injury. Ann Plast Surg 49: 369–374, 2002.

M

Further reading:

- Averbuch SD, Boldt M, Gaudiano G, et al: Experimental chemotherapy-induced skin nekrosis in swine. J Clin Invest 81: 142–148, 1988.
- Dorr RT, Soble MJ, Liddil JD, et al: Mitomycin C skin toxicity studies in mice: reduced ulceration and altered pharmacokinetics with topical dimethyl sulfoxide. J Clin Oncol 4: 1399–1404, 1986.
- Fenchel K, Karthaus M: Zytostatika-Paravasate – gibt es neue Empfehlungen zum therapeutischen Vorgehen? Wien Med Wochenschr 151: 44–46, 2001.
- Hahn SM, Sullivan FJ, De Luca AM, et al: Protection of mitomycin C induced skin extravasation with the nitroxide, 3-carbamoyl-proxyl (3-CP). Int J Oncol 10: 119–123, 1997.
- Ignoffo RJ, Tomlin W, Rubinstein E, et al: A model for skin toxicity of antineoplastic drugs: doxorubicin (DOX), mitomycin-C (MMC), and vincristine (VCR). Clin Res 29: 437A, 1981.

- Johnston-Early A, Cohen MH: Mitomycin C-induced skin ulceration remote from infusion site. Cancer Treat Rep 65: 529, 1981.
- Kassner E: Evaluation and treatment of chemotherapy extravasation injuries. J Pediatr Oncol Nurs 17: 135–148, 2000.
- Krämer I: Zehn Jahre Dokumentation von Zytostatika-Paravasat-Ereignissen: Auswertung von 175 Paravasate-Dokumentationen. Krankenhauspharmazie 23: 269–274, 2002.
- Krämer I: Onkologische Pharmazie. In: Jaehde U, Radziwill R, Mühlebach S, et al (eds) Lehrbuch der Klinischen Pharmazie. Wissenschaftliche Verlagsgesellschaft mbH, 2nd edition: 307–336, 2003.
- Kurul S, Saip P, Aydin T: Totally implantable venous-access ports: local problems and extravasation injury. Lancet Oncol 3: 684–692, 2002.
- Loth TS, Eversmann WW: Treatment methods for extravasations of chemotherapeutic agents: a comparative study. J Hand Surg 11A: 388–396, 1986.
- Otto J, Goebell PJ, Otto T: Urologischer Notfall in der Onkologie. Der Onkologe 10: 351–357, 2004.
- Rauh J, Pluntke S, Müller C: Paravenöse Zytostatikainjektion: Prophylaxe und Sofortmaßnahmen im Notfall. MMW Fortschr Med 146: 682–686, 2004.
- Schrijvers DL: Extravasation: a dreaded complication of chemotherapy. Ann Oncol 14: iii26–iii30, 2003.

Revisions by Elisabeth Nogler-Semenitz

Mitoxantrone

CONSENSUS

Type of damage: vesicant

Recommended treatment:

General measures:

1. Stop injection/infusion immediately
2. Get extravasation kit
3. Put on (sterile) gloves
4. Replace infusion lead or syringe with 5 ml disposable syringe and aspirate slowly as much as possible of the extravasated drug; **Cave!** do not exert pressure on extravasation area
5. Remove i.v. access while aspirating
6. If blisters occur: aspirate with 1 ml syringe and s.c. cannula, use new equipment for every new attempt at aspiration
7. Elevate limb and immobilise
8. Start **substance specific measures**
9. Ensure adequate analgesia
10. Complete extravasation documentation sheet (mention extent of extravasation)
11. Inform and instruct the patient and relatives
12. Regular control (aftercare)
13. Always consult a (plastic) surgeon within 24 hours

Substance specific measures:

DMSO:

1. Apply DMSO (99%) every 8 hours (e.g. with a sterile gauze pad) without pressure
2. Allow to air-dry – **Cave!** do not cover
3. Continue for a minimum of 7 days

Immediately afterwards topical cooling:

1. Apply cold, dry pack immediately for at least 1 hour (for example, using a cold-hot pack)
2. Continue several times daily for 15 minutes each time

Cave! after extravasation:

1. No flushing of i.v. access
2. No moist compresses
3. No alcohol compresses
4. No occlusive dressings

Type of damage reported in literature:

Non-vesicant [18]

Irritant [12] and/or weak vesicant in large amounts of high concentrations [16]

Irritant, rarely vesicant [15]

Exfoliant [13]

Low risk of necroses [11,14,22]

Vesicant [1,2,6,10,19]

Symptoms and clinical course reported in literature:

Initial symptoms: Oedema [2 (1 patient), 9], erythema [9]

Delayed-onset symptoms: One day after extravasation pain occurred, after 1 and 3 weeks (1 patient each) necroses developed [1, 2,6], reversible blueish skin discoloration [14 (1 patient), 8]

Residual findings: No data available

Single case report: No reaction in very low dosage of 1.2 mg/m^2 in a phase I study (1 patient) [7]

Measures reported in literature:

Successful treatment:
- 4 drops of DMSO (99%) per 10 cm^2 applied topically to an area twice the size of the affected area, repeat every 8 hours for 1 week or until symptoms have subsided; local cooling for 60 minutes, every 8 hours for 3 days (cold-hot pack); (12 patients [3] and 10 patients [4,10])

- 5–90 minutes after extravasation: infiltration of 500 mg hydrocortisone, application of betamethasone-gentamicin ointment every 12 hours for 2 days, then every 24 hours until healing is complete (5 patients) [5]; more than 5 days after extravasation: application of keratolytic ointment containing salicylic acid over 5 hours (2 patients) [5]

Unsuccessful treatment:
- Administration of 10 ml NaCl 0.9% through catheter in place (1 patient) [1]

- No measures; several weeks after extravasation surgical intervention became necessary [2,14]

- Ice pack (1 patient) [6]

Outcome of treatment not reported:
- 100 mg hydrocortisone s.c. and i.v., respectively, hydrocortisone applied topically, ice packs. DMSO 4 × daily over 5–7 days, can be alternated with topical hydrocortisone [13]

- If local symptoms develop, hydrocortisone (1%) or heparin to be applied topically combined with cold compresses (either once for 45 minutes or 20 minutes per day for 3 days) or warm compresses [19]

- Topical cooling 4 × daily for 20 minutes over 3–4 days [20]

- Apply dry cold immediately for 1 hour, followed by several times daily over 15 minutes; DMSO (99%) every 8 hours over 8 days; maintain treatment free interval between topical cooling and DMSO [21]

- Hydrocortisone i.v., s.c., and topically, topical cooling or DMSO applied locally, and intermittent topical cooling [12]

- No specific measures mentioned [11,14–16,18]

Particular remarks:

Occurrence of phlebitis is possible [7,17] but rare and is not associated with extravasation

Hypersensitivity reactions [23] are not associated with extravasation

Corticosteroids: positive effect is questionable, because extravasations are only rarely accompanied by inflammatory processes [10,11] (See chapter "Histopathological investigations")

DMSO and topical cooling: positive effects in preventing necroses have been reported [3,4] Cave! topical cooling alone is not sufficient [6]

Gentamicin: only for prophylaxis of secondary infection, no causal treatment of extravasation

M

Conclusion:

Mitoxantrone is controversially classified in the literature; in case of no therapeutic interventions [2] or inadequate measures [1,6] severe necroses have, however, been described; the substance is therefore classified as vesicant

Positive results using DMSO and topical cooling after extravasation with other DNA-intercalating substances are reported; therefore these non-invasive interventions are recommended

Original articles

[1] Levin M, Caravone D, Geiser C: Mitoxantrone extravasation and tissue necrosis. Am J Health-Syst Pharm 53: 1192–1194, 1996.

[2] Peters FT, Beijnen JH, Huinink WW: Mitoxantrone extravasation injury. Cancer Treat Rep 71: 992–993 1987.

[3] Bertelli G, Gozza A, Forno GB, et al: Topical dimethylsulfoxide for the prevention of soft tissue injury after extravasation of vesicant cytotoxic drugs: a prospective clinical study. J Clin Oncol 13: 2851–2855, 1995.

[4] Bertelli G, Dini D, Forno G, et al: Dimethylsulphoxide and cooling after extravasation of antitumour agents. Lancet 341: 1098–1099, 1993.

[5] Tsavaris NB, Karagiaouris P, Tzannou I, et al: Conservative approach to the treatment of chemotherapy-induced extravasation. J Dermatol Surg Oncol 16: 519–522, 1990.
[6] Kara M, Ross DC: Severe soft tissue necrosis after extravasation of mitoxantrone: case report. Can J Plast Surg 6: 204–206, 1998.
[7] Von Hoff DD, Pollard E, Kuhn J, et al: Phase I clinical investigation of 1,4-dihydroxy-5,8-bis {{{2-[(2-hydroxyethyl)amino]ethyl} amino}}-9,10-anthracenedione dihydrochloride (NSC 301739), a new anthracenedione. Cancer Res 40: 1516–1518, 1980.
[8] Alberts DS, Griffith KS, Goodman GE, et al: Phase I clinical trial of mitoxantrone: a new anthracenedione anticancer drug. Cancer Chemother Pharmacol 5: 11–15, 1980.

Secondary literature

[9] Posner LE, Dukart G, Goldberg J, et al: Mitoxantrone: an overview of safety and toxicity. Invest New Drugs 3: 123–132, 1985.
[10] Bertelli G: Prevention and management of extravasation of cytotoxic drugs. Drug Safety 12: 245–255, 1995.
[11] Schneider G: Paravasate von Zytostatika. Diagnostik und Therapie. Aina S. Schneider Verlag, 6th edition: 1–17, 1999.
[12] Gain M, Melzer S, Meyer-Jürshof A, et al: Mitoxantron: Behandlung von Paravasaten. In: Gain M, et al (eds) ADKA-Zytostatika-Handbuch, Pharmazeutisch-wissenschaftliche Monographien. Verlag Heiner Biller, vol 7, 38: 2003.
[13] Stanley A: Managing complications of chemotherapy administration. In: Allwood M, Stanley A, Wright P (eds) The Cytotoxics Handbook. Radcliffe Medical Press, 4th edition: 119–193, 2002.
[14] Dorr RT: Antidotes to vesicant chemotherapy extravasations. Blood Rev 4: 41–60, 1990.
[15] Mullin S, Beckwith MC, Tyler LS: Prevention and management of antineoplastic extravasation injury. Hosp Pharm 35: 57–76, 2000.
[16] Dorr RT: Pharmacologic management of vesicant chemotherapy extravasations. In: Dorr RT, Von Hoff DD (eds) Cancer Chemotherapy Handbook. Appleton & Lange, 2nd edition: 109–118, 1994.
[17] Dorr RT, Von Hoff DD: Drug monographs: mitoxantrone hydrochloride. In: Dorr RT, Von Hoff DD (eds) Cancer Chemotherapy Handbook. Appleton & Lange, 2nd edition: 730–735, 1994.
[18] Schneider SM, Distelhorst CW: Chemotherapy-induced emergencies. Semin Oncol 16: 572–578, 1989.
[19] Cox K, Stuart-Harris R, Abdini G, et al: The management of cytotoxic-drug extravasation: guide-lines drawn up by a working party for the Clinical Oncological Society of Australia. Med J Aust 148: 185–189, 1988.

[20] Krämer I, Stützle M: Zytostatika-Paravasation - Wie ist vorzugehen? Krankenhauspharmazie 23: 261–268, 2002.
[21] Jordan K, Grothe W, Schmoll HJ: Paravasation von Zytostatika: Prävention und Therapie. Dtsch Med Wochenschr 130: 33–37, 2005.
[22] Ener RA, Meglathery SB, Styler M: Extravasation of systemic hemato-oncological therapies. Ann Oncol 15: 858–862, 2004.
[23] Alley E, Green R, Schuchter L: Cutaneous toxicities of cancer therapy. Curr Opin Oncol 14: 212–216, 2002.

Further reading:

- Albanell J, Baselga J: Systemic therapy emergencies. Semin Oncol 27: 347–361, 2000.
- Dorr RT, Alberts DS, Soble M: Lack of experimental vesicant activity for the anticancer agents cisplatin, melphalan, and mitoxantrone. Cancer Chemother Pharmacol 16: 91–94, 1986.
- Fenchel K, Karthaus M: Zytostatika-Paravasate – gibt es neue Empfehlungen zum therapeutischen Vorgehen? Wien Med Wochenschr 151: 44–46, 2001.
- Koppel RA, Boh EE: Cutaneous reactions to chemotherapeutic agents. Am J Med Sci 321: 327–335, 2001.
- Krämer I: Zehn Jahre Dokumentation von Zytostatika-Paravasat-Ereignissen: Auswertung von 175 Paravasate-Dokumentationen. Krankenhauspharmazie 23: 269–274, 2002.
- Krämer I: Onkologische Pharmazie. In: Jaehde U, Radziwill R, Mühlebach S, et al (eds) Lehrbuch der Klinischen Pharmazie. Wissenschaftliche Verlagsgesellschaft mbH, 2nd edition: 307–336, 2003.
- Kurul S, Saip P, Aydin T: Totally implantable venous-access ports: local problems and extravasation injury. Lancet Oncol 3: 684–692, 2002.
- Rauh J, Pluntke S, Müller C: Paravenöse Zytostatikainjektion: Prophylaxe und Sofortmaßnahmen im Notfall. MMW Fortschr Med 146: 682–686, 2004.

Revisions by Elisbeth Nogler-Semenitz

Nimustine

CONSENSUS

Type of damage: non-vesicant

Recommended treatment:

General measures:

1. Stop injection/infusion immediately
2. Get extravasation kit
3. Put on (sterile) gloves
4. Replace infusion lead or syringe with 5 ml disposable syringe and aspirate slowly as much as possible of the extravasated drug; **Cave!** do not exert pressure on extravasation area
5. Remove i.v. access while aspirating
6. Elevate limb and immobilise
7. Complete extravasation documentation sheet (mention extent of extravasation)
8. Inform and instruct the patient and relatives
9. Regular control (aftercare)

Substance specific measures: none

Cave! after extravasation:

1. No flushing of i.v. access
2. No moist compresses
3. No alcohol compresses
4. No occlusive dressings

Type of damage reported in literature:

Unknown tissue toxic potential [2]

Non-vesicant [1,4]

Symptoms and clinical course reported in literature:

No data available

Measures reported in literature:

Successful treatment:
- No data available

Unsuccessful treatment:
- No data available

Outcome of treatment not reported:
- Topical cooling 4 × daily for 20 minutes over 3–4 days [2]

- No specific measures mentioned [4]

N

Particular remarks:

Results of literature search: no animal experiments or clinical studies regarding extravasation have been published

Irritations of the intima [3] are not associated with extravasation

Conclusion:

Since no clinical case of tissue damage after extravasation has been documented in the literature, nimustine is classified as non-vesicant

Owing to little or no experience with extravasations of nimustine, a final classification of the type of damage is not possible

No substance specific measures can be recommended

Original articles

–

Secondary literature

[1] Asta Medica, personal communication, November 1998.
[2] Krämer I, Stützle M: Zytostatika-Paravasation – Wie ist vorzugehen? Krankenhauspharmazie 23: 261–268, 2002.
[3] Summary of product characteristics ACNU® (Germany), Baxter, January 2002.
[4] Jordan K, Grothe W, Schmoll HJ: Paravasation von Zytostatika: Prävention und Therapie. Dtsch Med Wochenschr 130: 33–37, 2005.

Revisions by Patrizia Fürst-Weger

N

Oxaliplatin

CONSENSUS

Type of damage: vesicant

Recommended treatment:

General measures:

1. Stop injection/infusion immediately
2. Get extravasation kit
3. Put on (sterile) gloves
4. Replace infusion lead or syringe with 5 ml disposable syringe and aspirate slowly as much as possible of the extravasated drug; **Cave!** do not exert pressure on extravasation area
5. Remove i.v. access while aspirating
6. If blisters occur: aspirate with 1 ml syringe and s.c. cannula, use new equipment for every new attempt at aspiration
7. Elevate limb and immobilise
8. Start **substance specific measures**
9. Ensure adequate analgesia
10. Complete extravasation documentation sheet (mention extent of extravasation)
11. Inform and instruct the patient and relatives
12. Regular control (aftercare)
13. Always consult a (plastic) surgeon within 24 hours

Substance specific measures: not recommended on the basis of current data

Cave! no application of topical cooling

Cave! after extravasation:

1. No flushing of i.v. access
2. No moist compresses
3. No alcohol compresses
4. No occlusive dressings

Type of damage reported in literature:

Non-vesicant [9]

Non- or weak vesicant [11]

Irritant [15,18]

Exfoliant [14]

Low vesicant potential [16]

Vesicant [2,6,7,13]

Symptoms and clinical course reported in literature:

Initial symptoms: Pain, burning, and swelling (13 patients) [5–7]

Delayed-onset symptoms: Erythema (6 patients) [5,6], fever (1 patient) [5], inguinal abscess (1 patient) [3], paraesthesia (1 patient) [7], skin sclerosis (2 patients) [2,7], impaired movement in shoulder or arm (5 patients) [2,5–7], (muscle) necrosis (2 patients) [2,6]

Residual findings: Dumbness (1 patient) [7], scin fibrosis (1 patient) [7], residual necrosis (1 patient) [2]

Single case report: Immediately after extravasation of 104 mg oxaliplatin applied via Port-a-cath: swelling of the left breast; after 1 week: redness, swelling, and pain; after 2 weeks: progressive inflammation compatible with tissue necrosis but without skin lesions or fever; from the 3rd week pain and swelling subsided; during the following 4 months a plate-like induration developed which transformed into a nodular and streaky fibrosis (1 patient) [8]

Measures reported in literature:

Successful treatment:
- No data available

O

Unsuccessful treatment:

- Immediately after extravasation: flushing with NaCl 0.9%, cold pack, topical application of gel containing aescin and salicylic acid, analgesia p.o.; 9 days after extravasation: amoxicillin p.o., lymphatic drainage and physical therapy, curd cheese compresses [2]

- Topical cooling, oral indometacin (1 patient); topical cooling, oral indometacin, topical diclofenac, oral morphine, clindamycin (1 patient); oral dexamethasone, indometacin, topical cooling (2 patients); clindamycin, local DMSO (1 patient) [5]

- Ice packs immediately after extravasation; some days later: vancomycin i.v., physiotherapy, warm compresses and celecoxib (1 patient) [6]

- Cold compresses and 0.3% heparinoid cream, days later: antibiotic and anti-inflammatory medication (no data on application method) (1 patient) [7]

O

Outcome of treatment not reported:

- Warm compresses [9]

- 100 mg hydrocortisone s.c. and i.v., respectively, ice or cold pack 4 × daily over 15–20 minutes, topical hydrocortisone [11, 12]

- Topical cooling [13]

- 1500 IU hyaluronidase, subcutaneous infusion of 500 ml glucose 5% with 1500 IU hyaluronidase, heat [14]

- Topical glucocorticoids [15]

- No specific measures mentioned [16, 18]

Particular remarks: Results of literature search: no animal experiments regarding extravasation have been published

The harm of extravasation of even greater amounts of oxaliplatin is not comparable to that of classic vesicants like anthracyclines or vinca alkaloids [5]

Incidence of hypersensitivity reactions: 2% [1]

Corticosteroids: insufficient clinical evidence exists to support the use of oral steroids, which was rated positively in the recent literature [5,16,20]

Topical cooling: do not use because exposure to cold may cause sensory neuropathies [7,9,10,17]

NaCl 0.9%: instillation is not recommended as any mixture of NaCl 0.9% with oxaliplatin should be avoided [4] because of the risk of precipitation [14]

Conclusion: Considering several reports of documented necroses after extravasation, oxaliplatin is classified as vesicant

Positive results of substance specific measures have not been described so far; until further data become available no substance specific measures can be recommended

Original articles

[1] Tournigand C, Maindrault-Goebel F, Louvet C, et al: Severe anaphylactic reactions to oxaliplatin. Eur J Cancer 34: 1297–1298, 1998.
[2] Baur M, Kienzer HR, Rath T, et al: Extravasation of oxaliplatin (Eloxatin®) – clinical course. Onkologie 23: 468–471, 2000.
[3] Zelek L, Cottu P, Tubiana-Hulin M, et al: Phase II study of oxaliplatin and fluorouracil in taxane- and anthracycline-pretreated breast cancer patients. J Clin Oncol 20: 2551–2558, 2002.
[4] Kretzschmar A, Thuss-Patience PC, Pink D, et al: Extravasations of oxaliplatin. Proc Am Soc Clin Oncol 21: 270b, 2002.
[5] Kretzschmar A, Pink D, Thuss-Patience P, et al: Extravasations of oxaliplatin. J Clin Oncol 21: 4068–4069, 2003.

[6] Kennedy JG, Donahue JP, Hoang B, et al: Vesicant characteristics of oxaliplatin following antecubital extravasation. Clin Oncol 15: 237–239, 2003.
[7] Foo KF, Michael M, Toner G, et al: A case report of oxaliplatin extravasation. Ann Oncol 14: 961–962, 2003.
[8] Eckert R, Maier KP: Necrotizing panniculitis after extravasation of oxaliplatin. Ann Oncol 13 (Suppl 5): 29, 2002.

Secondary literature

[9] Sanofi-Whintrop, personal communication, November 1998.
[10] Dorr RT, Von Hoff DD: Drug monographs: oxaliplatin. In: Dorr RT, Von Hoff DD (eds) Cancer Chemotherapy Handbook. Appleton & Lange, 2nd edition: 758–761, 1994.
[11] Gain M, Melzer S, Meyer-Jürshof A, et al: Oxaliplatin: Behandlung von Paravasaten. In: Gain M, et al (eds) ADKA-Zytostatika-Handbuch, Pharmazeutisch-wissenschaftliche Monographien. Verlag Heiner Biller, Vol 4: 30, 2000.
[12] Gain M, Melzer S, Meyer-Jürshof A, et al: Allgemeiner Teil: Behandlung von Paravasaten. In: Gain M, et al (eds) ADKA-Zytostatika-Handbuch, Pharmazeutisch-wissenschaftliche Monographien. Verlag Heiner Biller, vol 1, 2nd edition : A42–44, 1997.
[13] Berdel WE, Schmoll HJ, Büchele T, et al: Prävention und Therapie von Paravasaten/Extravasaten. In: Schmoll HJ, Höffken K, Possinger K (eds) Kompendium Internistische Onkologie. Standards in Diagnostik und Therapie. Springer, vol 1, 3rd edition: 1689–1701, 1999.
[14] Stanley A: Managing complications of chemotherapy administration. In: Allwood M, Stanley A, Wright P (eds) The Cytotoxics Handbook. Radcliffe Medical Press, 4th edition: 119–193, 2002.
[15] Krämer I, Stützle M: Zytostatika-Paravasation – Wie ist vorzugehen? Krankenhauspharmazie 23: 261–268, 2002.
[16] Ener RA, Meglathery SB, Styler M: Extravasation of systemic hemato-oncological therapies. Ann Oncol 15: 858–862, 2004.
[17] Summary of product characteristics Eloxatin® (Germany), Sanofi-Synthelabo, September 2004.
[18] Jordan K, Grothe W, Schmoll HJ, et al: Paravasation von Zytostatika: Prävention und Therapie. Dtsch Med Wochenschr 130: 33–37, 2005.

Further reading:

- Cazin JL, Gosselin P, Demaille MC: Conduite à tenir devant une extravasation d'anticancéreux. J Pharm Clin 22: 5–7, 2003.

- Fenchel K, Karthaus M: Zytostatika-Paravasate – gibt es neue Empfehlungen zum therapeutischen Vorgehen? Wien Med Wochenschr 151: 44–46, 2001.
- Rauh J, Pluntke S, Müller C: Paravenöse Zytostatikainjektion: Prophylaxe und Sofortmaßnahmen im Notfall. MMW Fortschr Med 146: 682–686, 2004.
- Schrijvers DL: Extravasation: a dreaded complication of chemotherapy. Ann Oncol 14: iii26–iii30, 2003.

Revisions by Patrizia Fürst-Weger

O

Paclitaxel

CONSENSUS

Type of damage: vesicant

Recommended treatment:

General measures:

1. Stop injection/infusion immediately
2. Get extravasation kit
3. Put on (sterile) gloves
4. Replace infusion lead or syringe with 5 ml disposable syringe and aspirate slowly as much as possible of the extravasated drug; **Cave!** do not exert pressure on extravasation area
5. Remove i.v. access while aspirating
6. If blisters occur: aspirate with 1 ml syringe and s.c. cannula, use new equipment for every new attempt at aspiration
7. Elevate limb and immobilise
8. Start **substance specific measures**
9. Ensure adequate analgesia
10. Complete extravasation documentation sheet (mention extent of extravasation)
11. Inform and instruct the patient and relatives
12. Regular control (aftercare)
13. Always consult a (plastic) surgeon within 24 hours

Substance specific measures:

Hyaluronidase:

Inject up to 1500 IU hyaluronidase s.c. around the affected area depending on size of extravasation; **Cave!** local analgesia is recommended

Cave! after extravasation:

1. No flushing of i.v. access
2. No moist compresses
3. No alcohol compresses
4. No occlusive dressings

Type of damage reported in literature:

Non-vesicant [24]

Irritant [8,16,33,36]

Irritant/vesicant [31]

Vesicant after extravasations of large amounts and high concentrations [25,27]

Vesicant [3,5–7,9–11,14,17,22,23,26,28,30,32,38–40]

Symptoms and clinical course reported in literature:

Initial symptoms: Swelling with pain, erythema, hypersensitivity to touch (55 patients) [2,5–10,12,14,16,17,21], local hyperthermia (2 patients) [14,17], blister formation (17 patients) [5,10–12,16], fever and somnolence (1 patient) [11]

Delayed-onset symptoms: Increasing pain (2 patients) [11], cellulitis (9 patients) [5,7,12,14,16,17], hyperpigmentation (20 patients) [4,5,8,17], induration (18 patients) [4,8,9,12,16,17,20,21] and ulceration sometimes persisting for months, recall reaction (recurrence of or intensified initial symptoms after repeated administration of paclitaxel at a different site) (4 patients) [1,10,12,15], skin peeling (3 patients) [4,10,16]

Residual findings: Discolouration (16 patients) [4,5,11,17], induration (15 patients) [5,16,17], scarring (2 patients) [19,20], dysaesthesia (1 patient) [11], persistent lesion after 12 months (1 patient) [5]

Case reports:

- No immediate symptoms occurred, one week after extravasation: burning pain, paraesthesia, sensory loss, and motor weakness with increased symptoms in the subsequent week, in the third week symptoms gradually subsided in a cranio-caudal way; day 21: motor weakness with sensory deficit in the median nerve of the right arm persisted; three weeks later worsening of symptoms with lancinating pain, sensory loss, weakness, and severe functional deficit in terms of a local neurotoxicity (1 patient) [15]

- Extravasation after central venous application: within a few hours development of oedema, erythema, tenderness and local hyperthermia of the left breast, no necrosis; residual finding after 6 months: brown discolouration and thickened skin in the affected area with central scarring (1 patient) [19]

Measures reported in literature:

Successful treatment:

- No specific measures: complete healing within 10 days (1 patient) [3], and within 59–73 days (3 patients) [9], respectively
- 250 IU hyaluronidase in 6 ml NaCl 0.9% s.c. without topical cooling or application of heat (5 patients) [2,25]
- Local cooling for 3 hours (2 patients) [8] and hyaluronidase s.c. (2 patients) [8] (receding symptoms after combination treatment with hyaluronidase slower than in monotherapy with cooling alone)
- Topical application of corticosteroid cream and cooling, administration of analgesics, antibiotics, catecholamines, and G-CSF (1 patient) [11]
- 500 mg cloxacillin 4 × daily over 14 days, topical cooling (1 patient) [17]
- Animal experiment: hyaluronidase i.d. [18]

Unsuccessful treatment:

- Local moist heat resulted in blistering and hyperpigmentation (1 patient) [4]
- Topical cooling on day 1, on days 5 and 6 application of heat (1 patient) [6]
- 250 mg cephalexin 4 × daily, silver sulfadiazine applied topically 2 × daily, surgical intervention was required (1 patient) [7]
- Topical betamethasone (1 patient) [16]

P

- Alternating local application of heat and cold (1 patient) [17]

- Animal experiments: local application of heat or cold [18]

Outcome of treatment not reported:
- Application of heat [14,20,22,30,33,38], (17 patients) [5,21]

- Topical application of heat, topical and intradermal glucocorticoid (1 patient) [21]

- Topical cooling [23,38], (2 patients) [5]

- Local cooling (6 patients) with intradermal injection of a glucocorticoid (2 patients) or topically applied glucocorticoid (4 patients) [21]

- Non-steroidal anti-inflammatory medication (1 patient) [19]

- S.c. infiltration of 1–3 ml of a mixture of 100 mg hydrocortisone and 4 mg chlorpheniramine in 10 ml, 1500 IU hyaluronidase, warm compresses; subsequently alternating between warm compresses and topically applied mepyramine or another antihistamine (for 3 days); in severe cases administration of 1 g sodium cromoglycate p.o. followed by 200 mg 4 × daily over the following three days [26]

- 100 mg hydrocortisone s.c. and i.v., respectively, application of heat, topical hydrocortisone [32]

- S.c. administration of a mixture of 10 mg dexamethasone, 5 mg chlorpheniramine, 25 mg ranitidine, 1 g sodium cromoglycate p.o.; after 30 minutes 1500 IU hyaluronidase s.c., intermittently warm compresses for 20 minutes over 24 hours, 4 × daily hydrocortisone (1%) applied topically [36]

- 1500 IU hyaluronidase s.c., applied perilesionally, analgesia if required [39]
- 150-900 IU hyaluronidase i.v. or s.c.; repeated within the following 3–4 hours, topical cooling [40]
- No specific measure mentioned [28,31] or no local treatment (1 patient) [5]

Particular remarks:

A delay in the manifestation of symptoms of an extravasation is favoured by the high molecular weight, high protein binding, and the persistence of paclitaxel in the tissue that is associated with these factors[14]

The vesicant potential of paclitaxel is increased by the excipients that are classified as vesicants (e.g. Cremophor®)[14]

Phlebitis [5,41] and hypersensitivity reactions [5,13,29,33,41–43] are not associated with an extravasation; these symptoms are most likely to be due to the excipients in the formulation (Cremophor® EL and ethanol)

P

Recall phenomena have been described not only after radiation [34,41,42] but also after extravasation of paclitaxel [22,28–30,35,38,41,43], (1 patient each) [1,10,12,15]

Local ulcerations occur not only in cases of extravasation of large amounts or highly concentrated infusion solutions [25] but are likely to be indedependent of these [37]

Analgesics, C-CSF, and catecholamines: no causal treatment of extravasation

Antibiotics: only as secondary prophylaxis, no causal extravasation therapy

Corticosteroids: positive effect is questionable, because extravasations are only rarely accompanied by inflammatory processes (see chapter "Histopathological investigations")

Hyaluronidase: clinical reports about the positive effects in preventing necroses are available [2]; in animal experiments hyaluronidase was found to be clearly superior compared with exclusive use of topical hot or cold compresses

As the s.c. application of hyaluronidase is usually associated with severe pain for the patient, local analgesia is recommended [39]

Hyaluronidase and topical cooling: this combination does not make sense from a theoretical perspective [38]

Heat or cooling: neither positive nor negative effects observed in exclusive administration in animal experiments [18]; however, there are reports about the successful application of cold compresses

Conclusion: Although paclitaxel is classified as non-vesicant and irritant in some of the literature, several cases of necroses have been documented; the substance is therefore classified as vesicant

Monotherapy with hyaluronidase is recommended

Original articles

[1] Du Bois A, Kommoss FG, Pfisterer J, et al: Paclitaxel-induced "recall" soft tissue ulcerations occuring at the site of previous subcutaneous administration of paclitaxel in low doses. Gynecol Oncol 60: 94–96, 1996.

[2] Bertelli G, Cafferata MA, Ardizzoni A, et al: Skin ulceration potential of paclitaxel in a mouse skin model in vivo. Cancer 79: 2266–2268, 1997.

[3] Raymond E, Cartier S, Canuel C, et al: Extravasation de paclitaxel (Taxol®). Rev Méd Interne 16: 141–142, 1995.

[4] Goodman M, Stewart I, Lydon J, et al: Use caution when managing paclitaxel and taxotere infiltrations. Oncol Nurs Forum 23: 541–542, 1996.

[5] Bicher A, Levenback C, Burke TW, et al: Infusion site soft-tissue injury after paclitaxel administration. Cancer 76: 116–120, 1995.

[6] Kane MP, Medina PJ, Aisner J: Vesicant reaction to paclitaxel extravasation. J Oncol Pharm Practice 4: 45, 1998.
[7] Herrington JD, Figueroa JA: Severe necrosis due to paclitaxel extravasation. Pharmacotherapy 17: 163–165, 1997.
[8] Du Bois A, Fehr MK, Bochtler H, et al: Clinical course and management of paclitaxel extravasation. Oncol Rep 3: 973–974, 1996.
[9] Ajani JA, Dodd LG, Daugherty K, et al: Taxol-induced soft-tissue injury secondary to extravasation: characterization by histopathology and clinical course. J Natl Cancer Inst 86: 51–53, 1994.
[10] Meehan JL, Sporn JR: Case report of taxol administration via central vein producing a recall reaction at a site of prior taxol extravasation. J Natl Cancer Inst 86: 1250–1251, 1994.
[11] Riedel U, Serke M, Schönfeld N, et al: Extravasation of paclitaxel (Taxol®) – clinical course. Onkologie 22: 318–320, 1999.
[12] Shapiro J, Richardson GE: Paclitaxel-induced "recall" soft tissue injury occuring at the site of previous extravasation with subsequent intravenous treatment in a different limb. J Clin Oncol 12: 2237–2238, 1994.
[13] Panday VR, Huizing MT, Huinink WW, et al: Hypersensitivity reactions to the taxanes paclitaxel and docetaxel. Clin Drug Invest 14: 418–427, 1997.
[14] Stein ME, Drumea K, Abu-Rasmi R, et al: Taxol-induced cellulitis after extravasation: a rarely reported event. Am J Clin Oncol 20: 540, 1997.
[15] Hidalgo M, Benito J, Colomer R, et al: Recall reaction of a severe local peripheral neuropathy after paclitaxel extravasation. J Natl Cancer Inst 88: 1320, 1996.
[16] Berghmans T, Klastersky J: Paclitaxel-induced cutaneous toxicity. Support Care Cancer 3: 203–204, 1995.
[17] Bailey WL, Crump RM: Taxol extravasation: a case report. Can Oncol Nurs J 7: 96–99, 1997.
[18] Dorr RT, Snead K, Liddil JD: Skin ulceration potential of paclitaxel in a mouse skin model in vivo. Cancer 78: 152–156, 1996.
[19] Barutca S, Kadikoylu G, Bolaman Z, et al: Extravasation of paclitaxel into breast tissue from central catheter port. Support Cancer Care 10: 563–565, 2002.
[20] Link CJ, Sarosy GA, Kohn EC, et al: Cutaneous manifestations of Taxol® therapy. Investigational New Drugs 13: 261–261, 1995.
[21] Krämer I: Zehn Jahre Dokumentation von Zytostatika-Paravasat-Ereignissen: Auswertung von 175 Paravasate-Dokumentationen. Krankenhauspharmazie 23: 269–274, 2002.

Secondary literature

[22] van Gemmern R: Gewebstoxizität und Paravasatbehandlung neuer Zytostatika. Krankenhauspharmazie 17: 471–473, 1996.
[23] Bristol-Myers Squibb, personal communication, November 1998.
[24] Gain M, Melzer S, Meyer-Jürshof A, et al: Paclitaxel: Behandlung von Paravasaten. In: Gain M, et al (eds) ADKA-Zytostatika-Handbuch, Pharmazeutisch-wissenschaftliche Monographien. Verlag Heiner Biller, vol 3: 41, 1998.
[25] Dorr RT: Author reply to: Bertelli G, et al: Skin ulceration potential of paclitaxel in a mouse skin model in vivo. Cancer 79: 2268–2269, 1997.
[26] Stanley A: Managing complications of chemotherapy administration. In: Allwood M, Stanley A, Wright P (eds) The Cytotoxics Handbook. Radcliffe Medical Press, 4th edition: 119–193, 2002.
[27] Schneider G: Paravasate von Zytostatika. Diagnostik und Therapie. Aina S. Schneider Verlag, 6th edition: 1–17, 1999.
[28] Bertelli G: Prevention and management of extravasation of cytotoxic drugs. Drug Safety 12: 245–255, 1995.
[29] Bokemeyer C: Dermatoxizität antineoplastischer Substanzen. In: Schmoll HJ, Höffken K, Possinger K (eds) Kompendium Internistische Onkologie. Standards in Diagnostik und Therapie. Springer, vol 1, 3rd edition: 1411–1426, 1999.
[30] Berdel WE, Schmoll HJ, Büchele T, et al: Prävention und Therapie von Paravasaten/Extravasaten. In: Schmoll HJ, Höffken K, Possinger K (eds) Kompendium Internistische Onkologie. Standards in Diagnostik und Therapie. Springer, vol 1, 3rd edition: 1689–1701, 1999.
[31] Mullin S, Beckwith MC, Tyler LS: Prevention and management of antineoplastic extravasation injury. Hosp Pharm 35: 57–76, 2000.
[32] Gain M, Melzer S, Meyer-Jürshof A, et al: Allgemeiner Teil: Behandlung von Paravasaten. In: Gain M, et al (eds) ADKA-Zytostatika-Handbuch, Pharmazeutisch-wissenschaftliche Monographien. Verlag Heiner Biller, vol 1, 2nd edition: A42–44, 1997.
[33] Rogers BB: Nursing implications in the administration of paclitaxel (Taxol®). Semin Oncol Nurs 9: 11–15, 1993.
[34] Raghavan VT, Bloomer WD, Merkel DE: Taxol and radiation recall dermatitis. Lancet 341: 1354, 1993.
[35] Rowinsky EK, Eisenhauer EA, Chaudhry V, et al: Clinical toxicities encountered with paclitaxel (Taxol®). Semin Oncol 20 (Suppl 3): 1–15, 1993.
[36] Barth J: Paravasate und deren Behandlung. In: Barth J (ed) Zytostatika-Herstellung in der Apotheke. Deutscher Apotheker Verlag, chapter VI-3: 1–9, 2000.

[37] Stanford BL, Hardwicke F: A review of clinical experience with paclitaxel extravasations. Support Cancer Care 11: 270–277, 2003.
[38] Krämer I, Stützle M: Zytostatika-Paravasation – Wie ist vorzugehen? Krankenhauspharmazie 23: 261–268, 2002.
[39] Jordan K, Grothe W, Schmoll HJ: Paravasation von Zytostatika: Prävention und Therapie. Dtsch Med Wochenschr 130: 33–37, 2005.
[40] Ener RA, Meglathery SB, Styler M: Extravasation of systemic hemato-oncological therapies. Ann Oncol 15: 858–862, 2004.
[41] Koppel RA, Boh EE: Cutaneous reactions to chemotherapeutic agents. Am J Med Sci 321: 327–335, 2001.
[42] Alley E, Green R, Schuchter L: Cutaneous toxicities of cancer therapy. Curr Opin Oncol 14: 212–216, 2002.
[43] Summary of product characteristics Taxol® (Austria), Bristol-Myers Squibb, March 2005.

Further reading:

- Albanell J, Baselga J: Systemic therapy emergencies. Semin Oncol 27: 347–361, 2000.
- Fenchel K, Karthaus M: Zytostatika-Paravasate – gibt es neue Empfehlungen zum therapeutischen Vorgehen? Wien Med Wochenschr 151: 44–46, 2001.
- Khan MS, Holmes JD: Reducing the morbidity from extravasation injuries. Ann Plast Surg 48: 628–632, 2002.
- Krämer I: Onkologische Pharmazie. In: Jaehde U, Radziwill R, Mühlebach S, et al (eds) Lehrbuch der Klinischen Pharmazie. Wissenschaftliche Verlagsgesellschaft mbH, 2nd edition: 307–336, 2003.
- Langstein HN, Duman H, Seelig D, et al: Retrospective study of the management of chemotherapeutic extravasation injury. Ann Plast Surg 49: 369–374, 2002.
- Lorenz W, Reimann HJ, Schmal A, et al: Histamine release in dogs by cremophor EL and its derivatives: oxethylated oleic acid is the most effective constituent. Agents Actions 7: 63–67, 1977.
- Noone MH, McCabe MS, Denicoff AM, et al: Nursing management of the patient receiving taxol therapy. J Natl Cancer Inst Monogr 15: 149–154, 1993.
- Rauh J, Pluntke S, Müller C: Paravenöse Zytostatikainjektion: Prophylaxe und Sofortmaßnahmen im Notfall. MMW Fortschr Med 146: 682–686, 2004.
- Schrijvers DL: Extravasation: a dreaded complication of chemotherapy. Ann Oncol 14: iii26–iii30, 2003.

Revisions by Ines Mader

Pegaspargase

CONSENSUS

Type of damage: non-vesicant

Recommended treatment:

General measures:

1. Stop injection/infusion immediately
2. Get extravasation kit
3. Put on (sterile) gloves
4. Replace infusion lead or syringe with 5 ml disposable syringe and aspirate slowly as much as possible of the extravasated drug; **Cave!** do not exert pressure on extravasation area
5. Remove i.v. access while aspirating
6. Elevate limb and immobilise
7. Complete extravasation documentation sheet (mention extent of extravasation)
8. Inform and instruct the patient and relatives
9. Regular control (aftercare)

Substance specific measures: none

Cave! after extravasation:

1. No flushing of i.v. access
2. No moist compresses
3. No alcohol compresses
4. No occlusive dressings

Type of damage reported in literature:	No data available
Symptoms and clinical course reported in literature:	No data available
Measures reported in literature:	No data available
Particular remarks:	Results of literature search: no animal experiments or clinical studies regarding extravasation have been published Lower immunogenic potential than asparaginase because of binding to polyethyleneglycol [1–3]
Conclusion:	Since pegaspargase is also administered i.m. [3,4], a tissue-damaging effect is unlikely; the substance is therefore classified as non-vesicant No substance specific measures are required

P

Original articles

–

Secondary literature

[1] Fuxius S, Unger C: Pegaspargase. Arzneimitteltherapie 16: 170–173, 1998.
[2] Dorr RT, Von Hoff DD: Drug monographs: asparaginase. In: Dorr RT, Von Hoff DD (eds) Cancer Chemotherapy Handbook. Appleton & Lange, 2nd edition: 201–209, 1994.
[3] Albanell J, Baselga J: Systemic therapy emergencies. Semin Oncol 27: 347–361, 2000.
[4] Summary of product characteristics Oncaspar® (Germany), medac, May 2002.

Revisions by Patrizia Fürst-Weger

Pemetrexed

CONSENSUS

Type of damage: non-vesicant

Recommended treatment:

General measures:

1. Stop injection/infusion immediately
2. Get extravasation kit
3. Put on (sterile) gloves
4. Replace infusion lead or syringe with 5 ml disposable syringe and aspirate slowly as much as possible of the extravasated drug; **Cave!** do not exert pressure on extravasation area
5. Remove i.v. access while aspirating
6. Elevate limb and immobilise
7. Complete extravasation documentation sheet (mention extent of extravasation)
8. Inform and instruct the patient and relatives
9. Regular control (aftercare)

Substance specific measures: none

Cave! after extravasation:

1. No flushing of i.v. access
2. No moist compresses
3. No alcohol compresses
4. No occlusive dressings

Type of damage reported in literature:	No blister formation [1] Non-vesicant [2]
Symptoms and clinical course reported in literature:	No data available
Measures reported in literature:	**Successful treatment:** – No data available **Unsuccessful treatment:** – No data available **Outcome of treatment not reported:** – No specific measure mentioned [2]
Particular remarks:	Results of literature search: no animal experiments regarding extravasation have been published Up to January 2005, only one case of extravasation had been documented, which was assessed as not serious [2]
Conclusion:	Since no case of tissue damage after extravasation has been documented, pemetrexed is classified as non-vesicant Owing to little or no experience with extravasations of pemetrexed, a final evaluation of the type of damage is not possible No substance specific measures are required

Original articles

—

Secondary literature

[1] Summary of product characteristics Alimta® (Austria), Eli Lilly, October 2004.
[2] Lilly Research Laboratories, unpublished data, January 2005.

Revisions by Sabine Wassertheurer

Pentostatin

CONSENSUS

Type of damage: non-vesicant

Recommended treatment:

General measures:

1. Stop injection/infusion immediately
2. Get extravasation kit
3. Put on (sterile) gloves
4. Replace infusion lead or syringe with 5 ml disposable syringe and aspirate slowly as much as possible of the extravasated drug; **Cave**! do not exert pressure on extravasation area
5. Remove i.v. access while aspirating
6. Elevate limb and immobilise
7. Complete extravasation documentation sheet (mention extent of extravasation)
8. Inform and instruct the patient and relatives
9. Regular control (aftercare)

Substance specific measures: none

Cave! after extravasation:

1. No flushing of i.v. access
2. No moist compresses
3. No alcohol compresses
4. No occlusive dressings

Type of damage reported in literature:

Non-vesicant [3,4,6,8]

No tissue toxic potential [12]

Weak irritant (not vesicant) [9]

Irritant [5,7,10,11]

Vesicant [7]

Symptoms and clinical course reported in literature:

No data available

Measures reported in literature:

Successful treatment:
- No data available

Unsuccessful treatment:
- No data available

Outcome of treatment not reported:
- 1500 IU hyaluronidase s.c., application of heat and compression [4]
- Topical cooling [7] 4 × daily for 20 minutes over 3–4 days [12]
- No specific measures mentioned [3,5,8, 9–11]

Particular remarks:

Animal experiments: in weekly i.a. and i.v. application of 1 mg/ml and 5 mg/ml no vascular irritations occurred, in cases of several injections daily local irritations are possible [1,2]

In clinical studies no tissue damage after extravasation has been observed [6]

Reconstituted solutions of pentostatin have a maximum pH of 8.5; this can result in irritations with erythema, pain, and phlebitis [5]

Conclusion: Although pentostatin is classified as irritant/vesicant in some of the literature, no clinical case of tissue damage after extravasation has been documented; the substance is therefore classified as non-vesicant

No substance specific measures are required

Original articles

[1] Field KJ (Parke-Davis): Intraarterial irritation study in rabbits with Cl-825. Expert's Report RR 745–01429, 1989.
[2] Field KJ (Parke-Davis): Intravenous irritation study in rabbits with Cl-825. Expert's Report RR 745–01420, 1989.

Secondary literature

[3] Dorr RT: Pharmacologic management of vesicant chemotherapy extravasations. In: Dorr RT, Von Hoff DD (eds) Cancer Chemotherapy Handbook. Appleton & Lange, 2nd edition: 109–118, 1994.
[4] Stanley A: Managing complications of chemotherapy administration. In: Allwood M, Stanley A, Wright P (eds) The Cytotoxics Handbook. Radcliffe Medical Press, 4th edition: 119–193, 2002.
[5] van Gemmern R: Gewebstoxizität und Paravasatbehandlung neuer Zytostatika. Krankenhauspharmazie 17: 471–473, 1996.
[6] Summary of product characteristics Nipent® (Germany), Wyeth Pharma, November 2002.
[7] Berdel WE, Schmoll HJ, Büchele T, et al: Prävention und Therapie von Paravasaten/Extravasaten. In: Schmoll HJ, Höffken K, Possinger K (eds) Kompendium Internistische Onkologie. Standards in Diagnostik und Therapie. Springer, vol 1, 3rd edition: 1689–1701, 1999.
[8] Gain M, Melzer S, Meyer-Jürshof A, et al: Allgemeiner Teil: Behandlung von Paravasaten. In: Gain M, et al (eds) ADKA-Zytostatika-Handbuch, Pharmazeutisch-wissenschaftliche Monographien. Verlag Heiner Biller, vol 1, 2nd edition: A42–44, 1997.
[9] Barth J: Paravasate und deren Behandlung. In: Barth J (ed) Zytostatika-Herstellung in der Apotheke. Deutscher Apotheker Verlag, chapter VI-3: 1–9, 2000.
[10] Jordan K, Grothe W, Schmoll HJ: Paravasation von Zytostatika: Prävention und Therapie. Dtsch Med Wochenschr 130: 33–37, 2005.

[11] Ener RA, Meglathery SB, Styler M: Extravasation of systemic hemato-oncological therapies. Ann Oncol 15: 858–862, 2004.
[12] Krämer I, Stützle M: Zytostatika-Paravasation – Wie ist vorzugehen? Krankenhauspharmazie 23: 261–268, 2002.

Further reading:

- Fenchel K, Karthaus M: Zytostatika-Paravasate – gibt es neue Empfehlungen zum therapeutischen Vorgehen? Wien Med Wochenschr 151: 44–46, 2001.

Revisions by Sabine Wassertheurer

Raltitrexed

CONSENSUS

Type of damage: non-vesicant

Recommended treatment:

General measures:

1. Stop injection/infusion immediately
2. Get extravasation kit
3. Put on (sterile) gloves
4. Replace infusion lead or syringe with 5 ml disposable syringe and aspirate slowly as much as possible of the extravasated drug; **Cave!** do not exert pressure on extravasation area
5. Remove i.v. access while aspirating
6. Elevate limb and immobilise
7. Complete extravasation documentation sheet (mention extent of extravasation)
8. Inform and instruct the patient and relatives
9. Regular control (aftercare)

Substance specific measures: none

Cave! after extravasation:

1. No flushing of i.v. access
2. No moist compresses
3. No alcohol compresses
4. No occlusive dressings

Type of damage reported in literature:

Non-vesicant [2,6]

No tissue damaging potential [7]

Weak irritant (not vesicant) [3]

Inflammatory [1]

Symptoms and clinical course reported in literature:

No data available

Measures reported in literature:

Successful treatment:
- No data available

Unsuccessful treatment:
- No data available

Outcome of treatment not reported:
- 100 mg hydrocortisone iv. and s.c., respectively, additionally topical hydrocortisone, intermittent ice packs over 24 hours, after local reaction has receded, application of heat and compression [1]

- Topical cooling 4 × daily for 20 minutes over 3–4 days [7]

- No specific measure mentioned [6]

Particular remarks:

Results of literature search: no clinical studies regarding extravasation have been published

Animal experiments: in case of perivascular [2,4,5] and intra-arterial [2] application, no tissue irritations have been observed

Conclusion:

Although raltitrexed is classified as irritant in some of the literature, no clinical case of irritation of tissue after extravasation has been documented; the substance is therefore classified as non-vesicant

No substance specific measures are required

Original articles

–

Secondary literature

[1] Stanley A: Managing complications of chemotherapy administration. In: Allwood M, Stanley A, Wright P (eds) The Cytotoxics Handbook. Radcliffe Medical Press, 4th edition: 119–193, 2002.
[2] AstraZeneca, unpublished data, March 1999.
[3] Barth J: Paravasate und deren Behandlung. In: Barth J (ed) Zytostatika-Herstellung in der Apotheke. Deutscher Apotheker Verlag, chapter VI-3: 1–9, 2000.
[4] Stanley A: Chemotherapeutic agents: raltitrexed. In: Allwood M, Stanley A, Wright P (eds) The Cytotoxics Handbook. Radcliffe Medical Press, 4th edition: 403–404, 2002.
[5] Summary of product characteristics Tomudex® (Switzerland), AstraZeneca, October 2003.
[6] Jordan K, Grothe W, Schmoll HJ: Paravasation von Zytostatika: Prävention und Therapie. Dtsch Med Wochenschr 130: 33–37, 2005.
[7] Krämer I, Stützle M: Zytostatika-Paravasation – Wie ist vorzugehen? Krankenhauspharmazie 23: 261–268, 2002.

Further reading:

– Schrijvers DL: Extravasation: a dreaded complication of chemotherapy. Ann Oncol 14: iii26–iii30, 2003.

R

Revisions by Sabine Wassertheurer

Streptozocin

CONSENSUS

Type of damage: irritant

Recommended treatment:

General measures:

1. Stop injection/infusion immediately
2. Get extravasation kit
3. Put on (sterile) gloves
4. Replace infusion lead or syringe with 5 ml disposable syringe and aspirate slowly as much as possible of the extravasated drug; **Cave!** do not exert pressure on extravasation area
5. Remove i.v. access while aspirating
6. If blisters occur: aspirate with 1 ml syringe and s.c. cannula, use new equipment for every new attempt at aspiration
7. Elevate limb and immobilise
8. Complete extravasation documentation sheet (mention extent of extravasation)
9. Inform and instruct the patient and relatives
10. Regular control (aftercare)

Substance specific measures: none

Cave! after extravasation:

1. No flushing of i.v. access
2. No moist compresses
3. No alcohol compresses
4. No occlusive dressings

Type of damage reported in literature:	Irritant [2,6–8,12] Vesicant [3–5,9,13]
Symptoms and clinical course reported in literature:	**Initial symptoms:** No data available **Delayed-onset symptoms:** According to the summary of product characteristics severe tissue lesions and necrosis are possible [10] - but no further information available **Residual findings:** No data available
Measures reported in literature:	**Successful treatment:** – No data available **Unsuccessful treatment:** – No data available **Outcome of treatment not reported:** – On the first day DMSO every 2 hours, hydrocortisone (1%) applied topically, cold compresses for 30 minutes; followed by 7–10 days' alternating application of DMSO and hydrocortisone applied topically at 3 hourly intervals [3] – Optional local infiltration of corticosteroids, warm to hot compresses for 1 hour [4] – Topical cooling 4 × daily for 20 minutes over 3–4 days [5] – If local symptoms develop, hydrocortisone (1%) or heparin to be applied topically [7] – No specific measures mentioned [2,6,8,9,12,13]
Particular remarks:	Results of literature search: no animal experiments or clinical studies regarding extravasation have been published

S

Immediate burning along the vein during administration [1,11] and tissue irritation at the injection site [10] are not associated with extravasation; these reactions are likely to be a result of the acidic pH of 3.5–4.5 [10,11] of the reconstituted solution

Conclusion: Although streptozocin is classified as irritant/vesicant in the literature, no clinical case of tissue damage after extravasation has been documented; the classification as irritant is due to the acid pH of the reconstituted drug

The symptoms mentioned in the secondary literature–such as severe tissue damage or necroses–could not be verified by clinical case reports

Owing to little or no experience with extravasations of streptozocin, a final classification of the type of damage is not possible

Positive results of substance specific measures have not been described so far; until further data become available no substance specific measures can be recommended

Original articles

[1] DuPriest RW, Huntington MC, Massey WH, et al: Streptozotocin therapy in 22 cancer patients. Cancer 35: 358–367, 1975.

S

Secondary literature

[2] Ener RA, Meglathery SB, Styler M: Extravasation of systemic hemato-oncological therapies. Ann Oncol 15: 858–862, 2004.
[3] Stanley A: Managing complications of chemotherapy administration. In: Allwood M, Stanley A, Wright P (eds) The Cytotoxics Handbook. Radcliffe Medical Press, 4th edition: 119–193, 2002.
[4] Ignoffo RJ, Friedman MA: Therapy of local toxicities caused by extravasation of cancer chemotherapeutic drugs. Cancer Treat Rev 7: 17–27, 1980.
[5] Krämer I, Stützle M: Zytostatika-Paravasation – Wie ist vorzugehen? Krankenhauspharmazie 23: 261–268, 2002.

[6] Mullin S, Beckwith MC, Tyler LS: Prevention and management of antineoplastic extravasation injury. Hosp Pharm 35: 57–76, 2000.
[7] Cox K, Stuart-Harris R, Abdini G, et al: The management of cytotoxic-drug extravasation: guide-lines drawn up by a working party for the Clinical Oncological Society of Australia. Med J Aust 148: 185–189, 1988.
[8] Schneider SM, Distelhorst CW: Chemotherapy-induced emergencies. Semin Oncol 16: 572–578, 1989.
[9] Gain M, Melzer S, Meyer-Jürshof A, et al: Allgemeiner Teil: Behandlung von Paravasaten. In: Gain M, et al (eds) ADKA-Zytostatika-Handbuch, Pharmazeutisch-wissenschaftliche Monographien. Verlag Heiner Biller, vol 1, 2nd edition: A42–44, 1997.
[10] Summary of product characteristics Zanosar® (USA), Pharmacia & Upjohn, February 2003.
[11] Dorr RT, Von Hoff DD: Drug monographs: streptozocin. In: Dorr RT, Von Hoff DD (eds) Cancer Chemotherapy Handbook. Appleton & Lange, 2nd edition: 850–856, 1994.
[12] Holmes BC: Administration of cancer chemotherapy agents. In: Dorr RT, Von Hoff DD (eds) Cancer Chemotherapy Handbook. Appleton & Lange, 2nd edition: 57–94, 1994.
[13] Jordan K, Grothe W, Schmoll HJ: Paravasation von Zytostatika: Prävention und Therapie. Dtsch Med Wochenschr 130: 33–37, 2005.

Further reading:

- Fenchel K, Karthaus M: Zytostatika-Paravasate – gibt es neue Empfehlungen zum therapeutischen Vorgehen? Wien Med Wochenschr 151: 44–46, 2001.
- Rauh J, Pluntke S, Müller C: Paravenöse Zytostatikainjektion: Prophylaxe und Sofortmaßnahmen im Notfall. MMW Fortschr Med 146: 682–686, 2004.

S

Revisions by Patrizia Fürst-Weger

Teniposide

CONSENSUS

Type of damage: irritant

Recommended treatment:

General measures:

1. Stop injection/infusion immediately
2. Get extravasation kit
3. Put on (sterile) gloves
4. Replace infusion lead or syringe with 5 ml disposable syringe and aspirate slowly as much as possible of the extravasated drug; **Cave!** do not exert pressure on extravasation area
5. Remove i.v. access while aspirating
6. If blisters occur: aspirate with 1 ml syringe and s.c. cannula, use new equipment for every new attempt at aspiration
7. Elevate limb and immobilise
8. Complete extravasation documentation sheet (mention extent of extravasation)
9. Inform and instruct the patient and relatives
10. Regular control (aftercare)

Substance specific measures: none

Cave! after extravasation:

1. No flushing of i.v. access
2. No moist compresses
3. No alcohol compresses
4. No occlusive dressings

Type of damage reported in literature:

Non-vesicant [10]

Weak irritant (not vesicant) [15]

Irritant [2,6,9,11,13,14,16,22,24] and/or weak vesicant in large amounts and high concentrations [5]

No risk of necrosis [3, 4]

Vesicant [8,12]

Symptoms and clinical course reported in literature:

Initial symptoms: No data available

Delayed-onset symptoms: According to the summary of product characteristics rarely necroses [17]

Residual findings: No data available

Measures reported in literature:

Successful treatment:
- Animal experiments: NaCl 0.9% or hyaluronidase i.d. [1]

Unsuccessful treatment:
- No data available

Outcome of treatment not reported:
- 150 IU hyaluronidase in 1–3 ml NaCl 0.9% s.c. [2,3,14]

- Mild, dry heat over 1–2 hours, 150–900 IU hyaluronidase s.c., alternatively: DMSO every 3–4 hours for 1–3 days administered topically [4]

- Warm compresses immediately applied for 30–60 minutes, then for 24 hours alternating every 15 minutes (with/without compresses), 150 IU hyaluronidase s.c. [5]

- Locally applied mild heat for 1–2 hours, in severe cases additionally application of 150 IU hyaluronidase s.c. [6]

- 150–900 IU hyaluronidase s.c. or i.d. [8] and warm compresses [13]
- 150–900 IU hyaluronidase i.v. or s.c. applied several times over 3–4 hours, local application of heat [19]
- 150 IU hyaluronidase s.c. after extravasation of ≥50% of the planned total dose [20]
- Optional local infiltration of corticosteroids, warm to hot compresses for 1 hour [10]
- 100 mg hydrocortisone i.v. and s.c., respectively, hydrocortisone (1%) applied topically, ice pack [16]
- No specific measures mentioned [11, 15]

Particular remarks: Results of literature search: no clinical studies regarding extravasation have been published

Animal experiments: ulcerations in case of undiluted i.d. administration are due to the excipients of the formulation; lower ulcerogenic effect in diluted solutions observed [1, 3]

Phlebitis [3–5,16,24] and hypersensitivity reactions [7,17,18] are not associated with extravasation; these symptoms are likely to be due to the excipients in the formulation (Cremophor® EL, ethanol, and benzyl alcohol [17,18])

In formulations that contain benzyl alcohol, extravasation of teniposide may initially be painless and remain unnoticed (local anaesthetic effect) [6]

Hyaluronidase and NaCl 0.9%: positive effect has been described in animal experiment only [1]; disadvantage: invasive measure

There is no clinical evidence for the application of hyaluronidase after extravasation of teniposide, in spite of recent reports in the literature [6,16]

Conclusion:

Although teniposide is classified as vesicant in some of the literature, no clinical case of necrosis after extravasation has been documented; the substance is classified as irritant due to the excipients in the formulation

Symptoms mentioned in the secondary literature, such as necroses, could not be verified in clinical case reports

Positive results of substance specific measures have not been described so far; until further data become available no substance specific measures can be recommended

Original articles

[1] Dorr RT, Alberts DS: Skin ulceration potential without therapeutic anticancer activity for epipodophyllotoxin commercial diluents. Invest New Drugs 1: 151–159, 1983.

Secondary literature

[2] Gain M, Melzer S, Meyer-Jürshof A, et al: Teniposid: Behandlung von Paravasaten. In: Gain M, et al (eds) ADKA-Zytostatika-Handbuch, Pharmazeutisch-wissenschaftliche Monographien. Verlag Heiner Biller, vol 3: 34, 1998.
[3] Dorr RT: Antidotes to vesicant chemotherapy extravasations. Blood Rev 4: 41–60, 1990.
[4] Schneider G: Paravasate von Zytostatika. Diagnostik und Therapie. Aina S. Schneider Verlag, 6th edition: 1–17, 1999.
[5] Dorr RT: Pharmacologic management of vesicant chemotherapy extravasations. In: Dorr RT, Von Hoff DD (eds) Cancer Chemotherapy Handbook. Appleton & Lange, 2nd edition: 109–118, 1994.
[6] Krämer I, Stützle M: Zytostatika-Paravasation – Wie ist vorzugehen? Krankenhauspharmazie 23: 261–268, 2002.
[7] Bokemeyer C: Dermatoxizität antineoplastischer Substanzen. In: Schmoll HJ, Höffken K, Possinger K (eds) Kompendium Internistische Onkologie. Standards in Diagnostik und Therapie. Springer, vol 1, 3rd edition: 1411–1426, 1999.
[8] Bertelli G: Prevention and management of extravasation of cytotoxic drugs. Drug Safety 12: 245–255, 1995.

[9] Gain M, Melzer S, Meyer-Jürshof A, et al: Allgemeiner Teil: Behandlung von Paravasaten. In: Gain M, et al (eds) ADKA-Zytostatika-Handbuch, Pharmazeutisch-wissenschaftliche Monographien. Verlag Heiner Biller, vol 1, 2nd edition: A42–44, 1997.
[10] Ignoffo RJ, Friedman MA: Therapy of local toxicities caused by extravasation of cancer chemotherapeutic drugs. Cancer Treat Rev 7: 17–27, 1980.
[11] Mullin S, Beckwith MC, Tyler LS: Prevention and management of antineoplastic extravasation injury. Hosp Pharm 35: 57–76, 2000.
[12] Myers P: Investigational drugs: teniposide. In: Allwood M, Stanley A, Wright P (eds) The Cytotoxics Handbook. Radcliffe Medical Press, 4th edition: 407–409, 2002.
[13] Schneider SM, Distelhorst CW: Chemotherapy-induced emergencies. Semin Oncol 16: 572–578, 1989.
[14] Bristol-Myers Squibb, personal communication, January 1999.
[15] Barth J: Paravasate und deren Behandlung. In: Barth J (ed) Zytostatika-Herstellung in der Apotheke. Deutscher Apotheker Verlag, chapter VI-3: 1–9, 2000.
[16] Stanley A: Managing complications of chemotherapy administration. In: Allwood M, Stanley A, Wright P (eds) The Cytotoxics Handbook. Radcliffe Medical Press, 4th edition: 119–193, 2002.
[17] Summary of product characteristics VM 26-Bristol (Germany), Bristol-Myers Squibb, February 2005.
[18] Alley E, Green R, Schuchter L: Cutaneous toxicities of cancer therapy. Curr Opin Oncol 14: 212–216, 2002.
[19] Ener RA, Meglathery SB, Styler M: Extravasation of systemic hemato-oncological therapies. Ann Oncol 15: 858–862, 2004.
[20] Albanell J, Baselga J: Systemic therapy emergencies. Semin Oncol 27: 347–361, 2000.

Further reading:

- Fenchel K, Karthaus M: Zytostatika-Paravasate – gibt es neue Empfehlungen zum therapeutischen Vorgehen? Wien Med Wochenschr 151: 44–46, 2001.
- Jordan K, Grothe W, Schmoll HJ: Paravasation von Zytostatika: Prävention und Therapie. Dtsch Med Wochenschr 130: 33–37, 2005.
- Kassner E: Evaluation and treatment of chemotherapy extravasation injuries. J Pediatr Oncol Nurs 17: 135–148, 2000.
- Krämer I: Onkologische Pharmazie. In: Jaehde U, Radziwill R, Mühlebach S, et al (eds) Lehrbuch der Klinischen Pharmazie. Wissenschaftliche Verlagsgesellschaft mbH, 2nd edition: 307–336, 2003.

- Langstein HN, Duman H, Seelig D, et al: Retrospective study of the management of chemotherapeutic extravasation injury. Ann Plast Surg 49: 369–374, 2002.
- Lorenz W, Reimann HJ, Schmal A, et al: Histamine release in dogs by cremophor EL and its derivatives: oxethylated oleic acid is the most effective constituent. Agents Actions 7: 63–67, 1977.
- Rauh J, Pluntke S, Müller C: Paravenöse Zytostatikainjektion: Prophylaxe und Sofortmaßnahmen im Notfall. MMW Fortschr Med 146: 682–686, 2004.
- Whang SW, Lee SH, Elias PM, et al: Intralesional steroids reduce inflammation from extravasated chemotherapeutic agents. Br J Dermatol 145: 680–682, 2001.

Revisions by Ines Mader

Thiotepa

<u>CONSENSUS</u>

Type of damage: non-vesicant

Recommended treatment:

General measures:

1. Stop injection/infusion immediately
2. Get extravasation kit
3. Put on (sterile) gloves
4. Replace infusion lead or syringe with 5 ml disposable syringe and aspirate slowly as much as possible of the extravasated drug; **Cave!** do not exert pressure on extravasation area
5. Remove i.v. access while aspirating
6. Elevate limb and immobilise
7. Complete extravasation documentation sheet (mention extent of extravasation)
8. Inform and instruct the patient and relatives
9. Regular control (aftercare)

Substance specific measures: none

Cave! after extravasation:

1. No flushing of i.v. access
2. No moist compresses
3. No alcohol compresses
4. No occlusive dressings

Type of damage reported in literature:

Non-vesicant [1–3,6–8,10,14]

Irritant [4,5,9]

Symptoms and clinical course reported in literature:

No data available

Measures reported in literature:

Successful treatment:
- No data available

Unsuccessful treatment:
- No data available

Outcome of treatment not reported:
- 1500 IU hyaluronidase s.c., application of heat and compression [2]
- Optional local infiltration of corticosteroids, warm to hot compresses for 1 hour [4]
- If local symptoms develop, hydrocortisone (1%) or heparin to be applied topically [5]
- 100 mg hydrocortisone s.c. and i.v., respectively, ice or cold pack 4 × daily for 15–20 minutes, topical hydrocortisone [6, 7]
- Topical cooling 4 × daily for 20 minutes over 3–4 days [10]
- No specific measures mentioned [1,3,8, 9,14]

T

Particular remarks:

Results of literature search: no animal experiments or clinical studies regarding extravasation have been published

Pain and phlebitis are not to be expected if substance is applied i.v. [3]

Hypersensitivity reactions [11] and hyperpigmentation of the skin [11–13] are not associated with extravasation

Conclusion: Although thiotepa is classified as irritant in some of the literature, no clinical case of irritation of tissue after extravasation has been documented; since this substance can also be applied i.m. or s.c. [3], a tissue-damaging effect is unlikely; thiotepa is therefore classified as non-vesicant

No substance specific measures are required

Original articles

–

Secondary literature

[1] Wyeth-Lederle Pharma, personal communication, November 1998.

[2] Stanley A: Managing complications of chemotherapy administration. In: Allwood M, Stanley A, Wright P (eds) The Cytotoxics Handbook. Radcliffe Medical Press, 4th edition: 119–193, 2002.

[3] Dorr RT, Von Hoff DD: Drug monographs: thiotepa. In: Dorr RT, Von Hoff DD (eds) Cancer Chemotherapy Handbook. Appleton & Lange, 2nd edition: 898–905, 1994.

[4] Ignoffo RJ, Friedman MA: Therapy of local toxicities caused by extravasation of cancer chemotherapeutic drugs. Cancer Treat Rev 7: 17–27, 1980.

[5] Cox K, Stuart-Harris R, Abdini G, et al: The management of cytotoxic-drug extravasation: guide-lines drawn up by a working party for the Clinical Oncological Society of Australia. Med J Aust 148: 185–189, 1988.

[6] Gain M, Melzer S, Meyer-Jürshof A, et al: Thiotepa: Behandlung von Paravasaten. In: Gain M, et al (eds) ADKA-Zytostatika-Handbuch, Pharmazeutisch-wissenschaftliche Monographien. Verlag Heiner Biller, vol 3: 24, 1998.

[7] Gain M, Melzer S, Meyer-Jürshof A, et al: Allgemeiner Teil: Behandlung von Paravasaten. In: Gain M, et al (eds) ADKA-Zytostatika-Handbuch, Pharmazeutisch-wissenschaftliche Monographien. Verlag Heiner Biller, vol 1, 2nd edition: A42–44, 1997.

[8] Schneider SM, Distelhorst CW: Chemotherapy-induced emergencies. Semin Oncol 16: 572–578, 1989.

[9] Mullin S, Beckwith MC, Tyler LS: Prevention and management of antineoplastic extravasation injury. Hosp Pharm 35: 57–76, 2000.

[10] Krämer I, Stützle M: Zytostatika-Paravasation – Wie ist vorzugehen? Krankenhauspharmazie 23: 261–268, 2002.

[11] Koppel RA, Boh EE: Cutaneous reactions to chemotherapeutic agents. Am J Med Sci 321: 327–335, 2001.
[12] Alley E, Green R, Schuchter L: Cutaneous toxicities of cancer therapy. Curr Opin Oncol 14: 212–216, 2002.
[13] Summary of product characteristics Thiotepa "Lederle" (Germany), Riemser Arzneimittel, February 2003.
[14] Jordan K, Grothe W, Schmoll HJ: Paravasation von Zytostatika: Prävention und Therapie. Dtsch Med Wochenschr 130: 33–37, 2005.

Further reading:

- Rauh J, Pluntke S, Müller C: Paravenöse Zytostatikainjektion: Prophylaxe und Sofortmaßnahmen im Notfall. MMW Fortschr Med 146: 682–686, 2004.
- Schrijvers DL: Extravasation: a dreaded complication of chemotherapy. Ann Oncol 14: iii26–iii30, 2003.

Revisions by Patrizia Fürst-Weger

Topotecan

CONSENSUS

Type of damage: non-vesicant

Recommended treatment:

General measures:

1. Stop injection/infusion immediately
2. Get extravasation kit
3. Put on (sterile) gloves
4. Replace infusion lead or syringe with 5 ml disposable syringe and aspirate slowly as much as possible of the extravasated drug; **Cave!** do not exert pressure on extravasation area
5. Remove i.v. access while aspirating
6. Elevate limb and immobilise
7. Complete extravasation documentation sheet (mention extent of extravasation)
8. Inform and instruct the patient and relatives
9. Regular control (aftercare)

Substance specific measures: none

Cave! after extravasation:

1. No flushing of i.v. access
2. No moist compresses
3. No alcohol compresses
4. No occlusive dressings

Type of damage reported in literature:	Non-vesicant [1,2,7] Irritant [5,6] Exfoliant [8] Vesicant [4]
Symptoms and clinical course reported in literature:	**Initial symptoms:** Swelling and slight pain (2 patients) [1], slight inflammatory reaction (9 patients) [8] **Delayed-onset symptoms:** No data available **Residual findings:** No data available No ulceration [1]
Measures reported in literature:	**Successful treatment:** – Cooling (1 patient) [1] – No measures (1 patient) [1], (9 patients) [8] – Antibiotic treatment [2] **Unsuccessful treatment:** – No data available **Outcome of treatment not reported:** – Cooling [4,7] – Infiltration of sodium bicarbonate (1% or 2.1%) [8] – No specific measures mentioned [2,3,5,6]
Particular remarks:	Results of literature search: 11 clinical case reports have been published Antibiotics: only for prophylaxis of secondary infection, no causal treatment for extravasation

Conclusion: Although topotecan is classified as irritant/ vesicant in some of the literature, no clinical case of tissue damage after extravasation has been documented; the substance is therefore classified as non-vesicant

No substance specific measures – such as cooling – are required

Original articles

[1] Oostweegel LM, van Warmerdam LJ, Schot M, et al: Extravasation of topotecan, a report of two cases. J Oncol Pharm Practice 3: 115–116, 1997.

Secondary literature

[2] van Gemmern R: Gewebstoxizität und Paravasatbehandlung neuer Zytostatika. Krankenhauspharmazie 17: 471–473, 1996.
[3] Summary of product characteristics Hycamtin® (Austria), GlaxoSmithKline, July 2002.
[4] Berdel WE, Schmoll HJ, Büchele T, et al: Prävention und Therapie von Paravasaten/Extravasaten. In: Schmoll HJ, Höffken K, Possinger K (eds) Kompendium Internistische Onkologie. Standards in Diagnostik und Therapie. Springer, vol 1, 3rd edition: 1689–1701, 1999.
[5] Mullin S, Beckwith MC, Tyler LS: Prevention and management of antineoplastic extravasation injury. Hosp Pharm 35: 57–76, 2000.
[6] Gain M, Melzer S, Meyer-Jürshof A, et al: Allgemeiner Teil: Behandlung von Paravasaten. In: Gain M, et al (eds) ADKA-Zytostatika-Handbuch, Pharmazeutisch-wissenschaftliche Monographien. Verlag Heiner Biller, vol 1, 2nd edition: A42–44, 1997.
[7] Krämer I, Stützle M: Zytostatika-Paravasation – Wie ist vorzugehen? Krankenhauspharmazie 23: 261–268, 2002.
[8] Stanley A: Managing complications of chemotherapy administration. In: Allwood M, Stanley A, Wright P (eds) The Cytotoxics Handbook. Radcliffe Medical Press, 4th edition: 119–193, 2002.

Further reading:

- Ener RA, Meglathery SB, Styler M: Extravasation of systemic hemato-oncological therapies. Ann Oncol 15: 858–862, 2004.
- Fenchel K, Karthaus M: Zytostatika-Paravasate – gibt es neue Empfehlungen zum therapeutischen Vorgehen? Wien Med Wochenschr 151: 44–46, 2001.

- Jordan K, Grothe W, Schmoll HJ: Paravasation von Zytostatika: Prävention und Therapie. Dtsch Med Wochenschr 130: 33–37, 2005.
- Rauh J, Pluntke S, Müller C: Paravenöse Zytostatikainjektion: Prophylaxe und Sofortmaßnahmen im Notfall. MMW Fortschr Med 146: 682–686, 2004.

Revisions by Ines Mader

T

Treosulfan

CONSENSUS

Type of damage: irritant

Recommended treatment:

General measures:

1. Stop injection/infusion immediately
2. Get extravasation kit
3. Put on (sterile) gloves
4. Replace infusion lead or syringe with 5 ml disposable syringe and aspirate slowly as much as possible of the extravasated drug; **Cave!** do not exert pressure on extravasation area
5. Remove i.v. access while aspirating
6. If blisters occur: aspirate with 1 ml syringe and s.c. cannula, use new equipment for every new attempt at aspiration
7. Elevate limb and immobilise
8. Complete extravasation documentation sheet (mention extent of extravasation)
9. Inform and instruct the patient and relatives
10. Regular control (aftercare)

Substance specific measures: none

Cave! after extravasation:

1. No flushing of i.v. access
2. No moist compresses
3. No alcohol compresses
4. No occlusive dressings

Type of damage reported in literature:

Unknown tissue toxic potential [5]

Irritant [4,9,14]

Vesicant [3,8,12]

Symptoms and clinical course reported in literature:

Initial symptoms: No data available

Delayed-onset symptoms: According to the summary of product characteristics: pain, inflammation, destruction of tissue [8] - no further information available

Residual findings: No data available

Individual case reports:
- 1 week after extravasation of 50 ml treosulfan solution : erythema, swelling and pain, wound healing without scar formation (1 patient) [9]
- After extravasation of 100 ml treosulfan solution (4%): swelling, erythema, no necrosis (1 patient) [9]

Measures reported in literature:

Successful treatment:
- Topical cooling, cortisone s.c., dressings soaked with cortisone, heparin, NaCl, and scandicain (1 patient) [9]
- Application of DMSO every hour over 3.5 days, 2 × daily Topisolone-lotio®, cooling with gel pad, 24 mg Urbason® p.o. for 3 days, Fragmin® 1 × daily s.c. for prophylaxis of thrombosis (1 patient) [9]

Unsuccessful treatment:
- No data available

Outcome of treatment not reported:
- Cooling, optional topical DMSO [2]

- Infiltration of 1–3 ml sodium bicarbonate (1% or 2.1%), aspiration after 2 minutes, warm compresses [3]
- 100 mg hydrocortisone s.c. and i.v., respectively, ice or cold pack 4 × daily for 15–20 minutes, topical hydrocortisone [4, 7]
- Topical cooling 4 × daily for 20 minutes over 3–4 days [5]
- No specific measures reported [1 (1 patient), 14]

Particular remarks:

Results of literature search: no animal experiments regarding extravasation have been published

Acute adverse reactions are not to be expected as treosulfan is a cytotoxically ineffective prodrug [6,13]

Adverse reactions can occur after larger amounts of the extravasated drug [6]

Corticosteroids: positive effect is questionable, because extravasations are only rarely accompanied by inflammatory processes (see chapter "Histopathological investigations")

DMSO: positive effect not sufficiently confirmed (1 patient) [9]

Heparin: positive effect not sufficiently confirmed (1 patient) [9]

Topical cooling: positive effect not sufficiently confirmed (2 patients) [9]

Conclusion:

Although treosulfan is classified as vesicant in some of the literature, no clinical case of necroses after extravasation has been documented; only irritations of tissue have been reported, which are probably due to the acidic pH of 3.5 of the reconstituted solution [13]; the substance is therefore classified as irritant

Owing to little experience with extravasations of treosulfan, a final classification of the type of damage is not possible

Positive results of substance specific measures have not been sufficiently described so far (2 patients only); until further data become available no substance specific measures can be recommended

Original articles

[1] Krämer I: Zehn Jahre Dokumentation von Zytostatika-Paravasat-Ereignissen: Auswertung von 175 Paravasate-Dokumentationen. Krankenhauspharmazie 23: 269–274, 2002.

Secondary literature

[2] Torrex Pharma, personal communication, November 1998.
[3] Stanley A: Managing complications of chemotherapy administration. In: Allwood M, Stanley A, Wright P (eds) The Cytotoxics Handbook. Radcliffe Medical Press, 4th edition: 119–193, 2002.
[4] Donislawski S, Gain M, Meyer-Jürshof A, et al: Treosulfan: Behandlung von Paravasaten. In: Donislawski S, et al (eds) ADKA-Zytostatika-Handbuch, Pharmazeutisch-wissenschaftliche Monographien. Verlag Heiner Biller, vol 2: 17, 1994.
[5] Krämer I, Stützle M: Zytostatika-Paravasation – Wie ist vorzugehen? Krankenhauspharmazie 23: 261–268, 2002.
[6] Medac, personal communication, February 2000.
[7] Gain M, Melzer S, Meyer-Jürshof A, et al: Allgemeiner Teil: Behandlung von Paravasaten. In: Gain M, et al (eds) ADKA-Zytostatika-Handbuch, Pharmazeutisch-wissenschaftliche Monographien. Verlag Heiner Biller, vol 1, 2nd edition: A42–44, 1997.
[8] Summary of product characteristics Ovastat® (Germany), medac, January 2005.
[9] Medac, personal communication, March 2000.
[10] Schneider G: Paravasate von Zytostatika. Diagnostik und Therapie. Aina S. Schneider Verlag, 6th edition: 1–17, 1999.
[11] Bertelli G: Prevention and management of extravasation of cytotoxic drugs. Drug Safety 12: 245–255, 1995.
[12] Barth J: Paravasate und deren Behandlung. In: Barth J (ed) Zytostatika-Herstellung in der Apotheke. Deutscher Apotheker Verlag, chapter VI-3: 1–9, 2000.

[13] Information for hospital pharmacists Ovastat® (Germany), medac, January 1998.
[14] Jordan K, Grothe W, Schmoll HJ: Paravasation von Zytostatika: Prävention und Therapie. Dtsch Med Wochenschr 130: 33–37, 2005.

Further reading:

- Rauh J, Pluntke S, Müller C: Paravenöse Zytostatikainjektion: Prophylaxe und Sofortmaßnahmen im Notfall. MMW Fortschr Med 146: 682–686, 2004.

Revisions by Patrizia Fürst-Weger

Trimetrexate

CONSENSUS

Type of damage: irritant

Recommended treatment:

General measures:

1. Stop injection/infusion immediately
2. Get extravasation kit
3. Put on (sterile) gloves
4. Replace infusion lead or syringe with 5 ml disposable syringe and aspirate slowly as much as possible of the extravasated drug; **Cave!** do not exert pressure on extravasation area
5. Remove i.v. access while aspirating
6. If blisters occur: aspirate with 1 ml syringe and s.c. cannula, use new equipment for every new attempt at aspiration
7. Elevate limb and immobilise
8. Complete extravasation documentation sheet (mention extent of extravasation)
9. Inform and instruct the patient and relatives
10. Regular control (aftercare)

Substance specific measures: none

Cave! after extravasation:

1. No flushing of i.v. access
2. No moist compresses
3. No alcohol compresses
4. No occlusive dressings

Type of damage reported in literature:	Irritant [4]
Symptoms and clinical course reported in literature:	No data available
Measures reported in literature:	**Successful treatment:** – No data available **Unsuccessful treatment:** – No data available **Outcome of treatment not reported:** – No specific measure mentioned [4]
Particular remarks:	Results of literature search: no animal experiments or clinical studies regarding extravasation have been published Incidence of hypersensitivity reactions: 2% [1] Erythema, cellulitis [2], and phlebitis [3, 5] are not associated with extravasation; these local reactions, particularly if the drug is administered with a high infusion rate, are likely due to the acidic pH of 3.5–5.5 [1] of the reconstituted drug
Conclusion:	Although trimetrexate is classified as irritant in some of the literature, no clinical case of irritation of tissue after extravasation has been documented; the classification as irritant is due to the acid pH of the reconstituted drug Owing to little or no experience with extravasations of trimetrexate, a final classification of the type of damage is not possible Positive results of substance specific measures have not been described so far; until further data become available no substance specific measures can be recommended

Original articles

[1] Grem JL, King SA, Costanza ME, et al: Hypersensitivity reactions to trimetrexate. Invest New Drugs 8: 211–214, 1990.
[2] Weiss RB, James WD, Major WB, et al: Skin reactions induced by trimetrexate, an analog of methotrexate. Invest New Drugs 4: 159–163, 1986.
[3] Balis FM, Patel R, Luks E, et al: Pediatric phase I trial and pharmacokinetic study of trimetrexate. Cancer Res 47: 4973–4976, 1987.

Secondary literature

[4] Jordan K, Grothe W, Schmoll HJ: Paravasation von Zytostatika: Prävention und Therapie. Dtsch Med Wochenschr 130: 33–37, 2005.
[5] Dorr RT, Von Hoff DD: Drug monographs: trimetrexate. In: Dorr RT, Von Hoff DD (eds) Cancer Chemotherapy Handbook. Appleton & Lange, 2nd edition: 933–939, 1994.

Revisions by Sabine Wassertheurer

Vinblastine

CONSENSUS

Type of damage: vesicant

Recommended treatment:

General measures:

1. Stop injection/infusion immediately
2. Get extravasation kit
3. Put on (sterile) gloves
4. Replace infusion lead or syringe with 5 ml disposable syringe and aspirate slowly as much as possible of the extravasated drug; **Cave!** do not exert pressure on extravasation area
5. Remove i.v. access while aspirating
6. If blisters occur: aspirate with 1 ml syringe and s.c. cannula, use new equipment for every new attempt at aspiration
7. Elevate limb and immobilise
8. Start **substance specific measures**
9. Ensure adequate analgesia
10. Complete extravasation documentation sheet (mention extent of extravasation)
11. Inform and instruct the patient and relatives
12. Regular control (aftercare)
13. Always consult a (plastic) surgeon within 24 hours

Substance specific measures:

Hyaluronidase:

Inject up to 1500 IU hyaluronidase s.c. around the affected area depending on size of extravasation. **Cave!** local analgesia is recommended

Immediately afterwards dry heat:

Application of dry heat in a subjectively agreeable manner (e.g., cold-hot pack, hot water bottle) 4 × daily over 20 minutes

Cave! after extravasation:

1. No flushing of i.v. access
2. No moist compresses
3. No alcohol compresses
4. No occlusive dressings

Type of damage reported in literature:

High risk of necroses [11,14]

Vesicant [4,12,13,15–22,24–26]

Symptoms and clinical course reported in literature:

Initial symptoms: Pain, swelling, erythema (8 patients) [1,7,9], indurations (2 patients) [7]

Delayed-onset symptoms: Necroses (1 patient) [4,22], paraesthesias (4 patients) [9]

Residual findings: Contracture (1 patient) [9]

Individual case reports:

- 2 days after completion of the central venous vinblastine infusion: severe pleuritic-type right chest pain and fever; small pleural effusion showed on chest radiograph, which was the same as on previous examinations; after 9 days: firm masses supraclavicular fossae bilaterally, facial oedema, fever, and continued severe chest pain; mediastinitis and venous thrombosis of the superior vena cava diagnosed by computed tomography and contrast venography while blood cultures remained negative (1 patient) [6]

- During central venous application, needle dislodgment with subsequent extravasation of a small amount of drug. Symptoms limited to red-colored pinpoint area at the injection site, but the surrounding skin remained intact (1 patient) [8]

Measures reported in literature:

Successful treatment:
- 250 IU hyaluronidase in 6 ml NaCl 0.9% i.v. or s.c. in 6 single doses (1 patient) [1,19]
- Animal experiments: hyaluronidase i.d. once; NaCl 0.9% or calcium folinate i.d. 1 × daily for 5 days [2]
- Infiltration of 500 mg hydrocortisone, application of betamethasone-gentamicin ointment every 12 hours over 2 days, then every 12 hours until healing was complete (5 patients); additionally infiltration of sodium thiosulfate (2%) followed by rub in reduced the time of healing from 8 to 4 days (8 patients) [3]
- Analgesia, heparin and warfarin treatment, no surgical intervention after extravasation of central venous application (1 patient) [6]
- Animal experiments: hyaluronidase or NaCl 0.9% [5]

Unsuccessful treatment:
- Animal experiments: hydrocortisone, vitamin A-cream or cooling (increased ulcerations) [2]
- Animal experiments: application of heat for 45 minutes, single application of calcium folinate, sodium bicarbonate (no reduction of ulcerations) [2]
- Animal experiments: hydrocortisone applied topically (increased ulcerations) [5]

Outcome of treatment not reported:
- 500–1000 IU hyaluronidase s.c. [2]
- Cooling, glucocorticoid applied locally, hyaluronidase, and dry heat 6 days after the event (1 patient) [7]

- After extravasation in the context of combination therapy with vinblastine and MTX (extravasated substance not identified) hyaluronidase and dexamethasone applied intradermally, topical cooling (1 patient) [7]

- After simultaneous extravasation of vinblastine and doxorubicine: Phlogenzym® (trypsin, bromelin, rutin) 3 × daily 1 tablet over 1 month; in addition, patients, who were diagnosed within 24 hours, were given treatment according standard recommendations for extravasation such as warm compresses and hyaluronidase for vinca alkaloids and cold compresses and hydrocortisone for anthracyclines (5 patients) [9]

- After extravasation of vinblastine alone: Phlogenzym® (trypsin, bromelin, rutin) 3 × daily 1 tablet over 1 month; in addition patients, who were diagnosed within 24 hours, were given treatment according standard recommendations for extravasation such as warm compresses and hyaluronidase (1 patient) [9]

- Warm compresses over 24 hours (2 patients) [10]

- Mild, dry heat over 1–2 hours, 150–900 IU hyaluronidase s.c., alternatively DMSO every 3–4 hours for 1–3 days applied locally [11]

- 150 IU hyaluronidase in 1–3 ml NaCl 0.9% [14] or in 4 ml NaCl 0.9% [12] s.c. and application of local heat [12, 14]

- 300 IU hyaluronidase s.c., mild dry heat over 1-2 hours [13]

- Infiltration of 5 ml sodium bicarbonate (8.4%) or 150 IU hyaluronidase, optional local infiltration of corticosteroids, warm compresses for 1 hour [15]

- 150–900 IU hyaluronidase s.c. and 1–5 ml NaCl 0.9% s.c., repeated peri-/intralesional administration, local application of heat [16]
- 1500 IU hyaluronidase in single doses of 0.2 ml, application of heat over 24 hours, application of non-steroidal anti-inflammatory cream 4 × daily for 7 days [17]
- Warm compresses immediately applied for 30–60 minutes, then for 24 hours alternating every 15 minutes (with/without compresses), 150 IU hyaluronidase s.c. [19]
- Within 1 hour after extravasation: 150 IU hyaluronidase in 1 ml NaCl 0.9% s.c. or i.d. in 5 single doses of 0.2 ml, warm compresses over 15 minutes every 6 hours for 2–3 days [20]
- 150–900 IU hyaluronidase s.c. or i.d. [19] and warm compresses [21]
- 100 mg hydrocortisone s.c. and i.v., application of heat, topical hydrocortisone [22]
- Local injection of hyaluronidase, moderate heat [23]
- Perilesional application of 150 IU hyaluronidase in single doses of 0.1–0.2 ml, dry heat; never use cooling [24]
- Perilesional application of 1500 IU hyaluronidase s.c., analgesia if required, dry heat 4 × daily over 20 minutes [25]
- Application of 150–900 IU hyaluronidase i.v. or s.c., repeat within 3–4 hours, application of heat [26]
- Within 4 hours after extravasation: s.c. washout with 300–500 ml Ringer's solution; additionally intraoperative infiltration of 150-200 IU hyaluronidase, postoperative immobilisation for 3 days, followed by hydrocortisone (1%) applied locally over 2 months, and physiotherapeutic treatment [29]

Particular remarks:

Photosensitivity and recall phenomenon have been described for vinblastine [27,28]

Calcium folinate and NaCl 0.9%: positive effects observed in animal experiments only

Gentamicin: only for prophylaxis of secondary infection, no causal treatment of extravasation

Heparin, warfarin: only symptomatic treatment of thrombosis, no causal treatment of extravasation

Hyaluronidase: 1 case report about the positive effect in preventing necroses [1]; confirmed in animal experiments [2,5]

Since the s.c. application of hyaluronidase is usually associated with severe pain, local analgesia is recommended [25]

Hyaluronidase and DMSO without heat or cooling after simultaneous extravasation of vincristine and anthracyclines is recommended [13]; therefore it is also recommended after simultaneous extravasation of vinblastine and anthracyclines

Cooling and corticosteroids: no cooling and corticosteroids, as vesicant effect was increased in animal experiments [1,2,5,14]

Sodium thiosulfate: positive effect not sufficiently proved; disadvantage: invasive measure

Heat: neither positive nor negative effect observed in animal experiments [2]; theoretically it increases the effect of hyaluronidase [13]

Conclusion:

Vinblastine is classified exclusively as vesicant in the literature

Although the combined use of hyaluronidase and heat has been tested neither in a clinical study nor in animal experiments, this combination is established in clinical practice because of a putative synergistic mechanism (accelerated absorption of extravasated substance)

Original articles

[1] Bertelli G, Dini D, Forno GB, et al: Hyaluronidase as an antidote to extravasation of vinca alkaloids: clinical results. J Cancer Res Clin Oncol 120: 505–506, 1994.
[2] Dorr RT, Alberts DS: Vinca alkaloid skin toxicity: antidote and drug disposition studies in the mouse. J Natl Cancer Inst 74: 113–120, 1985.
[3] Tsavaris NB, Komitsopoulou P, Karagiaouris P, et al: Prevention of tissue necrosis due to accidental extravasation of cytostatic drugs by a conservative approach. Cancer Chemother Pharmacol 30: 330–333, 1992.
[4] Gill DP, Eakin DL, Weiss GB: Cutaneous necrosis from chemotherapy in a patient with an arteriovenous fistula. Cancer Treat Rep 65: 352–353, 1981.
[5] Dorr RT, Alberts DS, Woods MW: Vinca alkaloid ulceration: experimental mouse model and effects of local antidotes. Proc AACR 23: 109, 1982.
[6] Anderson JM, Walters RS, Hortobagyi GN: Mediastinitis related to probable central vinblastine extravasation in a woman undergoing adjuvant chemotherapy for early breast cancer. Am J Clin Oncol 19: 566–568, 1996.
[7] Krämer I: Zehn Jahre Dokumentation von Zytostatika-Paravasat-Ereignissen: Auswertung von 175 Paravasate-Dokumentationen. Krankenhauspharmazie 23: 269–274, 2002.
[8] Schulmeister L, Camp-Sorrell D: Chemotherapy extravasation from implanted ports. Oncol Nurs For 27: 531–538, 2000.
[9] Parikh PM, Ranjan S, Swami A, et al: Phlogenzym® is safe and effective in reducing morbidity of vesicant chemotherapy extravasation. A prospective study. Int J Immunother 17: 163–170, 2001.
[10] Langstein HN, Duman H, Seelig D, et al: Retrospective study of the management of chemotherapeutic extravasation injury. Ann Plast Surg 49: 369–374, 2002.

Secondary literature

[11] Schneider G: Paravasate von Zytostatika. Diagnostik und Therapie. Aina S. Schneider Verlag, 6th edition: 1–17, 1999.
[12] Gain M, Melzer S, Meyer-Jürshof A, et al: Vinblastin: Behandlung von Paravasaten. In: Gain M, et al (eds) ADKA-Zytostatika-Handbuch, Pharmazeutisch-wissenschaftliche Monographien. Verlag Heiner Biller, vol 4: 42–43, 2000.
[13] Krämer I, Stützle M: Zytostatika-Paravasation – Wie ist vorzugehen? Krankenhauspharmazie 23: 261–268, 2002. [14]

[14] Dorr RT: Antidotes to vesicant chemotherapy extravasations. Blood Rev 4: 41–60, 1990.
[15] Ignoffo RJ, Friedman MA: Therapy of local toxicities caused by extravasation of cancer chemotherapeutic drugs. Cancer Treat Rev 7: 17–27, 1980.
[16] Berdel WE, Schmoll HJ, Büchele T, et al: Prävention und Therapie von Paravasaten/Extravasaten. In: Schmoll HJ, Höffken K, Possinger K (eds) Kompendium Internistische Onkologie. Standards in Diagnostik und Therapie. Springer, vol 1, 3rd edition: 1689–1701, 1999.
[17] Stanley A: Managing complications of chemotherapy administration. In: Allwood M, Stanley A, Wright P (eds) The Cytotoxics Handbook. Radcliffe Medical Press, 4th edition: 119–193, 2002.
[18] Dorr RT: Pharmacologic management of vesicant chemotherapy extravasations. In: Dorr RT, Von Hoff DD (eds) Cancer Chemotherapy Handbook. Appleton & Lange, 2nd edition: 109–118, 1994.
[19] Bertelli G: Prevention and management of extravasation of cytotoxic drugs. Drug Safety 12: 245–255, 1995.
[20] Mullin S, Beckwith MC, Tyler LS: Prevention and management of antineoplastic extravasation injury. Hosp Pharm 35: 57–76, 2000.
[21] Schneider SM, Distelhorst CW: Chemotherapy-induced emergencies. Semin Oncol 16: 572–578, 1989.
[22] Gain M, Melzer S, Meyer-Jürshof A, et al: Allgemeiner Teil: Behandlung von Paravasaten. In: Gain M, et al (eds) ADKA-Zytostatika-Handbuch, Pharmazeutisch-wissenschaftliche Monographien. Verlag Heiner Biller, vol 1, 2nd edition: A42–44, 1997.
[23] Summary of product characteristics Vinblastinsulfat-Gry® (Germany), GRY-Pharma, September 2003.
[24] Barth J: Paravasate und deren Behandlung. In: Barth J (ed) Zytostatika-Herstellung in der Apotheke. Deutscher Apotheker Verlag, chapter VI-3: 1–9, 2000.
[25] Jordan K, Grothe W, Schmoll HJ: Paravasation von Zytostatika: Prävention und Therapie. Dtsch Med Wochenschr 130: 33–37, 2005.
[26] Ener RA, Meglathery SB, Styler M: Extravasation of systemic hemato-oncological therapies. Ann Oncol 15: 858–862, 2004.
[27] Koppel RA, Boh EE: Cutaneous reactions to chemotherapeutic agents. Am J Med Sci 321: 327–335, 2001.
[28] Alley E, Green R, Schuchter L: Cutaneous toxicities of cancer therapy. Curr Opin Oncol 14: 212–216, 2002.
[29] Giunta R, Akpaloo J, Kovacs L, et al: Technik der subcutanen Spülung bei hochtoxischen Paravasaten – Ein Kurzbeitrag. Handchir Mikrochir Plast Chir 34: 399–402, 2002.

Further reading:

- Albanell J, Baselga J: Systemic therapy emergencies. Semin Oncol 27: 347–361, 2000.
- Barr RD, Sertic J: Soft-tissue necrosis induced by extravasated cancer chemotherapeutic agents: a study of active intervention. Br J Cancer 44: 267–269, 1981.
- Bozkurt AK, Uzel B, Akman C, et al: Intrathoracic extravasation of antineoplastic agents: Case report and systematic review. Am J Clin Oncol 26: 121–123, 2003.
- Dorr RT: Extravasation of vesicant antineoplastics: clinical and experimental findings. Ariz Med 38: 271–275, 1981.
- Fenchel K, Karthaus M: Zytostatika-Paravasate – gibt es neue Empfehlungen zum therapeutischen Vorgehen? Wien Med Wochenschr 151: 44–46, 2001.
- Kassner E: Evaluation and treatment of chemotherapy extravasation injuries. J Pediatr Oncol 17: 135–148, 2000.
- Krämer I: Onkologische Pharmazie. In: Jaehde U, Radziwill R, Mühlebach S, et al (eds) Lehrbuch der Klinischen Pharmazie. Wissenschaftliche Verlagsgesellschaft mbH, 2nd edition: 307–336, 2003.
- Otto J, Goebell PJ, Otto T: Urologischer Notfall in der Onkologie. Der Onkologe 10: 351–357, 2004.
- Rauh J, Pluntke S, Müller C: Paravenöse Zytostatikainjektion: Prophylaxe und Sofortmaßnahmen im Notfall. MMW Fortschr Med 146: 682–686, 2004.
- Schrijvers DL: Extravasation: a dreaded complication of chemotherapy. Ann Oncol 14: iii26–iii30, 2003.
- Whang SW, Lee SH, Elias PM, et al: Intralesional steroids reduce inflammation from extravasated chemotherapeutic agents. Br J Dermatol 145: 680–682, 2001.
- Yap HJ, Blumenschein GR, Keating MJ, et al: Vinblastine given as a continuous 5-day infusion in the treatment of refractory advanced breast cancer. Cancer Treat Rep 64: 279–283, 1980.

Revisions by Ines Mader

Vincristine

CONSENSUS

Type of damage: vesicant

Recommended treatment:

General measures:

1. Stop injection/infusion immediately
2. Get extravasation kit
3. Put on (sterile) gloves
4. Replace infusion lead or syringe with 5 ml disposable syringe and aspirate slowly as much as possible of the extravasated drug; **Cave!** do not exert pressure on extravasation area
5. Remove i.v. access while aspirating
6. If blisters occur: aspirate with 1 ml syringe and s.c. cannula, use new equipment for every new attempt at aspiration
7. Elevate limb and immobilise
8. Start **substance specific measures**
9. Ensure adequate analgesia
10. Complete extravasation documentation sheet (mention extent of extravasation)
11. Inform and instruct the patient and relatives
12. Regular control (aftercare)
13. Always consult a (plastic) surgeon within 24 hours

Substance specific measures:

Hyaluronidase:

Inject up to 1500 IU hyaluronidase s.c. around the affected area depending on size of extravasation. **Cave!** local analgesia is recommended

Immediately afterwards dry heat:

Application of dry heat in a subjectively agreeable manner (e.g., cold-hot pack, hot water bottle) 4 × daily over 20 minutes

Substance specific measures after simultaneous extravasation of vincristine and anthracyclines (for example, in the context of the VAD protocol):

Hyaluronidase:

Inject up to 1500 IU hyaluronidase s.c. around affected area depending on the size of the extravasation. **Cave!** local analgesia is recommended

Immediately followed by DMSO:

1. Apply DMSO (99%) every 8 hours (e.g. with a sterile gauze pad) without pressure
2. Allow to air-dry – **Cave!** do not cover
3. Continue for a minimum of 7 days

Cave! no heat, no cooling

Cave! after extravasation:

1. No flushing of i.v. access
2. No moist compresses
3. No alcohol compresses
4. No occlusive dressings

Type of damage reported in literature:

High risk of necroses [18,21]

Vesicant [4,5,8,19,20,22–30,32–34]

Symptoms and clinical course reported in literature:

Peripheral venous application:
Initial symptoms: Pain, erythema, swelling (11 patients) [2,5,8,11,12], indurations (2 patients) [12], blistering (3 patients) [8,9,11]

Delayed-onset symptoms: Skin defect (1 patient) [11], painful ulcerations particularly accompanied by superinfection and exposed tendons (5 patients) [7]

Residual findings: Slight painful induration (1 patient) [3], hyperpigmented induration (1 patient) [5], scirrhous movable infiltration (1 patient) [12]

Central venous application:
Initial symptoms: Pain, swelling, and erythema (4 patients) [6,9,12,14], haematoma (1 patient) [6]

Delayed-onset symptoms: Fat tissue necrosis in the context of a VIE-regimen (1 patient) [6]; blistering in the context of a VAD regimen (1 patient) [9]

Residual findings: No data available

Individual case report:
Headache, pain in both arms and in the right shoulder, swollen, tender left neck and left upper chest, prominent venous pattern over the sternum, grunting respirations, substernal retractions, and decreased breath sounds bilaterally; fever; mediastinal widening, bilateral pleural effusions, diffuse interstitial pulmonary oedema; no superinfection; during the next 48 hours pain, tenderness, and chest-wall swelling subsided; after 4 days: only little remaining pleural fluid, mild interstitial oedema, and marked improvement in the superior mediastinum; clinical respiratory status returned to normal (1 child) [13]

Measures reported in literature:

Successful treatment:
- 50 mg hydrocortisone s.c. (2 patients) or 100 mg hydrocortisone immediately after accidental i.m. administration of vincristine (1 patient) [1]
- 50 mg or 100 mg hydrocortisone s.c. (1 patient each) [2]
- 250 IU hyaluronidase in 6 ml NaCl 0.9% i.v. or s.c. in 6 single doses (1 patient) [3,27]
- Animal experiments: hyaluronidase, calcium folinate (only effective if vincristine dosage is low) and local application of heat [4,21]

V

- 150 TRU chondroitin sulfatase in 3 ml NaCl 0.9% s.c., repeated after 24 hours, DMSO (90%) 4 × daily over 2 weeks (1 patient: VAD-regimen) [5]
- DMSO 4 × daily over 2 weeks and hydrocortisone (1%) applied topically, cold packs after application of DMSO (1 patient: VIE-regimen) [9]
- Repeated moist compresses (4 patients: combination therapy with mustine, bleomycin, and daunorubicin, respectively) [7]
- DMSO (99%) every 6 hours over 17 days (1 patient: VAD-regimen) [9]
- Animal experiment: débridement 1 hour after i.d. application or application of DMSO and α-tocopherol [10]
- Animal experiment: up to 6 × 300 IU hyaluronidase s.c. [15]

Unsuccessful treatment:

- Animal experiments: hydrocortisone, sodium bicarbonate, and cooling [4]
- Surgical intervention (1 patient) [7]
- Application of DMSO (99%) every 6 hours over 21 days with cold packs; on day 6 after surgical intervention additional whirlpool treatment 2 × daily for 20 minutes to promote granulation (1 patient: MOPP-regimen) [9]
- Animal experiments: administration of hydrocortisone s.c. [10]
- Immediately after extravasation: 50 mg prednisolone s.c. and topical cooling; after several days: antibiotics and analgesics; 10 days after extravasation: surgical intervention was necessary (1 patient) [11]

- After extravasation in the context of combination chemotherapy with vincristine and doxorubicin: oral dexamethasone over 2 days (1 patient) [12]

- Hydrocortisone s.c. and topical cooling, several surgical interventions over 6 months were unsuccessful; finally partial mastectomy with transplantation of muscle flap graft was required (1 patient) [14]

Outcome of treatment not reported:

- 500–1000 IU hyaluronidase s.c. [4]

- Hyaluronidase and heat [7,31]

- Hyaluronidase, heat, local glucocorticoid (1 patient) [12]

- Hyaluronidase, cooling, local glucocorticoid (1 patient) [12]

- After extravasation in the context of combination chemotherapy with vincristine and epirubicin: DMSO, local glucocorticoid (1 patient) [12]

- After extravasation in the context of combination chemotherapy with vincristine and doxorubicin: DMSO, cooling, intradermal glucocorticoid, hyaluronidase (1 patient) [12]

- After extravasation in the context of combination chemotherapy with vincristine and doxorubicin: DMSO, cooling, local glucocorticoid (1 patient) [12]

- Warm compresses over 24 hours (2 patients) [16]

- After simultaneous extravasation of vincristine and doxorubicin: Phlogenzym® (trypsin, bromelin, rutin) 3 × daily 1 tablet over 1 month; in addition, patients, who were diagnosed within 24 hours, were given treatment according standard recommendations for extravasation such as warm compresses and hyaluronidase for vinca alkaloids and cold compresses and hydrocortisone for anthracyclines (1 patient) [17]

- Phlogenzym® (trypsin, bromelin, rutin) 3 × daily 1 tablet over 1 month; in addition, patients, who were diagnosed within 24 hours, were given treatment according standard recommendations for extravasation such as warm compresses and hyaluronidase (4 patients) [17]

- Mild, dry heat for 1–2 hours, 150–900 IU hyaluronidase s.c., alternatively: DMSO every 3–4 hours over 1–3 days applied locally [18]

- 300 IU hyaluronidase s.c., dry and mild heat for 1–2 hours [20]

- After extravasation in the context of a VAD regimen: neither heat nor cooling but DMSO and hyaluronidase [20]

- 150 IU hyaluronidase in 1–3 ml NaCl 0.9% and application of local heat [21,30]

- Infiltration of 5 ml sodium bicarbonate (8.4%) or 150 IU hyaluronidase, optional local infiltration of corticosteroids, warm compresses for 1 hour [22]

- 150–900 IU hyaluronidase s.c. and 1–5 ml NaCl 0.9% s.c., repeated peri-/intralesional administration, local application of heat [23]

- 1500 IU hyaluronidase in single doses of 0.2 ml, application of heat over 24 hours, application of a non-steroidal anti-inflammatory cream 4 × daily for 7 days [24]
- Warm compresses immediately applied for 30–60 minutes, then for 24 hours alternating every 15 minutes (with/without compresses), 150 IU hyaluronidase s.c. [25]
- Within 1 hour after extravasation: 150 IU hyaluronidase in 1 ml NaCl 0.9% s.c. or i.d. in 5 single doses of 0.2 ml, warm compresses over 15 minutes every 6 hours for 2–3 days [26]
- 150–900 IU hyaluronidase s.c. or i.d. [21] and warm compresses [29]
- 100 mg hydrocortisone s.c. and i.v., application of heat, topical hydrocortisone [28], and 150–1500 IU hyaluronidase s.c. [19]
- Perilesional application of 150 IU hyaluronidase in single doses of 0.1–0.2 ml, dry heat; never use cooling [32]
- 1500 IU hyaluronidase s.c., applied perilesionally, analgesia if required, dry heat 4 × daily over 20 minutes [33]
- 150–900 IU hyaluronidase i.v. or s.c., repeated over the following 3–4 hours, application of heat [34]
- Within 4 hours after extravasation: s.c. washout with 300–500 ml Ringer's solution, additionally intraoperative infiltration of 150–200 IU hyaluronidase, postoperative immobilisation for 3 days, followed by hydrocortisone (1%) applied locally for 2 months, and physiotherapeutic treatment [36]

V

Particular remarks: Animal experiments: new formulation – vincristine liposomal — reduces toxicity in the event of an extravasation [35]

Calcium folinate: positive effects have been observed in animal experiments only

Chondroitin sulfatase: similar effect to hyaluronidase

Corticosteroids: some clinical reports about positive effect exist [1,2], but not successful in combination with cooling [11]; increased vesicant effect observed in animal experiments [3,4,21,30]; moreover: extravasations are only rarely accompanied by inflammatory processes (see chapter "Histopathological investigations")

DMSO: positive effect is associated with extravasation of anthracyclines (VAD/VIE-regimen)

Hyaluronidase: 1 case report about positive effect in preventing necrosis [3]; confirmed also in animal experiments [4,21]

Since the s.c. application of hyaluronidase is usually associated with severe pain for the patient, local analgesia is recommended [33]

α-tocopherol: positive effect observed in animal experiments only

Heat: positive effect observed in animal experiments [4]

After simultaneous extravasation of vincristine and anthracyclines: combination therapy with hyaluronidase and DMSO without application of heat of topical cooling is recommended [5,19]

Moist compresses can result in maceration of the skin and thus promote the development of necroses [33]

Conclusion:

Vincristine is classified exclusively as vesicant in the literature

Although the combined use of hyaluronidase and heat has been tested neither in a clinical study nor in animal experiments, this combination is established in clinical practice because of a putative synergistic mechanism (accelerated absorption of extravasated substance)

Original articles

[1] Choy DS: Effective treatment of inadvertent intramuscular administration of vincristine. JAMA 241: 695, 1979.
[2] Bellone JD: Treatment of vincristine extravasation. JAMA 245: 343, 1981.
[3] Bertelli G, Dini D, Forno GB, et al: Hyaluronidase as an antidote to extravasation of vinca alkaloids: clinical results. J Cancer Res Clin Oncol 120: 505–506, 1994.
[4] Dorr RT, Alberts DS: Vinca alkaloid skin toxicity: antidote and drug disposition studies in the mouse. J Natl Cancer Inst 74: 113–120, 1985.
[5] Comas D, Mateu J: Treatment of extravasation of both doxorubicin and vincristine administration in a y-site infusion. Ann Pharmacother 30: 244–246, 1996.
[6] Webster PJ, D'Souza D: Extravasation of epirubicin/vincristine and ifosfamide/mesna from a central venous catheter. J Oncol Pharm Practice 1: 41–44, 1995.
[7] Chait LA, Dinner MI: Ulceration caused by cytotoxic drugs. S Afr Med J 49: 1935–1936, 1975.
[8] James DH, George P: Vincristine in children with malignant solid tumors. J Pediatr 64: 534–541, 1964.
[9] Germain BS, Houlihan N, D'Amato S: Dimethyl sulfoxide therapy in the treatment of vesicant extravasation. J Intrav Nurs 17: 261–266, 1994.
[10] Loth TS, Eversmann WW: Treatment methods for extravasations of chemotherapeutic agents: a comparative study. J Hand Surg 11A: 388–396, 1986.
[11] Larson DL: Treatment of tissue extravasation by antitumor agents. Cancer 49: 1796–1799, 1982.
[12] Krämer I: Zehn Jahre Dokumentation von Zytostatika-Paravasat-Ereignissen: Auswertung von 175 Paravasate-Dokumentationen. Krankenhauspharmazie 23: 269–274, 2002.

V

[13] Watterson J, Heisel M, Cich J, et al: Intrathoracic extravasation of sclerosing agents associated with central venous catheters. Am J Pediatr Hematol Oncol 10: 249–251, 1988.
[14] Schulmeister L, Camp-Sorrell D: Chemotherapy extravasation from implanted ports. Oncol Nurs For 27: 531–538, 2000.
[15] Spugnini E: Use of hyaluronidase for the treatment of extravasation of chemotherapeutic agents in six dogs. JAVMA 221: 1437–1440, 2002.
[16] Langstein HN, Duman H, Seelig D, et al: Retrospective study of the management of chemotherapeutic extravasation injury. Ann Plast Surg 49: 369–374, 2002.
[17] Parikh PM, Ranjan S, Swami A, et al: Phlogenzym® is safe and effective in reducing morbidity of vesicant chemotherapy extravasation. a prospective study. Int J Immunother 17: 163–170, 2001.

Secondary literature

[18] Schneider G: Paravasate von Zytostatika. Diagnostik und Therapie. Aina S. Schneider Verlag, 6th edition: 1–17, 1999.
[19] Gain M, Melzer S, Meyer-Jürshof A, et al: Vincristin: Behandlung von Paravasaten. In: Gain M, et al (eds) ADKA-Zytostatika-Handbuch, Pharmazeutisch-wissenschaftliche Monographien. Verlag Heiner Biller, vol 3: 44–45, 1998.
[20] Krämer I, Stützle M: Zytostatika-Paravasation - Wie ist vorzugehen? Krankenhauspharmazie 23: 261–268, 2002.
[21] Dorr RT: Antidotes to vesicant chemotherapy extravasations. Blood Rev 4: 41–60, 1990.
[22] Ignoffo RJ, Friedman MA: Therapy of local toxicities caused by extravasation of cancer chemotherapeutic drugs. Cancer Treat Rev 7: 17–27, 1980.
[23] Berdel WE, Schmoll HJ, Büchele T, et al: Prävention und Therapie von Paravasaten/Extravasaten. In: Schmoll HJ, Höffken K, Possinger K (eds) Kompendium Internistische Onkologie. Standards in Diagnostik und Therapie. Springer, vol 1, 3rd edition: 1689–1701, 1999.
[24] Stanley A: Managing complications of chemotherapy administration. In: Allwood M, Stanley A, Wright P (eds) The Cytotoxics Handbook. Radcliffe Medical Press, 4th edition: 119–193, 2002.
[25] Dorr RT: Pharmacologic management of vesicant chemotherapy extravasations. In: Dorr RT, Von Hoff DD (eds) Cancer Chemotherapy Handbook. Appleton & Lange, 2nd edition: 109–118, 1994.
[26] Mullin S, Beckwith MC, Tyler LS: Prevention and management of antineoplastic extravasation injury. Hosp Pharm 35: 57–76, 2000.

[27] Bertelli G: Prevention and management of extravasation of cytotoxic drugs. Drug Safety 12: 245–255, 1995.
[28] Gain M, Melzer S, Meyer-Jürshof A, et al: Allgemeiner Teil: Behandlung von Paravasaten. In: Gain M, et al (eds) ADKA-Zytostatika-Handbuch, Pharmazeutisch-wissenschaftliche Monographien. Verlag Heiner Biller, vol 1, 2nd edition: A42–44, 1997.
[29] Schneider SM, Distelhorst CW: Chemotherapy-induced emergencies. Semin Oncol 16: 572–578, 1989.
[30] Bristol-Myers Squibb, personal communication, November 1998.
[31] Summary of product characteristics Vincristin "Pfizer" CS (Austria), Pfizer, April 2004.
[32] Barth J: Paravasate und deren Behandlung. In: Barth J (ed) Zytostatika-Herstellung in der Apotheke. Deutscher Apotheker Verlag, chapter VI-3: 1–9, 2000.
[33] Jordan K, Grothe W, Schmoll HJ: Paravasation von Zytostatika: Prävention und Therapie. Dtsch Med Wochenschr 130: 33–37, 2005.
[34] Ener RA, Meglathery SB, Styler M: Extravasation of systemic hemato-oncological therapies. Ann Oncol 15: 858–862, 2004.
[35] Boman NL, Tron VA, Bally MB, et al: Vincristine-induced dermal toxicity is significantly reduced when the drug is given in liposomes. Cancer Chemother Pharmacol 37: 351–355, 1996.
[36] Giunta R, Akpaloo J, Kovacs L, et al: Technik der subcutanen Spülung bei hochtoxischen Paravasaten – Ein Kurzbeitrag. Handchir Mikrochir Plast Chir 34: 399–402, 2002.

Further reading:

- Albanell J, Baselga J: Systemic therapy emergencies. Semin Oncol 27: 347–361, 2000.
- Alley E, Green R, Schuchter L: Cutaneous toxicities of cancer therapy. Curr Opin Oncol 14: 212–216, 2002.
- Barr RD, Sertic J: Soft-tissue necrosis induced by extravasated cancer chemotherapeutic agents: a study of active intervention. Br J Cancer 44: 267–269, 1981.
- Bozkurt AK, Uzel B, Akman C, et al: Intrathoracic extravasation of antineoplastic agents: Case report and systematic review. Am J Clin Oncol 26: 121–123, 2003.
- Buchanan GR, Buchsbaum HJ, O'Banion K, et al: Extravasation of dactinomycin, vincristine, and cisplatin: studies in an animal model. Med Pediatr Oncol 13: 375–380, 1985.
- Ignoffo RJ, Tomlin W, Rubinstein E, et al: A model for skin toxicity of antineoplastic drugs: doxorubicin (DOX), mitomycin-C (MMC), and vincristine (VCR). Clin Res 29: 437A, 1981.

- Fenchel K, Karthaus M: Zytostatika-Paravasate – gibt es neue Empfehlungen zum therapeutischen Vorgehen? Wien Med Wochenschr 151: 44–46, 2001.
- Kassner E: Evaluation and treatment of chemotherapy extravasation injuries. J Pediatr Oncol 17: 135–148, 2000.
- Krämer I: Onkologische Pharmazie. In: Jaehde U, Radziwill R, Mühlebach S, et al (eds) Lehrbuch der Klinischen Pharmazie. Wissenschaftliche Verlagsgesellschaft mbH, 2nd edition: 307–336, 2003.
- Otto J, Goebell PJ, Otto T: Urologischer Notfall in der Onkologie. Der Onkologe 10: 351–357, 2004.
- Rauh J, Pluntke S, Müller C: Paravenöse Zytostatikainjektion: Prophylaxe und Sofortmaßnahmen im Notfall. MMW Fortschr Med 146: 682–686, 2004.
- Raderer M, Chott A, Drach J, et al: Chemotherapy for management of localised high-grade gastric B-cell lymphoma: how much is necessary? Ann Oncol 13: 1094–1098, 2002.
- Schrijvers DL: Extravasation: a dreaded complication of chemotherapy. Ann Oncol 14: iii26–iii30, 2003.
- Whang SW, Lee SH, Elias PM, et al: Intralesional steroids reduce inflammation from extravasated chemotherapeutic agents. Br J Dermatol 145: 680–682, 2001.

Revisions by Ines Mader

Vindesine

CONSENSUS

Type of damage: vesicant

Recommended treatment:

General measures:

1. Stop injection/infusion immediately
2. Get extravasation kit
3. Put on (sterile) gloves
4. Replace infusion lead or syringe with 5 ml disposable syringe and aspirate slowly as much as possible of the extravasated drug; **Cave!** do not exert pressure on extravasation area
5. Remove i.v. access while aspirating
6. If blisters occur: aspirate with 1 ml syringe and s.c. cannula, use new equipment for every new attempt at aspiration
7. Elevate limb and immobilise
8. Start **substance specific measures**
9. Ensure adequate analgesia
10. Complete extravasation documentation sheet (mention extent of extravasation)
11. Inform and instruct the patient and relatives
12. Regular control (aftercare)
13. Always consult a (plastic) surgeon within 24 hours

Substance specific measures:

Hyaluronidase:

Inject up to 1500 IU hyaluronidase s.c. around the affected area depending on size of extravasation. **Cave!** local analgesia is recommended

Immediately afterwards dry heat:

Application of dry heat in a subjectively agreeable manner (e.g., cold-hot pack, hot water bottle) 4 × daily over 20 minutes

Cave! after extravasation:

1. No flushing of i.v. access
2. No moist compresses
3. No alcohol compresses
4. No occlusive dressings

Type of damage reported in literature:

High risk of necroses [7,10]

Vesicant [2,8,9,11–16,19–21]

Symptoms and clinical course reported in literature:

Initial symptoms: (Severe) pain, swelling, erythema (5 patients) [2,3,6,18]

Delayed-onset symptoms: Increased or delayed pain (3 patients) [2,3], induration (3 patients) [2,6], blistering (2 patients) [3,6], ulceration [1 patient) [3], eschar formation [18]

Residual findings: Slight painful induration (1 patient) [2], scarring (1 patient) [3], local paraesthesia (1 patient) [2]

Measures reported in literature:

Successful treatment:

- Animal experiments: hyaluronidase or NaCl 0.9% i.d. [1]
- 34 hours after extravasation: 150 TRU chondroitin sulfatase s.c. and dry heat over 20 minutes, repeated after 12 and 24 hours (1 patient) [2]
- Animal experiments: hyaluronidase, NaCl 0.9%, or isoproterenol [5]

Unsuccessful treatment:

- Animal experiments: hydrocortisone, isoprotenerol i.d., vitamin-A applied topically and, cooling (increased ulceration), heat (no reduction in ulceration) [1]
- 50 mg hydrocortisone i.v. before and after administration of vindesine, 100 mg hydrocortisone s.c., hydrocortisone applied topically, ice packs (1 patient) [3]

- Immediate administration of hydrocortisone s.c., ice packs (1 patient) [3]
- Ice packs for 2 days (1 patient) [3]
- Hot or cold compresses (depending on patient's preference) (1 patient) [3]
- Animal experiments: hydrocortisone applied topically [5]

Outcome of treatment not reported:

- 500–1000 IU hyaluronidase s.c. [1]
- Hyaluronidase (no further details reported) (1 patient) [6]
- After extravasation in the context of combination chemotherapy with cisplatin, etoposide, and vindesine (extravasated substance not identified) local application of glucocorticoid (1 patient) [6]
- Mild, dry heat over 1–2 hours, 150–900 IU hyaluronidase s.c., alternatively: DMSO every 3–4 hours for 1–3 days applied locally [7]
- 100 mg hydrocortisone s.c. and i.v., application of heat, topical hydrocortisone [8]
- 300 IU hyaluronidase s.c., dry and mild heat over 1–2 hours [9]
- 150–900 IU hyaluronidase s.c. and 1–5 ml NaCl 0.9% s.c., repeated peri-/intralesional administration, local application of heat [11]
- 1500 IU hyaluronidase in single doses of 0.2 ml, application of heat over 24 hours, application of non-steroidal anti-inflammatory cream 4 × daily for 7 days [12]
- 150–900 IU hyaluronidase s.c. or i.d. [14] and warm compresses [16]
- Local injection of hyaluronidase, moderate heat [18]

- Perilesional application of 150 IU hyaluronidase in single doses of 0.1–0.2 ml, dry heat; never use cooling [19]
- 1500 IU hyaluronidase s.c., applied perilesionally; analgesia if required, dry heat 4 × daily over 20 minutes [20]
- 150-900 IU hyaluronidase i.v. or s.c., repeated within 3–4 hours, application of heat [21]
- Within 4 hours after extravasation: s.c. washout with 300–500 ml Ringer's solution; additionally intraoperative infiltration of 150–200 IU hyaluronidase, postoperative immobilisation for 3 days, followed by hydrocortisone (1%) applied locally over 2 months, and physiotherapeutic treatment [22]

Particular remarks:

Phlebitis and/or cellulites (5–20%) [1,3,17] are not associated with extravasation

Chondroitin sulfatase and heat: the positive effect in preventing necrosis has been reported once; for reasons of commercial availability chondroitin sulfatase was used to substitute hyaluronidase [2]

Corticosteroids and cooling: corticosteroids and/or cooling seemed to increase toxicity [16]; confirmed in animal experiments for cooling [1] and hydrocortisone [5]

Hyaluronidase: clinical reports about the positive effect in preventing necroses are available for the vinca alkaloids vinblastine, vincristine, and vinorelbine [4]; for vindesine this has been observed in animal experiments only [1,10]

Since s.c. application of hyaluronidase is usually associated with severe pain for the patient, local analgesia is recommended [20]

Isoproterenol: positive effects observed in animal experiments only

NaCl 0.9%: positive effects observed in animal experiments only [1,5]

	Heat: 1 clinical report about positive effects of heat in combination with chondroitin sulfatase is available [2]
Conclusion:	Vindesine is classified exclusively as vesicant in the literature
	Although the combined use of hyaluronidase and heat has been tested neither in a clinical study nor in animal experiments, this combination is established in clinical practice because of a putative synergistic mechanism (accelerated absorption of extravasated substance)

Original articles

[1] Dorr RT, Alberts DS: Vinca alkaloid skin toxicity: antidote and drug disposition studies in the mouse. J Natl Cancer Inst 74: 113–120, 1985.
[2] Mateu J, Llop C: Delayed treatment of vindesine extravasation. Ann Pharmacother 28: 967–968, 1994.
[3] Dorr RT, Jones SE: Inapparent infiltrations associated with vindesine administration. Med Pediatr Oncol 6: 285–288, 1979.
[4] Bertelli G, Dini D, Forno GB, et al: Hyaluronidase as an antidote to extravasation of vinca alkaloids: clinical results. J Cancer Res Clin Oncol 120: 505–506, 1994.
[5] Dorr RT, Alberts DS, Woods MW: Vinca alkaloid ulceration: experimental mouse model and effects of local antidotes. Proc AACR 23: 109, 1982.
[6] Krämer I: Zehn Jahre Dokumentation von Zytostatika-Paravasat-Ereignissen: Auswertung von 175 Paravasate-Dokumentationen. Krankenhauspharmazie 23: 269–274, 2002.

Secondary literature

[7] Schneider G: Paravasate von Zytostatika. Diagnostik und Therapie. Aina S. Schneider Verlag, 6th edition: 1–17, 1999.
[8] Gain M, Melzer S, Meyer-Jürshof A, et al: Allgemeiner Teil: Behandlung von Paravasaten. In: Gain M, et al (eds) ADKA-Zytostatika-Handbuch, Pharmazeutisch-wissenschaftliche Monographien. Verlag Heiner Biller, vol 1, 2nd edition: A42–44, 1997.
[9] Krämer I, Stützle M: Zytostatika-Paravasation – Wie ist vorzugehen? Krankenhauspharmazie 23: 261–268, 2002.
[10] Dorr RT: Antidotes to vesicant chemotherapy extravasations. Blood Rev 4: 41–60, 1990.

[11] Berdel WE, Schmoll HJ, Büchele T, et al: Prävention und Therapie von Paravasaten/Extravasaten. In: Schmoll HJ, Höffken K, Possinger K (eds) Kompendium Internistische Onkologie. Standards in Diagnostik und Therapie. Springer, vol 1, 3rd edition: 1689–1701, 1999.
[12] Stanley A: Managing complications of chemotherapy administration. In: Allwood M, Stanley A, Wright P (eds) The Cytotoxics Handbook. Radcliffe Medical Press, 4th edition: 119–193, 2002.
[13] Dorr RT: Pharmacologic management of vesicant chemotherapy extravasations. In: Dorr RT, Von Hoff DD (eds) Cancer Chemotherapy Handbook. Appleton & Lange, 2nd edition: 109–118, 1994.
[14] Bertelli G: Prevention and management of extravasation of cytotoxic drugs. Drug Safety 12: 245–255, 1995.
[15] Donislawski S, Gain M, Meyer-Jürshof A, et al: Vindesin: Behandlung von Paravasaten. In: Donislawski S, et al (eds) ADKA-Zytostatika-Handbuch, Pharmazeutisch-wissenschaftliche Monographien. Verlag Heiner Biller, vol 2: 20, 1994.
[16] Schneider SM, Distelhorst CW: Chemotherapy-induced emergencies. Semin Oncol 16: 572–578, 1989.
[17] Dorr RT, Von Hoff DD: Drug monographs: vindesine. In: Dorr RT, Von Hoff DD (eds) Cancer Chemotherapy Handbook. Appleton & Lange, 2nd edition: 957–966, 1994.
[18] Summary of product characteristics Eldisin® (Austria), Stada, September 2002.
[19] Barth J: Paravasate und deren Behandlung. In: Barth J (ed) Zytostatika-Herstellung in der Apotheke. Deutscher Apotheker Verlag, chapter VI-3: 1–9, 2000.
[20] Jordan K, Grothe W, Schmoll HJ: Paravasation von Zytostatika: Prävention und Therapie. Dtsch Med Wochenschr 130: 33–37, 2005.
[21] Ener RA, Meglathery SB, Styler M: Extravasation of systemic hemato-oncological therapies. Ann Oncol 15: 858–862, 2004.
[22] Giunta R, Akpaloo J, Kovacs L, et al: Technik der subcutanen Spülung bei hochtoxischen Paravasaten – Ein Kurzbeitrag. Handchir Mikrochir Plast Chir 34: 399–402, 2002.

Further reading:

- Albanell J, Baselga J: Systemic therapy emergencies. Semin Oncol 27: 347–361, 2000.
- Fenchel K, Karthaus M: Zytostatika-Paravasate – gibt es neue Empfehlungen zum therapeutischen Vorgehen? Wien Med Wochenschr 151: 44–46, 2001.

- Krämer I: Onkologische Pharmazie. In: Jaehde U, Radziwill R, Mühlebach S, et al (eds) Lehrbuch der Klinischen Pharmazie. Wissenschaftliche Verlagsgesellschaft mbH, 2nd edition: 307–336, 2003.
- Langstein HN, Duman H, Seelig D, et al: Retrospective study of the management of chemotherapeutic extravasation injury. Ann Plast Surg 49: 369–374, 2002.
- Rauh J, Pluntke S, Müller C: Paravenöse Zytostatikainjektion: Prophylaxe und Sofortmaßnahmen im Notfall. MMW Fortschr Med 146: 682–686, 2004.
- Whang SW, Lee SH, Elias PM, et al: Intralesional steroids reduce inflammation from extravasated chemotherapeutic agents. Br J Dermatol 145: 680–682, 2001.

Revisions by Ines Mader

Vinorelbine

CONSENSUS

Type of damage: vesicant

Recommended treatment:

General measures:

1. Stop injection/infusion immediately
2. Get extravasation kit
3. Put on (sterile) gloves
4. Replace infusion lead or syringe with 5 ml disposable syringe and aspirate slowly as much as possible of the extravasated drug; **Cave!** do not exert pressure on extravasation area
5. Remove i.v. access while aspirating
6. If blisters occur: aspirate with 1 ml syringe and s.c. cannula, use new equipment for every new attempt at aspiration
7. Elevate limb and immobilise
8. Start **substance specific measures**
9. Ensure adequate analgesia
10. Complete extravasation documentation sheet (mention extent of extravasation)
11. Inform and instruct the patient and relatives
12. Regular control (aftercare)
13. Always consult a (plastic) surgeon within 24 hours

Substance specific measures:

Hyaluronidase:

Inject up to 1500 IU hyaluronidase s.c. around the affected area depending on size of extravasation. **Cave!** local analgesia is recommended

Immediately afterwards dry heat:

Application of dry heat in a subjectively agreeable manner (e.g., cold-hot pack, hot water bottle) 4 × daily over 20 minutes

Cave! after extravasation:

1. No flushing of i.v. access
2. No moist compresses
3. No alcohol compresses
4. No occlusive dressings

Type of damage reported in literature:

Vesicant [4–6,11–18,20–23]

Symptoms and clinical course reported in literature:

Initial symptoms: Pain, swelling, erythema (7 patient) [6, 7, 9]

Delayed-onset symptoms: Erythema and swelling (3 patients) [5–7], blistering and ulceration (2 patients) [7,9], development of necroses with eschar formation [6,9], hyperpigmentation, induration [9]

Residual findings: Induration of subcutaneous fatty tissues and paraesthesia (1 patient) [6], epithelial defect (1 patient) [8]

Individual case reports:

- Day 1: 14 cm × 5 cm erythematous lesion with slight induration, burning pains; day 4: slight reduction in erythema, longitudinal size 12 cm, pain not reported; day 12: further reduction of erythema, affected area 7 cm × 3 cm, scaly skin with onset of maceration (DMSO); day 21: eschar formation of affected area, induration reducing; day 36: slightly hyperpigmented area of 3 cm × 3 cm, no functional impairment of the limb after therapeutic intervention (1 patient) [4]

- Within a few hours extensive erythema with induration and pain, after 1 week black discoloration of the lesion with central blister formation, burning and stabbing pain, central ulceration within a few days, complete healing with eschar formation within 3 months after therapeutic intervention (1 patient) [5]

Measures reported in literature:

Successful treatment:

- 250 IU hyaluronidase in 6 ml NaCl 0.9%

- i.v. or s.c. in 6 single doses (4 patients); also effective in delayed administration 10 days after extravasation (1 patient) [2]

- 1500 IU hyaluronidase s.c., accompanied by sedative if required, days 1–3: DMSO 80% applied locally every 4 hours; days 4–14: additionally mometasone cream applied locally every 6 hours (1 patient) [4]

- Glucocorticoid administered locally and systemically, analgesia (2 patients) [5]

- Within 4 hours after extravasation: s.c. wash-out with 300–500 ml Ringer's solution, additionally intraoperative infiltration of 150–200 IU hyaluronidase, postoperative immobilisation for 3 days, followed by hydrocortisone (1%) applied locally over 2 months, and physiotherapeutic treatment [6]

- After injection of 1500 IU hyaluronidase, s.c. wash-out with 500 NaCl under local anaesthesia (1 patient) [7]

- 2 × intralesional application of triamcinolone acetonide 7–8 ml (10 mg/l) at a week's interval, healing within 4–5 weeks (4patients) [7]

- After extravasation in the context of combination chemotherapy with cisplatin, ifosfamide und vinorelbine (extravasated substance not identified) intralesional steroid injections (5 patients) [9]

- Animal experiments: hyaluronidase i.d. [1]

Unsuccessful treatment:
- Animal experiments: NaCl 0.9% and hydrocortisone i.d., cooling or application of heat [1]

- After injection of 1500 IU hyaluronidase, s.c. wash-out with 500 ml NaCl under local anaesthesia, 2 × daily dressings with betadine soaked gauze over 2 months; because of ulceration further antibiotic treatment until the cellulitis healed (1 patient) [7]

- Heat (1 patient) [8]

Outcome of treatment not reported:
- Hyaluronidase (no further details reported) (2 patients) [8]

- Warm compresses over 24 hours (3 patients) [10]

- Perilesional application of 150 IU hyaluronidase in single doses of 0.1–0.2 ml, dry heat; never use cooling [11, 18]

- 150–900 IU hyaluronidase s.c. and 1–5 ml NaCl 0.9% s.c., repeated peri-/intralesional administration, local application of heat [12]

- Local infiltration of hyaluronidase [13,17]

- Within 1 hour after extravasation: 150 IU hyaluronidase in 1 ml NaCl 0.9% s.c. or i.d. in 5 single doses of 0.2 ml, warm compresses over 15 minutes every 6 hours for 2–3 days [14]

- 150–900 IU hyaluronidase s.c. or i.d. [15]
- 100 mg hydrocortisone s.c. and i.v., application of heat, topical hydrocortisone [16]
- 300 IU hyaluronidase s.c., mild and dry heat over 1–2 hours [20]
- 1500 IU hyaluronidase given as single doses of 0.2 ml, application of heat over 24 hours; 4 × daily over 7 days application of non-steroidal anti-inflammatory cream [21]
- 1500 IU hyaluronidase s.c. given perilesionally, analgesia if required, dry heat 4 × daily over 20 minutes [22]
- 150–900 IU hyaluronidase i.v. or s.c., repeated application within 3–4 hours, application of heat [23]

Particular remarks: Local reactions at the injection site (up to 12%) [1,3] and phlebitis [13] are not associated with extravasation

Animal experiments: lower ulcerogenic effect than the other vinca alkaloids in same dosage [1]

Since the routinely applied dosage of vinorelbine is higher than that of the other vinca alkaloids the advantage of the lower tissue toxicity disappears and the sequelae after extravasation of vinorelbine are similar to those of the other vinca alkaloids [5]

Corticosteroids: positive effects questionable as extravasations are only rarely accompanied by inflammatory processes (see chapter "Histopathological investigations")

DMSO: positive effects not sufficiently proved

Hyaluronidase: clinical reports about the positive effect in preventing necroses are available [2,4,7]

Since s.c. application of hyaluronidase is usually associated with severe pain for the patient, local analgesia is recommended [22]

Heat: no positive effect in animal experiments [1]; however, in theory heat supports the effect of hyaluronidase [20]

There is insufficient clinical evidence for the flushout technique mentioned in the recent literature; further trauma to the affected tissue is possible [19]

Conclusion: Vinorelbine is classified exclusively as vesicant in the literature

Although the combined use of hyaluronidase and heat has been tested neither in a clinical study nor in animal experiments, this combination is established in clinical practice because of a putative synergistic mechanism (accelerated absorption of extravasated substance)

Original articles

[1] Dorr RT, Bool KL: Antidote studies of vinorelbine-induced skin ulceration in the mouse. Cancer Chemother Pharmacol 36: 290–292, 1995.

[2] Bertelli G, Dini D, Forno GB, et al: Hyaluronidase as an antidote to extravasation of vinca alkaloids: clinical results. J Cancer Res Clin Oncol 120: 505–506, 1994.

[3] Le Chevalier T, Brisgand D, Douillard JY, et al: Randomized study of vinorelbine and cisplatin versus vindesine and cisplatin versus vinorelbine alone in advanced non-small-cell lung cancer: results of a european multicenter trial including 612 patients. J Clin Oncol 12: 360–367, 1994.

[4] Barth J, Bildat S: Empfehlungen zur Behandlung von Paravasaten mit Vinorelbin. Krankenhauspharmazie 12: 622–624, 2000.

[5] Moreno de Vega MJ, Dauden E, Abajo P, et al: Skin necrosis from extravasation of vinorelbine. JEADV 16: 488–490, 2002.

[6] Giunta R, Akpaloo J, Kovacs L, et al: Technik der subcutanen Spülung bei hochtoxischen Paravasaten – Ein Kurzbeitrag. Handchir Mikrochir Plast Chir 34: 399–402, 2002.
[7] Cicchetti S, Jemec B, Gault DT: Two cases of vinorelbine extravasation: management and review of the literature. Tumori 86: 289–292, 2000.
[8] Krämer I: Zehn Jahre Dokumentation von Zytostatika-Paravasat-Ereignissen: Auswertung von 175 Paravasate-Dokumentationen. Krankenhauspharmazie 23: 269–274, 2002.
[9] Whang SW, Lee SH, Elias PM, et al: Intralesional steroids reduce inflammation from extravasated chemotherapeutic agents. Br J Dermatol 145: 680–682, 2001.
[10] Langstein HN, Duman H, Seelig D, et al: Retrospective study of the management of chemotherapeutic extravasation injury. Ann Plast Surg 49: 369–374, 2002.

Secondary literature

[11] Gain M, Melzer S, Meyer-Jürshof A, et al: Vinorelbin: Behandlung von Paravasaten. In: Gain M, et al (eds) ADKA-Zytostatika-Handbuch, Pharmazeutisch-wissenschaftliche Monographien. Verlag Heiner Biller, vol 4: 39, 2000.
[12] Berdel WE, Schmoll HJ, Büchele T, et al: Prävention und Therapie von Paravasaten/Extravasaten. In: Schmoll HJ, Höffken K, Possinger K (eds) Kompendium Internistische Onkologie. Standards in Diagnostik und Therapie. Springer, vol 1, 3rd edition: 1689–1701, 1999.
[13] Summary of product characteristics Navelbine® (Switzerland), Robapharm, April 2004.
[14] Mullin S, Beckwith MC, Tyler LS: Prevention and management of antineoplastic extravasation injury. Hosp Pharm 35: 57–76, 2000.
[15] Bertelli G: Prevention and management of extravasation of cytotoxic drugs. Drug Safety 12: 245–255, 1995.
[16] Gain M, Melzer S, Meyer-Jürshof A, et al: Allgemeiner Teil: Behandlung von Paravasaten. In: Gain M, et al (eds) ADKA-Zytostatika-Handbuch, Pharmazeutisch-wissenschaftliche Monographien. Verlag Heiner Biller, vol 1, 2nd edition: A42–44, 1997.
[17] Dorr RT, Von Hoff DD: Drug monographs: vinorelbine. In: Dorr RT, Von Hoff DD (eds) Cancer Chemotherapy Handbook. Appleton & Lange, 2nd edition: 966–969, 1994.
[18] Barth J: Paravasate und deren Behandlung. In: Barth J (ed) Zytostatika-Herstellung in der Apotheke. Deutscher Apotheker Verlag, chapter VI-3: 1–9, 2000.

[19] Bertelli G, Garrone O, Bighin C, et al: Correspondence re: Cicchetti S, Jemec B, Gault DT: Two case reports of vinorelbine extravasation: management and review of the literature. Tumori 86: 289–292, 2000. Tumori 87: 112–113, 2001.
[20] Krämer I, Stützle M: Zytostatika-Paravasation – Wie ist vorzugehen? Krankenhauspharmazie 23: 261–268, 2002.
[21] Stanley A: Managing complications of chemotherapy administration. In: Allwood M, Stanley A, Wright P (eds) The Cytotoxics Handbook. Radcliffe Medical Press, 4th edition: 119–193, 2002.
[22] Jordan K, Grothe W, Schmoll HJh: Paravasation von Zytostatika: Prävention und Therapie. Dtsch Med Wochenschr 130: 33–37, 2005.
[23] Ener RA, Meglathery SB, Styler M: Extravasation of systemic hemato-oncological therapies. Ann Oncol 15: 858–862, 2004.

Further reading:

- Albanell J, Baselga J: Systemic therapy emergencies. Semin Oncol 27: 347–361, 2000.
- Alley E, Green R, Schuchter L: Cutaneous toxicities of cancer therapy. Curr Opin Oncol 14: 212–216, 2002.
- Fenchel K, Karthaus M: Zytostatika-Paravasate – gibt es neue Empfehlungen zum therapeutischen Vorgehen? Wien Med Wochenschr 151: 44–46, 2001.
- Krämer I: Onkologische Pharmazie. In: Jaehde U, Radziwill R, Mühlebach S, et al (eds) Lehrbuch der Klinischen Pharmazie. Wissenschaftliche Verlagsgesellschaft mbH, 2nd edition: 307–336, 2003.
- Rauh J, Pluntke S, Müller C: Paravenöse Zytostatikainjektion: Prophylaxe und Sofortmaßnahmen im Notfall. MMW Fortschr Med 146: 682–686, 2004.
- Schrijvers DL: Extravasation: a dreaded complication of chemotherapy. Ann Oncol 14: iii26–iii30, 2003.

Revisions by Ines Mader

Subject Index

MIX
Papier aus verantwortungsvollen Quellen
Paper from responsible sources
FSC® C105338

If you have any concerns about our products,
you can contact us on
ProductSafety@springernature.com

In case Publisher is established outside the EU,
the EU authorized representative is:
Springer Nature Customer Service Center GmbH
Europaplatz 3, 69115 Heidelberg, Germany

Printed by Libri Plureos GmbH
in Hamburg, Germany